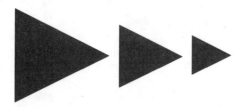

Nutrition, Diet Modifications and Meal Patterns

Second Edition

Ruby P. Puckett MA, RD, LD/N, FCSI
Sherryl E. Danks RD, LD/N

 KENDALL/HUNT PUBLISHING COMPANY
4050 Westmark Drive   Dubuque, Iowa 52002

Cover design by Laurel P. Brown

▶ CONTENTS ◀

▶ SECTION 1 ◀

Module 1: Nutrition

Module 2: Nutrition Through the Life Cycle

Module 2: Modification for Seasoning

Module 3: Modification for Calories

Module 4: Modification for Nutrients

Module 5: Other Modification

Module 6: Modification for Special Needs

Module 7: Modification for Test Diets

Appendices

▶ FOREWORD ◀

Cardiovascular disease continues to be the number one cause of death in the United States. Cancer and HIV infections are increasingly adding to the death rate. Due to inactivity and poor nutritional habits children and youth are facing obesity and in general more Americans have a weight problem than in previous decades. Female teenagers fall prey to the "perfect body image" that can lead to bulimia and anorexia nervosa. The majority of U.S. citizens are now middle-aged. As this group ages, the ratio of old people to young will grow larger. The fastest growing age group is people over 85 years of age. There are many healthy elderly people who continue to function independently until late in life, but others face complications of disease, environmental and lifestyle factors. Malnutrition is still a factor in healthcare facilities and adds to the cost of the care.

Healthcare providers and especially nutrition care "experts" must become more proactive in developing ways to assist the patient to meet optimal nutrition throughout the life cycle. Nutrition plays a major role in the prevention and curative effects of therapy. Diet histories, assessment, screening and care plans can effectively identify those persons who are at a high risk of malnutrition. Once the assessment is completed the nutrition care and interdisciplinary teams need to seek input from the patient and family to individualize the care to meet the needs of the patient.

This book provides information and references that will enable the nutrition care team to enhance the nutrition therapy of the patient. The material on diet modification and meal patterns can he used in menu planning and education of the patient. Section I can be modified to conduct in-service educational programs for the staff. Most of the information can be adopted to meet JCAHO and OBRA standards.

▶ PREFACE ◀

Nutrition, Diet Modifications and Meal Patterns is a concise, practical guide to normal nutrition and diet modification. It was written to assist the nutrition care and interdisciplinary teams who are employed in extended care facilities, home health, clinics, hospitals, physician's offices, as well as an educational guide for students. The material in the text is the latest available references of nutrition related materials.

The text of *Nutrition, Diet Modifications and Meal Patterns* is divided into two sections and within these sections there are modules. Section 1, Module 1 contains information on dietary guidelines, nutrient requirements, digestion and absorption. Module 2 is on nutrition through the life cycle including physical fitness and sports medicine as well as cultural, religious, lifestyles and folk lore. Module 3 concerns healthcare food and nutrition services. It contains charts that can be used for screening, documentation in the medical history, standards of care and other useful information on providing care to the patient. There is a major section on drug and nutrient interaction including a chart on psychoactive drugs, nutrition support and information on other healthcare services.

Section 2 contains healthcare diet modification and meal patterns. The major modules are modification for consistency/texture, seasoning, calories, nutrients, special needs and test diets. References and suggestions for additional information are also included.

The Appendix contains a variety of data that includes the latest published (1989) Recommended Dietary Allowances, caffeine content of various beverages, alcohol, kilocalories and carbohydrates of beverages as well as other data to assist the user.

The information follows the recommendations from the Surgeon General. The meal patterns meet the Recommended Dietary Allowances of the National Research Council, 1989 wherever applicable. The text contains lists of foods that are allowable and those that are discouraged for a restricted diet. List may not be all inclusive and may vary from facility to facility. The lists vary with the complexity of the diet modification. Because infant formulas and enteral and parenteral formulations are subject to change a list of formulas is not included. Brand names are used to assist the user and do not imply endorsement of one product over and equivalent product.

If you have comments and/or recommendations on how to improve this book please contact:

Ruby P. Puckett, MA, RD, LD/N, FCSI
President/owner
Food Service Management Consultant
5200 NW 43rd Street, Suite 102-302
Gainesville, FL 32606-4482

Telephone: 352-371-6160
FAX: 352-371-7622
E-Mail: puckerp@juno.com

▶ ACKNOWLEDGMENTS ◀

A special acknowledgment is given to Laurel P. Brown who designed the cover and page layouts, to Gwen Love, Corner Drug Store, Gainesville for information on psychoactive drugs, to all the clinical dietitians and other clinical providers, in a variety of states, especially those who we have worked with for many years as they strive to provide optimal nutritional care for their patients; to all the dietitians who so willingly answered questions posed on the dietetic 1-serve, and to the staff at the American Dietetic Association who provided information on a variety of topics to all the individual researchers and companies who granted us permission to reprint a variety of information, to Judy Perkin, DrPH, RD, LD, Associate Dean, Health Related Professions the North Florida University Jacksonville, FL., for her input and knowledge on HIV infections; and to all those individuals and companies who strive to improve the nutritional health of Americans through their product development and research, and Kendall Hunt for their support in making this book a reality. We also thank Larry W. Puckett and Doug Danks for their support, encouragement, and understanding.

We dedicate this book to all food and nutrition workers in all healthcare facilities whose important and essential efforts often go unappreciated.

Ruby P. Puckett, MA, RD, LD/N
Sherryl E. Danks, RD, LD/N
2000

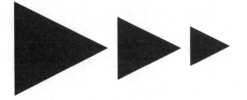

SECTION 1

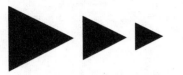

Module 1

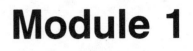

Nutrition

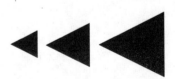

▶ INTRODUCTION TO SECTION 1 ◀

You are a product of what you eat. Most people make decisions several times a day concerning the kind and amount of food they will consume. This wide variety of food supplies many materials to the body to insure good health. It is vitally important that the food selected each day be the food that is needed to produce and maintain a healthy body and not be chosen for faddist or pseudo-scientific reasons.

Nutrition is the study of food and its contribution to individual health and growth. *Food* is nutritive material that is taken into the body, which: (1) furnishes energy; (2) builds and repairs tissues; and (3) regulates body process.

Food substances are *proteins, carbohydrates, lipids, vitamins, minerals* and *water.*

▶ NUTRITIONAL RECOMMENDATIONS ◀

An adequate diet for a healthy individual should include a variety of foods in appropriate amounts to provide all necessary nutrients and to maintain ideal body weight. The six classes of nutrients are carbohydrates, proteins, fats, vitamins, minerals, and water.

Dietary adequacy may be determined by comparing nutrient intake to the Recommended Dietary Allowances (RDA) 1989, dietary guidelines established by the Food and Nutrition Board of the National Research Council. "Recommended Dietary Allowances (RDA) are the levels of intake of essential nutrients considered, in the judgment of the Committee on Dietary Allowances of the Food and Nutrition Board on the basis of available scientific knowledge, to be adequate to meet the known nutritional needs of practically all healthy persons."[1] First published in 1943 and periodically revised since then, the purpose of these figures is to "provide for individual variations among most normal persons as they live in the United States under usual environmental stress."[1] Allowances are recommended for each sex and for different age groups. See Appendix for 10th Edition Recommended Daily Dietary Allowances, Revised 1989.

The major changes are as follows:

Age Groupings: Because peak bone mass is not attained before 25 years, the age group of 19 to 22 years was extended through age 24 for men and women.[1]

Reference Individuals: The heights and weights of reference adults in each age-sex class are the medians for the United States population, rather than arbitrary ideal standards used in the previous edition.[1]

Nutrients: RDAs during pregnancy and lactation are expressed as absolute figures, rather than as additions to the baseline allowance. Also, RDAs for lactating women have been provided, which reflect changes in milk production from the first 6 months to the second 6-month period. Previous editions only provided a single allowance for lactating women.[1]

Energy: With the change to using actual medians as reference weights instead of arbitrary ideals, previous recommended allowances cannot be directly compared to current RDAs. Energy allowances for adults, based on light to moderate exercise, range from 2,300 to 2,900 Kcal/day for men and 1,900 to 2,200 Kcal/day for women. Recommended energy allowances are very similar to previous editions despite the higher weights of reference adults and different methods used to estimate energy expenditure.[1]

Protein: Different methods are now used to derive the RDAs for protein, but the recommended allowance for adults remains at 0.8 g/kg of body to account for the 70% efficiency in the conversion of dietary protein to milk protein. The RDA of additional protein is 15 g/day during the first 6 months of lactation and 12 g/day during the second 6 months. The decreased requirement in the second 6 months is related to a 20% decrease in the volume of milk produced during this period.[1]

Calcium: A calcium intake of 1,200 mg/day is recommended during pregnancy and lactation for all age groups.[1]

Other Nutrients: Lactation increases the requirements for almost all nutrients, however, these increased needs can be supplied with a well-balanced diet, and nutritional supplements are unnecessary under normal circumstances. For specific 1989 RDA recommendations, see the *Appendix*.

Fluid: An increased fluid requirement of 1,000 ml/day is necessary to replace water secreted in milk and maintain normal maternal fluid balance.[1]

Contaminants: Substances, such as drugs, alcohol, caffeine, nicotine, food allergens, environmental pollutants, and viruses, may be passed into the breast milk. Although moderate amounts of these substances may not be harmful to the breast-fed infant, some drugs may cause adverse effects and are contraindicated during lactation.[2]

Human Immunodeficiency Virus (HIV): Breast-feeding is contraindicated in HIV-positive women. The virus can be transmitted in breast milk. The Centers for Disease Control and the US Public Health Service recommend that these women abstain from breast-feeding to prevent potential HIV transmission.[3] See Module 6, *Nutrition and HIV Infection*.

Vitamin K: For the first time, RDAs for Vitamin K have been established. The RDA for adults and children is set at approximately 1 μg/kg, with no increase during pregnancy and lactation.[1]

Vitamin C: The incremental increase in the RDA during pregnancy has been reduced to 10 mg/day, half of the recommended increase in previous additions. The RDA for vitamin C for cigarette smokers was set at 100 mg/day, as smoking may increase the metabolic turnover of vitamin C and therefore decrease the concentration in the blood.[1]

Vitamin B: The RDA for vitamin B_6 has been reduced to 2.0 mg/day and 1.6 mg/day for men and women respectively. This is equivalent to approximately 0.016 mg of vitamin B_6/g of protein.[1]

Folate: Folate allowances are lower in all categories, often by 50% or more. The recommended folate allowance of 3 μg/kg for adults and adolescents is equivalent to 200 μg/day for adult men, 180 μg/day for adult women, and 400 μg/day for women during pregnancy. It was determined that adequate folate status and liver stores are maintained on diets containing less than the previous RDA levels.[1]

Vitamin B_{12}: Vitamin B_{12} allowances were decreased by as much as one half of the previous RDAs for all age-sex groups. Recent data indicate that adequate metabolic function can be sustained with lower intakes of vitamin B_{12}.[1]

Calcium: The RDA for calcium for adolescents, which was 1,200 mg/day for ages 11 to 18, has been extended through age 24 for both sexes. The RDA for older adults did not change from 800 mg/day. According to the 1989 RDA committee, there was insufficient evidence to indicate that an increased calcium intake after age 25 would reduce the risk of osteoporosis. It is believed that the best way to reduce the risk of osteoporosis later in life is to promote the development of peak bone mass. For this reason, increased emphasis has been placed on ensuring adequate calcium intake prior to age 25. However individuals diagnosed with osteoporosis may require increased levels of calcium. RDAs for phosphorous and calcium are parallel except in infancy. The RDA for vitamin D remains at 10 μg/day through age 25.[1]

Magnesium: The incremental increase in magnesium during pregnancy and lactation was reduced significantly. In pregnancy, the allowance was reduced from +150 to +20 mg/day and to +75 mg/day during the first 6 months of lactation and to +60 mg/day during the second 6 months. These levels were determined to be adequate to support growth and maintenance of fetal and maternal tissues. Allowances for children 1 through 15 years of age were also reduced to 6.0 mg/kg/day.[1]

Iron: The RDA for iron for healthy adolescent and adult women was reduced from 18 mg/day to 15 mg day. The allowance for postmenopausal women and adult men remains at 10 mg/day. During pregnancy, an increase of 15 mg/day was recommended with no additional recommendation during lactation. Iron supplementation during pregnancy is still recommended, however it is not necessary to continue using supplements after childbirth as previously recommended.[1]

Zinc: The daily allowance for zinc remains at 15 mg/day for adult men but has been reduced to 12 mg/day for adult women because of their lower body weight.[1]

Selenium: RDAs for selenium have been established for the first time. The allowances were set at 70 μg/day for adult men and 55 μg/day for adult women. The adult RDAs were used to extrapolate values for infants, children, and adolescents, based on body weight and a growth factor.[1]

Estimated Safe and Adequate Daily Dietary Intakes (ESADDIs): The previous edition included a category for essential nutrients for which data were insufficient for establishing RDAs. This is also included in this edition, however several changes have been made. Vitamin K and selenium have been removed from the table and RDAs have been set for them. Estimated minimum requirements have been provided for sodium, potassium, and chloride, rather than estimated safe and adequate ranges of intake. For adults and adolescents, the estimated ranges of safe and adequate intakes for the following trace elements were reduced to 30 to 100 μg/day for biotin, 1.5 to 3 mg/day for copper, 2 to 5 mg/day for manganese, and 75 to 250 μg/day for molybdenum.[1] For listing of ESADDIs, see the *Appendix*.

Although there is some evidence suggesting that elderly persons have altered nutritional requirements for some nutrients, there is no evidence that increased levels of nutrients above the RDAs would be beneficial. Because there are insufficient data to support a separate RDA for people over 70 years of age, the 1989 RDAs divide adults into two age categories as in previous editions.[1]

▶ DIETARY GUIDELINES FOR AMERICANS ◀

The Dietary Guidelines for Americans were first issued in 1980 and revised in 1985, 1990, and 1995 by the Department of Agriculture and the Department of Health and Human Sciences.

The 1995 Guidelines emphasizes the importance of eating a varied diet, exercising and consuming alcohol in moderation. These Guidelines also recommend choosing a diet low in saturated fat, cholesterol, salt, sodium, and sugar. It further promotes a diet rich in grain products, such as pasta and other whole grain foods fruits, and vegetables. These Guidelines also recognize the role of the vegetarian diet, noting through the consumption of milk products and eggs persons on a vegetarian regime can meet the RDAs for nutrients; For the first time the Guidelines advocate exercising 30 minutes a day to help maintain a healthy weight.

In April 1992, the U.S. Department of Agriculture and the Department of Health and Human Sciences introduced the *Food Guide Pyramid*. The *Pyramid* graphically depicts daily food choices, emphasizing the increased use of breads, cereal, rice and pasta group. The Daily Guidelines and the pyramid are closely interrelated in the following ways:

▶ THE FOOD GUIDE ◀ PYRAMID—PUTTING THE DIETARY GUIDELINES INTO ACTION

Learning to eat right is now made simpler with the new Food Guide Pyramid by the U.S. Department of Agriculture (USDA). The Pyramid is a graphic description of what registered dietitians and other nutrition experts have been advising for years: Build your diet on a base of grains, vegetables, and fruits. Add moderate quantities of lean meat (poultry, fish, eggs, legumes) and dairy products, and limit the intake of fats and sweets. The Food Guide Pyramid illustrates how to turn the Dietary Guidelines for Americans (issued by USDHHS/USDA in 1990) into real food choices.

The Dietary Guidelines—and their relationship to the Food Guide Pyramid—are as follows:

▶ *Eat a variety of foods*. The body needs more than 40 different nutrients for good health, and since no single food can supply all these nutrients, variety is crucial. Variety can be assured by choosing foods each day from the five major groups shown in the Pyramid: (1) Breads, Cereals, Rice & Pasta (6–11 servings); (2) Vegetables (3–5 servings); (3) Fruits (2–4 servings);

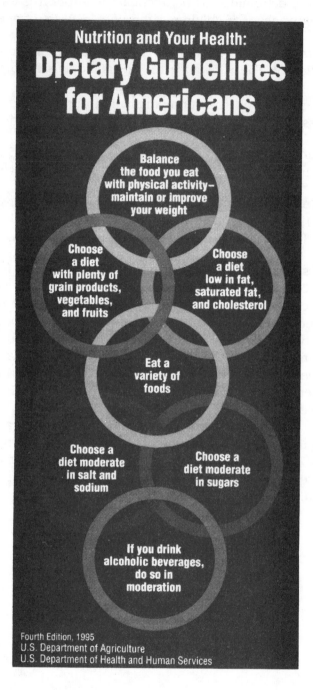

Nutrition and Your Health:
Dietary Guidelines for Americans

Balance the food you eat with physical activity—maintain or improve your weight

Choose a diet with plenty of grain products, vegetables, and fruits

Choose a diet low in fat, saturated fat, and cholesterol

Eat a variety of foods

Choose a diet moderate in salt and sodium

Choose a diet moderate in sugars

If you drink alcoholic beverages, do so in moderation

Fourth Edition, 1995
U.S. Department of Agriculture
U.S. Department of Health and Human Services

(4) Milk, Yogurt & Cheese (2–3 servings); (5) Meat, Poultry, Fish, Dry Beans, Eggs & Nuts (2–3 servings) and (6) Fats, Oils and Sweets (use sparingly).

▶ *Maintain healthy weight.* Being overweight or underweight increases the risk of developing health problems, so it is important to consume the right amount of calories each day. The number of calories needed for ideal weight (which varies according to height, frame, age, and activity) will generally determine how many servings in the Pyramid are needed.

▶ *Choose a diet low in fat, saturated fat, and cholesterol.* As shown in the Pyramid, fats and oils should be used sparingly, since diets high in fat are associated with obesity, certain types of cancer, and heart disease. A diet low in fat also makes it easier to include a variety of foods, because fat contains more than twice the calories of an equal amount of carbohydrates or protein.

▶ *Choose a diet with plenty of vegetables, fruits, and grain products.* Vegetables, fruits, and grains provide the complex carbohydrates, vitamins, minerals, and dietary fiber needed for good health. Also, they are generally low in fat. To obtain the different kinds of fiber contained in these foods, it is best to eat a variety.

▶ *Use sugars only in moderation.* Sugars, and many foods containing large amounts of sugars, supply calories but are limited in nutrients. Thus, they should be used in moderation by most healthy people and sparingly by those with low calorie needs. Sugars, as well as foods that contain starch (which breaks down in sugars), can also contribute to tooth decay. The longer foods containing sugars or starches remain in the mouth before teeth are brushed, the greater the risk for tooth decay. Some examples of foods that contain starches are milk, fruits, some vegetables, breads, and cereals.

▶ *Use salt and sodium only in moderation.* Table salt contains sodium and chloride, which are essential to good health. However, most Americans eat more than they need. Much of the sodium in people's diets comes from salt they add while cooking and at the table. Sodium is also added during food processing and manufacturing.

▶ *If you drink alcoholic beverages, do so in moderation.* Alcoholic beverages contain calories but little or no nutrients. Consumption of alcohol is linked with many health problems, causes many accidents, and can lead to addiction. Therefore, alcohol consumption is not recommended.

Reference: Nutrition Screening Initiative, Executive Summary Manual. Greer, Margolis, Mitchell, Grunwald & Associates, Inc., pg. 36. 1992.

▶ THE FOOD GUIDE PYRAMID ◀
A Guide to Daily Food Choices

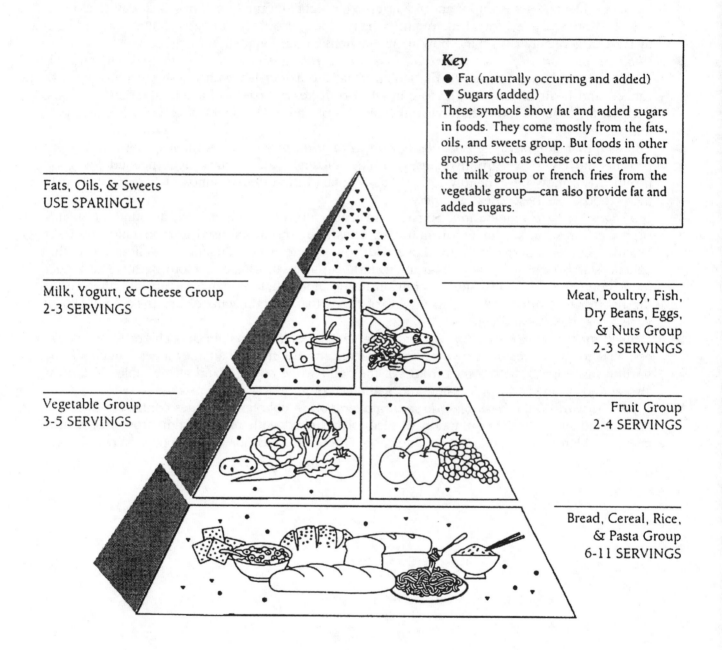

Key
● Fat (naturally occurring and added)
▼ Sugars (added)
These symbols show fat and added sugars in foods. They come mostly from the fats, oils, and sweets group. But foods in other groups—such as cheese or ice cream from the milk group or french fries from the vegetable group—can also provide fat and added sugars.

Fats, Oils, & Sweets
USE SPARINGLY

Milk, Yogurt, & Cheese Group
2-3 SERVINGS

Meat, Poultry, Fish,
Dry Beans, Eggs,
& Nuts Group
2-3 SERVINGS

Vegetable Group
3-5 SERVINGS

Fruit Group
2-4 SERVINGS

Bread, Cereal, Rice,
& Pasta Group
6-11 SERVINGS

Looking at the Pieces of the Pyramid

The Food Guide Pyramid emphasizes foods from the five major food groups shown in the three lower sections of the Pyramid. Each of these food groups provides some, but not all, of the nutrients you need. Foods in one group can't replace those in another. No one of these major food groups is more important than another—for good health, you need them all.

The U.S. Department of Health and Human Services published *Healthy People 2000: National Health Promotion and Disease Prevention Objectives,* in 1990, that included 21 objectives to improve the health of Americans. These objectives were divided into three sections: disease-related, nutrient and food, and nutrition information and service objectives. The objectives correlate with the Food Guide Pyramid and the 1995 Guidelines. They all have the same objective of eating healthier through reduction of various food, therefore reducing the possibility of various diseases. Education and exercise complete the overall objectives.

Nutrition-Related Health Objectives for the Nation, Year 2000

Disease-Related Objectives:

1. Reduce *heart disease* deaths.
2. Reverse the rise in *cancer* deaths.
3. Reduce the prevalence of *overweight.*
4. Reduce *growth retardation* among low-income children.

Nutrient and Food Objectives:

5. Reduce dietary *fat* intake.*
6. Increase intakes of complex *carbohydrates* and *fiber* containing foods.**
7. Increase the proportion of *overweight* people taking effective steps to control their weight.
8. Increase *calcium* intake among teenagers, pregnant women, women who are breastfeeding their infants, and adults in general.
9. Reduce *salt* intakes and purchases of food high in salt.
10. Remedy *iron* deficiencies in children and women.
11. Encourage *breastfeeding* of infants immediately after birth and the continuation of breastfeeding for at least six months after birth.
12. Teach parents *infant-feeding practices* that will minimize the chances of tooth decay.

Nutrition Information and Service Objectives:

13. Promote people's learning how to best use *food labels* to correctly select nutritious foods.
14. Make food labels more informative and complete.
15. Make more low-fat, low-saturated fat foods available.
16. Encourage more restaurants and institutions to serve low-fat, low-calorie foods.
17. Improve the nutrition quality of school lunches and breakfasts and child-care foodservice meals.
18. Make sure as many elderly people as possible receive home food services.
19. Offer nutrition education to more schools from preschool through 12th grade.
20. Encourage workplaces to provide nutrition education and/or weight-management programs for their employees.
21. Support healthcare providers in offering nutrition assessment, nutrition counseling, and referrals to qualified nutrition experts as part of their services.

---

*The exact objective is to reduce fat intake to an average of 30 percent of calories or less, and saturated fat intake to less than 10 percent of calories.
**The objective is spelled out: increase these intakes in diets of adults to five or more daily servings of vegetables (including legumes) and fruits and to six or more daily servings of grain products.
Source: *Healthy People 2000: National Health Promotion and Disease Prevention Objectives* (Washington DC: U.S. Department of Health and Human Services, 1990).

▶ HEALTHY PEOPLE 2010* ◀

On January 25, 2000 the U.S. Department of Health and Human Service (HHS) launched its initiative Healthy People 2010. This initiative is a road map showing opportunities for improvements in health that is grounded in science, built through public consensus, and designed to measure progress.

The Healthy People 2010 has established two preeminent goals:

1. Increase quality and years of healthy life
2. Eliminate health disparities

The four enabling goals are:

1. Promote healthy behaviors
2. Promote healthy and safe communities
3. Improve systems for personal and public health
4. Prevent and reduce diseases and disorders

There are twenty-six health focus areas which are organized under the four enabling goals. There are more than 500 objectives for the 26 focus areas. Objectives will be measurable as well as developmental.

Nutrition focus areas contains 20 objectives as well as nine other objectives from other focus areas.

The following list contains 28 focus areas. Several of these have been combined to equal 26

Focus Areas

1. Access to Quality Health Services
2. Arthritis, Osteoporosis and Chronic Back Conditions
3. Cancer
4. Chronic Kidney Disease
5. Diabetes
6. Disability and Secondary Conditions
7. Educational and Community-Based Programs
8. Environmental Health
9. Family Planning
10. Food Safety
11. Health Communication
12. Heart Disease and Stroke
13. HIV
14. Immunizations and Infectious Diseases
15. Injury/Violence Prevention
16. Maternal, Infant, and Child Health
17. Medical Product Safety
18. Mental Health and Mental Disorders
19. Nutrition/Overweight
20. Occupational Safety and Health
21. Oral Health
22. Physical Activity and Fitness
23. Public Health Infrastructure
24. Respiratory Diseases
25. Sexually Transmitted Diseases
26. Substance Abuse
27. Tobacco Use
28. Vision and Hearing

*See Journal of the American Dietitic Assoc. For your information Vol. 99 Number 4 pp 415–420 or check out website: www.odphp.osophs.dhhs.gov and www.health.gov/healthypeople

▶ NUTRIENT REQUIREMENTS ◀

Caloric Allowances

The energy exchange of the body and the potential energy value of foods is called calories. One calorie is the amount of heat required to raise the temperature of 1 kg of water 1° Centigrade.

The carbohydrate, fat, protein, and alcohol content of food provides the energy for all body activities. The energy value of these nutrients is:

Nutrient	KCAL/CM
Carbohydrate	4
Fat	9
Protein	4
Alcohol	7

The RDA for energy is an estimate of the calories needed for healthy persons living in an environment with an annual mean temperature of 68°–77°F (20°–25°C), leading moderately active lives and moderate physical activity. See Appendix for Median Heights and Weights and Recommended Energy Intake.

It should be noted that various factors affect the daily allowance for calories, such as climate, activity, sex, body size, and age of the individual. For example, with advancing age, the need for calories decreases. Periods of rapid growth, such as infancy and adolescence, require high caloric allowances in proportion to body size.

The balance between energy input (calories from food) and energy output (activity) determines an individual's weight. Calories in excess of body needs are stored as fat.

▶ EXAMPLES OF DAILY ENERGY EXPENDITURES OF ◀ MATURE WOMEN AND MEN IN LIGHT OCCUPATIONS

Active Category	Time (hr)	Man, 70kg Rate (kcal/min)	Total (kcal)	Woman, 58kg Rate (kcal/min)	Total (kcal)
Sleeping, reclining	8	1.0–1.2	540	0.9–1.1	440
Very light	12	up to 2.5	1300	up to 2.0	900
Seated and standing activities, painting trades, auto and truck driving, laboratory work, typing, playing musical instruments, sewing, ironing					
Light	3	2.5–4.9	600	2.0–3.9	450
Walking on level, 2.5–3 mph, tailoring, garage work, electrical trades, carpentry, restaurant trades, cannery workers, washing clothes, shopping with light load, golf, sailing, table tennis, volleyball					
Moderate	1	5.0–7.4	300	4.0–5.9	240
Walking 3.5–4 mph, plastering, weeding and hoeing, loading and stacking bales, scrubbing floors, shopping with heavy load, cycling, skiing, tennis, dancing					
Heavy	0	7.5–12.0		6.0–10.0	
Walking with load uphill, tree felling, work with pick and shovel, basketball, swimming, climbing, football					
TOTAL	24		2740		2030

The daily energy expenditures contains variation as the results of different investigators. Ranges vary and categories include the major forms of energy expenditure.

Carbohydrates

People the world over depend on carbohydrates as the principle source of calories. In the United States, carbohydrates furnish about half of the total daily intake; in some other parts of the world carbohydrates furnish approximately eighty percent (80%) of the calories. Carbohydrate foods are easily grown, are inexpensive, are easily digested, and are used by the body for energy.

Sugars, cereal grains, roots and legumes are the principle sources of carbohydrates in the United States. During the past decade, there has been a steady decline in the use of cereal grains and potatoes, with a gradual increase of sugars.

All carbohydrates contain carbon, hydrogen, and oxygen. Carbohydrates are classified as monosaccharides (simple sugars), disaccharides (double sugars) and polysaccharides (complex sugars). The chief function of carbohydrate is to provide energy to the body to carry on its work and to maintain the body's temperature.

All carbohydrates furnish four (4) calories per gram. Fifty eight (58) percent of the protein intake and ten (10) percent of the fat intake is converted to carbohydrates in the body. Ten (10) grams of carbohydrates is the minimum required to supply sufficient glucose to the brain.

There is no RDA for carbohydrates, generally the diet should contain at lease 50–100 grams of carbohydrates. Researchers suggest that carbohydrates should provide about 58% of the calories with complex carbohydrates and natural sugars providing 45–55% of calories and the added sweeteners providing 10% or less. The intake of fiber should be 27–40 grams per day.

Digestibility of carbohydrates varies with sources, but for most foods is 90–98%. Cellulose is insoluble; man unlike animal, cannot utilize its carbohydrate content as there are no enzymes in the body that can digest it. The value of cellulose in nutrition is for its roughage that is necessary for gastrointestinal health.

Although not a true carbohydrate, alcohol contains seven (7) calories per gram, which is ultimately used in the form of glucose.

Carbohydrates, particularly sucrose, have been directly linked to the frequency of dental caries—the most prevalent chronic disease known. It occurs in all parts of the world and no racial group is exempt from its damages.

Digestion of Carbohydrates

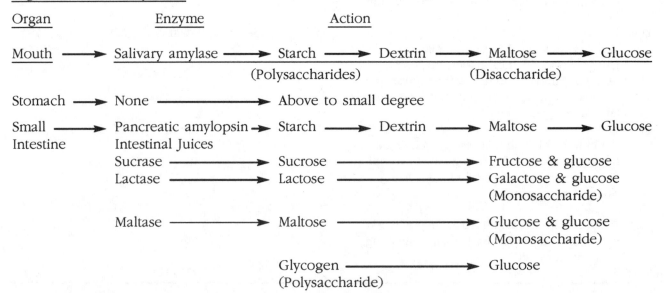

Organ	Enzyme	Action			
Mouth	Salivary amylase	Starch (Polysaccharides)	Dextrin	Maltose (Disaccharide)	Glucose
Stomach	None	Above to small degree			
Small Intestine	Pancreatic amylopsin Intestinal Juices	Starch	Dextrin	Maltose	Glucose
	Sucrase	Sucrose		Fructose & glucose	
	Lactase	Lactose		Galactose & glucose (Monosaccharide)	
	Maltase	Maltose		Glucose & glucose (Monosaccharide)	
		Glycogen (Polysaccharide)		Glucose	

Studies have shown dietary intake to be closely related to tooth malformation and decay. Sticky, readily fermented sweets cling to tooth surfaces and encourage bacterial growth and acid formation. Examples of these foods include pastries, cake icings, candies (caramels are the worst) and sweet cookies. The carbohydrate foods least likely to cause decay are fresh fruits, vegetables and hard breads.

Frequency of eating sugar-containing foods is another factor influencing the number of caries produced. Sweets eaten with a meal cause less acid formation and thus less tooth enamel destruction, than do between-meal snacks.

Typical American diets furnish 46% of calories from digestible carbohydrates, 35% from complex carbohydrates and naturally occurring sugars in milk, fruit, and vegetables and 11% from added sweeteners

Most nutritionists suggest about 58% of the calories should come from carbohydrates with complex carbohydrates and natural occurring sugars furnishing 48-50% of the calories and 10% or less from added sweeteners. Carbohydrates are made up of mono-, di- and polysaccharides. Monosaccharide are the most common single sugars found in nature—with fructose and glucose being the most common. Disaccharides include sucrose (table sugar), powdered sugar, and brown sugar. Polysaccharides include dextrin, starch, cellulose and glycogen.

Dietary fiber is an important carbohydrate and are the parts of plants that are not digested by enzymes and juices in the human digestive tract. Fiber is a polysaccharide which includes cellulose, pectin, hemocellous, gums, mucilages and ligins. Some of the dietary fibers are soluble in water. Since dietary fibers are indigestible, they do not provide any nutrients to the diet but add bulk or roughage to the diet. Some fiber is changed by the intestinal bacteria into products that are absorbed however, most fiber passes through the digestive tract unchanged. (see chapter on gastrointestinal for diets low and high in fiber)

Functions of Carbohydrates:
▶ Provide energy to carry on the body's work.
▶ Heat to maintain the body's temperature.
▶ Spare protein so protein can be used for building and repairing cells.
▶ Assist the body in the utilization of fat.
▶ Encourage growth of useful bacteria.
▶ Promote normal functioning of the lower intestinal tract.

Common Sources of Carbohydrates:
▶ cereals, grains
▶ fruits, vegetables
▶ sugar, sweets, (cookies, candy, cake, etc.)
▶ jelly, jam, syrup, honey
▶ milk and milk products

Possible Nutrition Problems:
▶ dental problems, especially dental caries
▶ decreased fiber intake due to increase intake of refine foods
▶ diabetes mellitus where the body cannot use carbohydrates normally
▶ lactose intolerance deficiency of lactose enzyme which is necessary for digestion of lactose (milk sugar)
▶ obesity due to the increase consumption of sugar (For example, drinking one 12 ounce can of regular soda per day for 30 days will add 4350 calories/month or 52,925 calories/year!)

▶ CARBOHYDRATES OF IMPORTANCE IN NUTRITION ◀

Carbohydrate	Chief Food Sources	Results of Digestion	Characteristics
Monosaccharides $(C_6H_{12}O_6)$			
Glucose	Fruit, honey, corn syrup	Glucose	More or less sweet, water soluble, not affected by digestive enzymes.
Fructose	Fruit, honey, corn syrup	Fructose	Same as above.
Galactose		Galactose	Do not occur in free forms of food.
Mannose		Mannose	
Disaccharides $(C_{12}H_{22}O_{11})$			
Sucrose	Cane and beet sugar, molasses, maple syrup	Glucose and Fructose	Water soluble, diffusible, crystallizable and variable in sweetness.
Maltose	Malt products	Glucose	Does not occur in free form. Manufactured from starch.
Lactose	Milk and milk products	Glucose and Galactose	Produced only by mammals.
Polysaccharides $(C_6H_{10}O_5)$			
Starch	Grain, seeds, roots, potatoes, legumes	Glucose	Complex compounds with relatively high molecular weight. Amorphous, not sweet, generally insoluble and are digested in the body with varying degrees of completeness.
Glycogen	Meat products and seafood	Glucose	
Cellulose	Stalks and leaves of vegetables, outer covering of seeds	0	

Sugar Substitute (Artificial Sweeteners)

The use of *cyclamates* was banned in the United States in 1970 as it was suspected to cause cancer in humans. Canada still allows its use as a tabletop sweetener on the advice of a physician and as a sweetening additive in medicines.

Saccharin is an artificial sweetener that has been in existence for almost a 100 years and is presently used by over 50 million Americans mostly in soft drinks and as a tabletop sweetener. In 1977 it was thought to cause bladder cancer in rats. Due to this controversy a warning label is on all diet beverages that states: "Use of this product may be hazardous to your health. This product contains saccharin, which has been determined to cause cancer in laboratory animals.".

Aspartame (EQUAL or *NUTRA-SWEET)* are artificial sweeteners used in a variety of foods especially canned drinks, chewing gum, candies, gelatins, puddings, and some presweetened cereals. Aspartame sales almost equal the sales of table sugar. Individuals who inherit a condition known as *phenylketonuria* should avoid products that contain aspartame. People with PKU must know what foods contain. Products with aspartame now carry a warning label.

Many healthy people poorly absorb sorbitol and mannitol found in some sugar-free foods such as candies and gums. In some individuals ingestion of these products can cause gas and diarrhea.

There are other artificial sweeteners coming out. There are several that are awaiting FDA approval.

Proteins

Food proteins are organic substances composed of carbon, hydrogen, oxygen, and nitrogen. Other elements such as sulphur, phosphorous, and iron are also found in minute amounts. Intact proteins cannot be absorbed as such, they must be broken down into their component amino acids for absorption and transport to the liver via the portal vein. All tissues use amino acids for the anabolic needs of the body such as the synthesis of plasma proteins and new cells, and the repair and maintenance of existing cells. Amino acids in excess of daily needs are used for energy.

The requirement for protein is actually the requirement for amino acids. There are approximately *twenty* amino acids needed, nine of these are considered "essential" due to the fact that they cannot be synthesized by the body but must be provided through the diet. The other "nonessential" amino acids are synthesized in adequate amounts by the body. For maximal absorption to occur, a constant and optimal mixture of amino acids must be present in the gut simultaneously. If an essential amino acid is lacking then protein synthesis will be quantitatively limited; non-essential amino acids not provided by diet will be supplied from the metabolic pool of the body.

Proteins have been classified as complete, partially incomplete and incomplete. Complete proteins are those that contain the essential amino acids in the correct ratio and amount to maintain life and support growth. They are said to have a "high biologic value." When protein intake is limited, emphasis should be given to foods high in biological value.

Partially incomplete proteins are those that contain enough essential amino acids to maintain life, but will not provide for growth.

Incomplete proteins can not provide for life or growth. Because they lack many essential amino acids, they have a "low biologic value".

Animal sources supply proteins of high biological value. Milk, eggs, cheese, meat, poultry, and fish are examples of high biological value proteins. Other foods are partially or completely lacking in the essential amino acids and, thus, have a lower biological value.

Proteins are organic substances that, when digested, are converted to amino acids. There are approximately twenty-three known amino acids that have varying nutritive value.

Amino Acids (from Protein)

**Essential amino acids in human nutrition

L-phenylalanine
L-methionine
L-leucine
L-valine
L-lysine
L-isoleucine
L-threonine
L-tryptophan

Essential only for young children
Histidine
Arginine

Nonessential amino acids

Glycine	Tyrosine	Citrulline
Alanine	Aspartic acid	Norleucine
Serine	Glutamic acid	Hydroxyglutamic acid
Cysteine	Proline	Argintine
Cystine	Hydroxyproline	

**These are "essential", simply because the human animal is incapable of manufacturing them metabolically—they must be supplied in the diet. In addition, the ratio of amino acids must be proper, for maximal absorption to occur. A mixed, varied diet supplies this ratio. An animal protein (milk, meat, egg, etc.) should be included with cereal or gelatin foods for best utilization of the latter proteins.

Protein is essential for growth, formation of essential body compounds and regulation of water balance. Approximately 15–20 percent of the human body is protein. About one-third is in the muscle, one-fifth in the cartilage. Protein is found in every cell; it is an essential component of enzymes, body secretions, hormones, blood and antibodies.

Digestion of Protein

Organ	Enzyme	Action
Mouth		Mechanical
↓		
Stomach ——→	Gastric Protease ——→	Proteoses & peptones
↓		
Small Intestine ——→	Pancreatic protease ——→	Dipeptides, Polypeptides, Amino Acids
↓		
Wall of Intestine ——→	Intestinal dipeptidose ——→	Amino Acids, Smaller Peptides

Amino Acids

↓ enter

Portal Blood

↓ enter

Liver

↓ enter

Body Tissue

Kwashiorkor is a disease resulting from inadequate amounts of protein in the diet. It is commonly found in young children in underdeveloped countries and in very poor American homes. It usually occurs when a child is weaned from mother's milk to starches. This induces acute protein deficiency with lack of most essential amino acids in the presence of adequate or even excess calories. Since protein is needed for growth and development, these children suffer multiple symptoms of body and brain damage.

Marasmus is a term used for another form of severe malnutrition, in which the child lacks adequate protein, calories and other nutrients most often seen in infants and is characterized by muscle wasting, loss of subcutaneous fat reserves and very low bodyweight. Mortality rates for Marasmus are high and surviving children are often mentally retarded.

Functions of Proteins:
▶ Aids tissue maintenance and growth.
▶ Helps fight disease.
▶ Regulates fluid balance of cells.
▶ Provides for regulatory function.
▶ Maintains blood at nearly neutral, or slightly alkaline state.
▶ Provides energy.

Common Source of Proteins:
Animal:
▶ meat, fish, poultry
▶ milk and milk products
▶ eggs
Plant:
▶ most vegetables
  • legumes
  • nuts, seeds, peanut butter
▶ bread, cereals, pasta
▶ textured vegetable protein (TVP) [foods manufactured by extraction of protein from certain oilseeds, such as soybean, peanuts, and cottonseed. These extracts contain no cholesterol and are low in saturated fats.]

Possible Nutrition Problems:
▶ Protein loss during illness, surgery, stress and injury may lead to wasting of muscle tissue, weight loss, possible edema, more susceptible to infection nutritional marasmus.
▶ Kwashiorkor
▶ In some instances infants are born with the inability to produce enzymes that are necessary for normal metabolism of certain amino acids.
▶ High protein diets may increase risk of heart disease.

Protein Substitute

Due to the continued increase of heart disease and cancer many individuals are reducing their intake of animal protein and increasing the intake of plant protein since plant protein is lower in lipids (fat). Vegetarian diets may include only protein from plants or may include milk and milk products, eggs, and fish. (see chapter on vegetarian diets.)

Many vegetarian diets include a *textured vegetable protein (soy protein)* [TVP] that has been formulated to look and taste like meat, fish or poultry. *Tofu,* another form of soybean curd is used in some diets and is a staple in many Asian dishes. In using TVP or tofu it is a wise ideas to combine them with a variety of foods to ensure a balanced protein diet.

Lipids

Lipid, or fats, are the most concentrated energy group in the diet, and furnish nine (9) calories per gram. Fats have been steadily increasing in the American diet, and now account for 40–45% of the total caloric intake. Animal sources account for two thirds of the available fats in the diet and one third from vegetable sources. The fat intake in the American diet has increased to approximately 145 grams per day.

Lipids, like carbohydrates, are made up of carbon, hydrogen and oxygen, which are linked together in chains. The shorter the chain, the faster the rate of digestion. The degree of saturation in the chain is also important and affects the level of serum cholesterol. Saturated fats elevate the level of serum cholesterol; monosaturated fats have a neutral effect; and polyunsaturated fats tend to lower cholesterol levels.

Lipids are an inclusive term for fats and fat-like substances. Within this category are triglycerides, compound lipids (phospho-, glyco- and lipoproteins), steroids and sterols (cholesterol), and other derived lipids (free fatty acids). Nutritionally, triglycerides, cholesterol, and the essential fatty acids are of greatest importance.

Most of the fat in foods occur as triglycerides (98–99%) which are composed of 1 molecule of glycerol and 3 molecules of fatty acids. The physical, chemical, and biochemical activities of these compounds are determined by the length of the carbon chain and the degree of saturation of the fatty acid components. Short and medium-chain triglycerides are more rapidly digested than long-chain triglycerides. However, most food fats predominantly contain long-chain triglycerides. Although triglycerides in the pure state are relatively tasteless, they readily absorb and retain flavor thus enhancing the palatability of the diet.

Three essential fatty acids have been identified: linoleic, linolenic, and arachadonic acid. They are found in a variety of foods of both plant and animal origins; vegetable oils are the richest source.

Cholesterol is the most abundant sterol found in man. It is synthesized by most tissues of the body (approximately 100 mg/day) with the liver being the most active site. Cholesterol functions as a structural component of cells and plasma lipoproteins, and is the source of bile acids and steroid hormones. Dietary intake of cholesterol also contributes to the body pool; the intake of cholesterol in the American diet ranges from 500–1000 mg/day, with approximately one-third absorbed. Serum cholesterol levels appear to be altered by the degree of saturation of triglycerides. Saturated fats elevate the level of serum cholesterol; monosaturated fats have a neutral effect, and polyunsaturated fats ten to lower cholesterol levels.

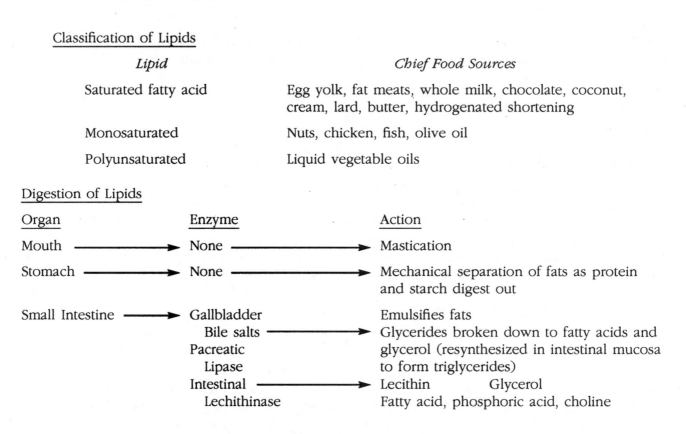

Classification of Lipids

Lipid	Chief Food Sources
Saturated fatty acid	Egg yolk, fat meats, whole milk, chocolate, coconut, cream, lard, butter, hydrogenated shortening
Monosaturated	Nuts, chicken, fish, olive oil
Polyunsaturated	Liquid vegetable oils

Digestion of Lipids

Organ	Enzyme	Action
Mouth →	None →	Mastication
Stomach →	None →	Mechanical separation of fats as protein and starch digest out
Small Intestine →	Gallbladder	Emulsifies fats
	Bile salts →	Glycerides broken down to fatty acids and
	Pacreatic	glycerol (resynthesized in intestinal mucosa
	Lipase	to form triglycerides)
	Intestinal →	Lecithin Glycerol
	Lechithinase	Fatty acid, phosphoric acid, choline

Medium chain triglycerides require less enzymes and bile acids for digestion than conventional food fats. They are predominantly transported directly by the portal circulation while conventional food fat requires the more complex intestinal micellar formation and chylomicron transport system. Thus usual result is a markedly increased availability of fat calories.

MCT oil® (a liquid), Portagen® and Pregestimal® (lactose-free powders substituting MCT oil for conventional fats) are useful methods of adding additional medium and short chain fats to the diet. The products are made by Mead Johnson; Evansville, Indiana.

Functions of Lipids:
▶ Provides energy reserves furnishing 9 kcal/gram.
▶ Lends satiety to a meal (sometimes call "ribsticking").
▶ Enhances food's aroma and flavor.
▶ Cushions vital organs.
▶ Helps maintain a constant body temperature.
▶ Enhances absorption of fat soluble vitamins.
▶ Provides the major material of which cell membranes are made.

Common Sources of Lipids:**

▶ oil, lard, animal fat, margarine, butter
▶ meats such as heavily marbled beef, bacon, fatty fish, sausage, pate
▶ fried foods especially fast foods such as French fries, onion rings
▶ duck, goose
▶ cold cuts, hot dogs
▶ cheddar cheese, sour cream, whole milk, heavy cream, creamed cottage cheese
▶ eggs, hollandaise sauces, butter sauces, commercial salad dressings
▶ butter cream fillings in desserts, gooey triple rich chocolate cake

**Many of the high fat products are now available in low-to-no-fat products. Careful reading of labels is necessary to determine which product will best meet the needs of each individual.

Possible Nutritional Problems:

▶ atherosclerosis
▶ hyperlipoptoteinemias
▶ obesity
▶ gastrointestinal and other disorder such as, gallbladder disease, pancreatitis, and cystic fibrosis
▶ seizure disorders for example the ketogenic diet which is high in fat and restricted in carbohydrates and protein

Fat Substitutes[1,2,3]

For decades researchers have been working on ways to reduce the fat in food. There are many low fat, lite fat, no fat food items available to consumers. Some of these products have met with poor acceptance because they taste "different". Many scientists and food manufacturing companies are developing artificial fats. *Olestra,* is a synthetic combination of fatty acids and sucrose, which is indigestible. *Olestra* feels, tastes and looks like dietary fat. It can be used in food preparation especially "frying", ice cream, and other desserts. In 1996 the FDA approved the use of *Olestra* in certain snack foods such as potato chips. The package must carry a warning label about the possible effects from ingesting the product.

Another fat substitute is *Simplesse* which is made from protein. The FDA has approved the use of *Simplesse* for use in such products as mayonnaise, frozen desserts, salad dressing. The protein is from egg whites or milk. If there is a food allergy to eggs or milk it may be prudent to forgo the use of this product. As always READ the label. *Olestra* and *Simplesse* differ in composition and use. *Simplesse* is digested and absorbed, provides 1⅓ calories per gram. *Olestra* passes through the body unchanged and provides zero calories. *Simplesse* is unsuitable for frying or baking. *Olestra* is heat stable and can be used in cooking and frying.

Scientists are still researching a fat replacement that tastes, looks, smells and cooks like fat, contains no calories, has no side effects, is well accepted by the public and is inexpensive. It may take decades before all of this criteria is met. Recently, two new fat replacements have received FDA approval. They are basically soy based.

Breakdown of Triglycerides

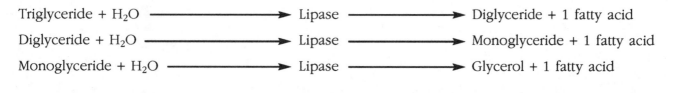

Triglyceride + H_2O ⟶ Lipase ⟶ Diglyceride + 1 fatty acid

Diglyceride + H_2O ⟶ Lipase ⟶ Monoglyceride + 1 fatty acid

Monoglyceride + H_2O ⟶ Lipase ⟶ Glycerol + 1 fatty acid

---

[1]Position of the American Dietetic Association: Fat replacements, J. of the American Dietetic Association, 91, 1285–1288 1991

[2]Drewnowski, A. Sensory properties of fat and fat replacements, Nutrition Reviews 50, 1117–1120 1992

[3]Jan. 8, 1996 Time Magazine—excellent information for the layperson

▶ SATURATED AND UNSATURATED FATS ◀

Fat Source and Type	Percent		
		Unsaturated	
	Saturated	Poly	Mono
Saturated			
Egg, Chicken	37	11	52
Sheep	52	6	42
Beef	53	6	41
Pig	44	11	45
Cow Milk	60	4	36
Cocoa bean	51–66	2–3	41–47
Coconut	94	1	5
Lard	39	13	48
Tallow	52–60	3–5	37–43
Monosaturated			
Olive Oil	7–24	5–15	65–86
Polyunsaturated			
Peanut (groundnut)	15–24	19–37	39–66
Linseed	6–16	13–36	55–70
Pecan	5–7	16–25	71–78
Walnut	5–11	60–80	9–35
Safflower	5–10	57–59	13–37
Corn (maize)	11–15	34–61	24–50
Sunflower	8–15	33–73	10–58
Sesame seed	12–16	38–48	35–49
Cotton seed	27	53	20
Barley	12	55	33
Rice	18	35	47
Wheat	15	59	26

Vitamins

Vitamins are chemical compounds that occur in minute quantities in food and are necessary for growth and life. Vitamins are either fat soluble or water soluble. Fat soluble vitamins are:

	Precursors
Vitamin A	Axerophtal
	Dehydronetinal
	Retenoic acid
	Retinal
	Retinol
Vitamin D	Antirachitic factor
	Cholecalciferal
	Ergocalciferal
Vitamin E	Tocopherol
	Antisterility factor
Vitamin K	Phylloguinone
	Antihemorrhogic factor
	Menadione (synthetic)

Properties of Fat Soluble Vitamins

1. Soluble in fat and fat solvents.
2. Not excreted.
3. Excessive intake stored in body.
4. Symptoms of deficiency slow to develop.
5. Need not be taken in diet daily.
6. Have precursors.
7. Made up of carbon, hydrogen and oxygen.

Mineral oil will interfere with absorption of fat soluble vitamins and should be avoided.

Properties of Water Soluble Vitamins

1. Soluble in water.
2. Minimum storage.
3. Excreted in urine.
4. Deficiency symptoms often develop rapidly.
5. Must be supplied in diet every day.
6. Generally no precursors.
7. Contains carbon, hydrogen, oxygen and nitrogen, and in some cases, cobalt and sulphur.

The water soluble vitamins are Vitamin C (ascorbic acid), B_2 (thiamine), B_1 (riboflavin), niacin, folic acid and pyridoxine (B_6), and other vitamins of the B complex.

▶ FAT SOLUBLE VITAMINS ◀

Vitamin	Function	Deficiency or Excess	Source	Recommended* Dosage
Vitamin A: (Precursors Carotenes)	Maintains function of epithelial & mucous membranes, skin, bone, vision in dim light. *Stored* in liver. Bile needed for absorption of carotenes.	*Deficiency:* Night blindness; lowered resistance to infection; Changes in genitourinary tract; changes in gastrointestinal tract. *Severe:* drying and scaling of skin, eye infection and blindness. *Overdose* is toxic.	Liver, egg yolks, kidney, butter, fortified margarine, whole milk, cream cheese, dark leafy and deep yellow vegetables. Deep yellow fruits.	Adults: Males 1,000 µg Females 800 µg Pregnancy 800 µg IU 1300 µg Lactation 1200 µg
Vitamin D: (Precursors Ergosterol in plants; 7-dehydrocholesterol in skin)	Aids in absorption of calcium and phosphorus. Calcification of bones, teeth. Some stored in liver.	*Deficiency:* Rickets, Osteomalacia in adults. *Small* excess is toxic.	Fortified milk, fish, liver, oils. Exposure to the ultraviolet rays of sun.	5–10µg infants, children, adolescents and pregnant women.
Vitamin E	Protects red blood cells. Antioxidants for both animal and plant tissue. Limited amount *stored* in body. Needs bile for absorption.	Rarely seen in humans.	Wheat germ, oil, vegetable oils, egg yolk, beef liver, peanuts, margarine, nuts, dark leafy vegetables.	Variable depending on age.
Vitamin K	Forms prothrombin for normal blood clotting.	*Deficiency:* Low prothrombin levels. Hemorrhage.	Dark green leafy vegetables. Synthesized in intestine.	Variable depending on age.

*For more detailed information see the 1989 RDAs in the Appendix. Carefully review for children and pregnant and lactating females. Age also makes a difference in requirements.

Vitamins, beta carotene, Vitamin C and Vitamin E are rich in antioxidants which may reduce the risk of cancer. Oxygen damage (oxidation) to cells may be partly responsible for the effects of aging and certain diseases. There are on-going studies on antioxidation in food that may protect against this damage. Cells make toxic molecules called "free radicals"—(a damaged cell—one that is missing an electron). This "free radical" molecule wants its electron—it will react with any molecule from which it can take an electron. By taking an electron from certain key compotents in the cell, free radicals damage cells. Antioxidants may block some of the damage by donating electrons to stabilize and neutralize the harmful effects of free radicals. Eventually free radicals may overwhelm the body's natural defense, it may contribute to aging and certain diseases.

▶ WATER SOLUBLE VITAMINS ◀

Vitamin	Function	Deficiency or Excess	Source	Recommended Dosage
Vitamin C: (Ascorbic Acid)	Healing wounds, dentin formation, tyrosine metabolism, utilization of calcium, protein, folic acid. Resistance to infection.	*Deficiency:* Loose teeth, bleeding gums, bruising, hemorrhaging, scurvy.	Citrus fruits, strawberries, cantaloupe, tomatoes, broccoli, sweet peppers, potatoes, kale, parsley, turnip greens.	Males, 60 mg Females, 55 mg Pregnancy, 70 mg Lactation, 90 mg
Vitamin B_1: (Thiamine)	Good digestion, healthy nerves, normal appetite, metabolism of carbohydrates, Coenzyme from cocarboxylase.	*Deficiency:* Fatigue, mental depression, poor appetite, neuritis of legs, decreased muscle tone. Beriberi.	Pork, liver, organ meat, whole grain or enriched cereal products, nuts, legumes, milk, eggs.	Males, 1.3 mg Females, 1.1 mg
Vitamin B_2: (Riboflavin)	Healthy skin, metabolism of carbohydrate fats, protein. Coenzyme from FMN and FAD.	*Deficiency:* Cheilosis. Cracked lips, scaling skin, burning, itching eyes.	Liver, milk, meat, eggs, enriched cereal products, green leafy vegetables.	Males, 1.7 mg Females, 1.3 mg
Niacin (Nicotine Acid)	All living cells. Metabolism of carbohydrates, fats and proteins. Active coenzyme from NAD and NADP. 60 mg. tryptophan = 1 unit niacin.	*Deficiency:* Pellegra. Dermatitis, sore mouth, diarrhea, mental depression, disorientation, delirium.	Meat, fish, liver, poultry, dark green leafy vegetables, whole-grain or enriched bread, cereal.	Males, 19 mg NE Females, 15 mg NE Pregnancy, 17 mgNE Lactation, 20 mgNE
Folic Acid (Folacin)	Growth, blood formation, choline, synthesis, amino acid metabolism.	*Deficiency:* Toxemia of pregnancy, megaloblastic anemia.	Pork, liver and other organ meats: eggs, asparagus.	Males, 200 μg Females, 180 μg Increased with pregnancy and lactation
Vitamin B_6: (Pyridoxine Pyridoxal)	Metabolism of amino acid. Coenzyme PALD	*Deficiency:* Adults–microcytic hypochromic anemia, irritability.	Pork, beef liver, bananas, ham, egg yolks.	Males, 2.0 mg Females, 1.6 mg

Minerals

Minerals are inorganic substances and are found in all body tissue and fluids. Four percent of the body's weight is made up of 15 or more mineral elements. Calcium makes up one half of all the mineral matter in the body. An absence of any of the minerals can cause serious problems; an excess of some can be toxic.

▶ MINERAL COMPOSITION OF THE ADULT BODY ◀ AND DIETARY ALLOWANCES

	Approximate Amount in Adult Body 70 kg	Adult Dietary Allowances
Minerals for which an RDA has been set		
Calcium	1200 g	800 mg
Phosphorus	750 g	800 mg
Magnesium	30 g	280 mg (females) 350 mg (males)
Iron	4 g	15 mg (females) 10 mg (males)
Zinc	2 g	12 mg (females) 15 mg (males)
Iodine	30 mg	150 μg
Selenium	2 g	55 μg (females) 70 μg (males)
Minerals for which an estimated safe and adequate intake has been set		
Molybdenum	3 g	75-250 μg
Fluoride	1 g	1.5-4.0 mg
Copper	150 mg	1.5-3.0 mg
Manganese	150 mg	2.0-5.0 mg
Chromium	5 mg	50-200 μg
Minerals with estimated minimum requirements		
Potassium	245 g	2000 mg
Sodium	105 g	500 mg
Chlorine	105 g	750 mg
Minerals for which no allowances have been set		
a. Essential as parts of other nutrients		
Sulfur	175 g	
Cobalt	5 mg	
b. Present in the body and possibly essential: arsenic, cadmium, nickel, silicon, rin, vanadium		
c. Present in the body but no known function: aluminum, barium, boron, bromine, gold, lead, mercury, strontium		

Robinson/Weigley/Mueller. BASIC NUTRITION AND DIET THERAPY. 7.e, c 1992, p. 151. Reprinted by permission of Prentice Hall, Upper Saddle River, New Jersey.

▶ INORGANIC ELEMENTS IN HUMAN NUTRITION ◀

(Known or Believed to be Essential)

Mineral/ Body Content	Location in Body and Some Biological Functions	Estimated Daily Requirement for Adult	Food Source	Comments of Likelihood of a Deficiency
Macrominerals				
Calcium	90% in bones and teeth. Ionic calcium in body fluids essential for ion transport across cell membranes. Calcium is also bound to protein, citrate, or inorganic acids.	Recommended Dietary Allowance: 1200 mg-1500 mg for 11-24 yr. 1,000-1500 to prevent osteoporosis	Best: milk, hard cheese, grains, turnips, collards, kale, mustard, broccoli Good: ice cream, cottage cheese, oysters, shrimp, salmon, clams	Dietary surveys indicate that many diets do not meet recommended Dietary allowances for calcium. Since bone serves as a homeostatic mechanism to maintain calcium level in blood, many essential functions are maintained, regardless of diet. Long-term dietary deficiency is probably one of the factors responsible for osteoporosis (bone thinning), a significant clinical problem.
Phosphorus	About 85% in inorganic phase of bones and teeth. Phosphorus is a component of every cell and of highly metabolites, including DNA, RNA, ATP (high energy compound), phospholipids.	In ordinary diets, phosphorus intake of adults is approx. 11/2 times that of calcium. On an intake of 800 mg. calcium, phosphorus intake is approx. 1200 mg.	Milk, cheese, egg yolk, meat, fish, fowl, legumes, nuts, whole grain cereals	Dietary deficiency not likely to occur if protein and calcium intake is adequate. However, increased need for phosphorus is postulated with diet leading to acid urine and during prolonged therapy with certain antacids.
Potassium	Major cation of intracellular fluid, with only small amounts in extracellular fluid. Functions in regulating pH and osmolarity, cell membrane transfer. Ion is necessary for carbohydrate and protein metabolism.	Usual diet in U.S. contains from 0.8 to 1.5 gm potassium/1000 calories.	Meat, fish, fowl, cereals, fruits, vegetables	Dietary deficiency unlikely but conditioned deficiency may be found in kidney disease, diabetic acidosis, excessive vomiting or diarrhea, hyperfunction of adrenal cortex, etc. potassium excess may be a problem in renal failure and sever acidosis.
Sulfur	Bulk of dietary sulfur is present in sulfur-containing amino acids needed for synthesis of essential metabolites; functions in oxidation-reduction reactions. Sulfur also functions in thiamine, biotin, and as inorganic sulfur.	Need for sulfur is satisfied by estimated daily requirements for essential amino acids and vitamins.	Eggs, cheese, milk, meat, nuts, legumes	Dietary intake is chiefly from sulfur containing amino acids and adequacy is related to protein intake

INORGANIC ELEMENTS IN HUMAN NUTRITION—Continued

Mineral/ Body Content	Location in Body and Some Biological Functions	Estimated Daily Requirement for Adult	Food Source	Comments of Likelihood of a Deficiency
Macrominerals				
Iron	About 60% is in hemoglobin; about 26% stored in liver, spleen and bone. Iron is component of hemoglobin and myoglobin, important in oxygen transfer; also present in serum transferrin and certain enzymes. Almost none in ionic form.	Recommended dietary allowance: 12 mg for adult man; 15 mg for premenopausal woman with an additional 5 mg during pregnancy and lactation.	Best: liver Good: meat, egg yolk, enriched bread and cereal, dark green vegetables, molasses, legumes	Iron-deficiency anemia occurs in women in reproductive years and infants and preschool children. May be associated with unusual blood loss, parasites, malabsorption (in some cases).
Magnesium	About 50% in bone. Remaining 50% is almost entirely inside body cells with only about 1% in extracellular fluid. Ionic Mg functions as an activator of many enzymes and must influence almost all processes.	Males, 350 mg Females, 280 mg	Whole grain cereal, legumes, nuts, dark green vegetables	Dietary deficiency considered unlikely, but conditioned deficiency is often seen in clinical medicine, associated with surgery, malabsorption, loss of body fluids, certain hormone and renal diseases, etc. Magnesium deficiency has a profound effect on other minerals.
Sodium	30–45% in bone. Major cation of extracellular fluid and only a small amount is inside cell. Regulates body fluid osmolarity, pH and body fluid volume.	About 10 gm NaCl/day usual intake in U.S.	Table salt, meat, fish, fowl, milk, eggs, sodium compounds, such as baking soda and baking powder	Dietary deficiency probably never occurs, although low blood sodium requires treatment in certain disorders. Evidence is accumulating that requirements increase during pregnancy. Sodium restriction is practiced in certain cardiovascular disorders.
Chloride	Major anion of extracellular fluid, functions in combination with sodium; serves as a buffer, enzyme activator; component of gastric hydrochloric acid. Mostly present in extracellular fluid; less than 15% inside cells.	(Included under sodium)	Table salt, meat, milk, eggs	In most cases, dietary intake is of little significance except in presence of vomiting, diarrhea or profuse sweating.

INORGANIC ELEMENTS IN HUMAN NUTRITION—Continued

Mineral/ Body Content	Location in Body and Some Biological Functions	Estimated Daily Requirement for Adult	Food Source	Comments of Likelihood of a Deficiency
Microminerals				
Zinc	Present in most tissues, with higher amounts in liver, voluntary muscle, and bone. Constituent of essential enzymes and insulin. May be of importance in nucleic acid metabolism.	Males, 15 mg Females, 12 mg	Widely distributed, oysters, seafood, liver, wheat germ, yeast	Zinc deficiency has been demonstrated in Iran and Egypt in certain patients whose diet is also deficient in protein and iron. Possibility of dietary deficiency in this country considered remote, but conditioned deficiency may be seen in systemic childhood illnesses; and in patients who are nutritionally depleted or have been subjected to severe stress such as surgery.
Copper	Found in all body tissues, larger amounts in liver, brain, heart and kidney. Constituent of enzymes; of ceruloplasm and erythrocubre in blood. May be integral part of DNA or RNA molecule.	Daily intake of 2 mg appears to maintain balance; ordinary diets provide 2-5 mg/day.	Liver, shellfish, meat, fish, nuts, legumes, whole grain cereal	No evidence that specific dietary deficiencies of copper in the human.
Iodine	Constituent of thyroxine and related compounds synthesized by thyroid gland. Thyroxine function in control of reactions involving cellular energy.	150 micrograms.	Iodized salt is best protection	Iodization of table salt is recommended especially in areas where food is low in iodine. Certain foods contain goitrogens which may accentuate effect of low dietary iodine.
Manganese	Highest concentration is in bone, also relatively high concentrations in pituitary, liver, pancreas, and gastrointestinal tissue. Constituent of essential enzyme systems; rich in mitochondria of liver cells.	3-9 mg for children: 0.2 mg/kg.	Whole grain cereal, legumes, meat, fish, fowl, green leafy vegetables	Unlikely that dietary deficiency occurs in humans.
Fluorine	Present in bone. In optimal amounts in water and diet, reduces dental caries and may minimize bone loss. This effect appears to be due to it combining with bone crystal to form a more stable compound.	Essentially not established, but appears to be necessary for optimal health of bones and teeth.	Water with 1 ppm fluoride	In areas where fluorine content of water is low, fluoridation of water (1 ppm) has been found beneficial in reducing incidence of dental caries. (Excess may be toxic)

INORGANIC ELEMENTS IN HUMAN NUTRITION—Continued

Mineral/ Body Content	Location in Body and Some Biological Functions	Estimated Daily Requirement for Adult	Food Source	Comments of Likelihood of a Deficiency
Microminerals				
Molybdenum	Constituent of essential enzyme (xanthine oxidase) and of flavo proteins.	Little quantitative evidence of requirement.	————	No information.
Cobalt	Constituent of cyanocobalamin (vitamin B_{12}), occurring bound to protein in foods of animal origin. Essential to normal function of all cells, particularly cells of bone marrow, nervous system and gastrointestinal system.	3-5 micrograms Vitamin B_{12}	Must be supplied as Vitamin B_{12}	Primary dietary deficiency is rare except when no animal products are consumed. Deficiency may be found in such conditions as lack of gastric intrinsic factor, gastrectomy, and malabsorption syndrome.

Adapted from a vary of sources.

Water

It is impossible to survive without the intake of water. Water constitutes 60% of the total body weight, and should not be severely restricted without medical advice.

Water that is present in the arteries, veins and capillaries acts as a solvent for nutrients and for hormones secreted by the glands. This fluid also acts as a transporter of wasted material of metabolism. Within the cell, intracellular water is used as a body builder. Water is essential to digestion and it controls body temperature.

About 40% of the water ingested comes from tap water. The rest comes from milk, other beverages, and food.

Solid foods contain approximately 70% water. Protein contains .41 grams water per gram protein; carbohydrate has 0.60 gram water per gram carbohydrate; fat has 1.07 grams of water per gram fat.

Balance—in normal circumstances, the amounts should balance; that is, the amount lost should equal amount taken in.

Dehydration—the removal of water from the body through breathing, sweat, feces, urine. Abnormal losses occur through vomiting, diarrhea, fever and blood loss.

Edema—is the accumulation of fluids in body spaces. This results in swelling of the extremities, usually in the feet and ankles, hands and face. It is a common symptom in pregnancy and in a number of diseases, indicating that the water balance has been disturbed.

▶ APPROXIMATE DAILY ADULT INTAKE AND OUTPUT OF WATER ◀

Sources of Water	Ml.	Losses of Water	Ml.
Solid foods	500–1000	Urine	100–1400
Liquid foods	1100	Insensible perspiration (skin)	500
Water of oxidation (metabolism)	300–400	Lungs	300–500
		Feces	100
Total	1900–2500	Total	1900–2500

▶ FLUID REQUIREMENT PER KILOGRAM OF BODY WEIGHT ◀

	Ml./Kg.
Infants	110
10 year old children	40
Adults	
72 F	22
100 F	38

▶ DIGESTION AND ABSORPTION OF FOOD ◀

Digestion is the process whereby food is broken down into simple, soluble materials (nutrients) which can be absorbed through the gastrointestinal mucosa into the blood and lymph streams. It occurs by both mechanical (mastication and peristalsis) and chemical action (hydrolysis, enzymatic breakdown) beginning in the mouth and ending in the small intestine.

The food is taken into the mouth where it is broken into small pieces by the teeth and mixed with saliva, mucous, and digestive enzymes. Saliva softens and lubricates food and starts the breakdown of starch with the enzyme salivary amylase. Food then moves down the esophagus to the stomach, a temporary storage pouch, where peristalsis softens the food as it combines with gastric juices. Hydrochloric acid and pepsin begin the breakdown of protein in the stomach. Very little digestion of carbohydrates and fats occur here. The food, now called chyme, is slowly emptied into the small intestines where most of the digestive activity takes place. Bile from the liver, and digestive enzymes from the pancreas and the walls of the intestines break protein, carbohydrates, and fats down to their simplest forms for absorption. The final end products of digestion are simple sugars, fatty acids and glycerol, and amino acids.

Simple carbohydrates, minerals, and water are absorbed directly into the bloodstream from the stomach mucosa due to their elemental chemical structures. Absorption of most other nutrients occurs in the small intestine, specifically through the villi, fingerlike projections lining the small intestine. Each villi is composed of a lymph vessel surrounded by capillaries. Nutrients absorbed into the lymph vessel pass into the lymphatic system and those absorbed via the capillaries enter portal circulation and go directly to the liver.

The sugars are absorbed directly through the capillaries and are carried to the liver where they are stored as glycogen if not needed for energy. The end products of fat digestion pass into the lymphatic system and are transported directly to the tissues where they are used for energy or stored as body fat. Amino acids are absorbed via the capillaries and pass to the liver through portal circulation and then disseminated to the tissues to be used in protein metabolism. Vitamins, minerals and fluids are also absorbed through the intestinal mucosa along with the end products of carbohydrate, protein, and fat digestion.

Unabsorbed food enters into the large intestines. As water and digestive juice are reabsorbed, the waste (feces) takes on a solid consistency and is eliminated through the rectum and anus.

The speed of digestion varies widely, from 9 to 48 hours, depending on the size and composition of the meal and certain psychological factors. Carbohydrates are digested most rapidly, proteins next and fats last. Enzymes are the primary substances that are involved in the process of digestion (See the following chart). Other chemical substances, besides enzymes, that aid in digestion are:

1. Hydrochloric acid secreted by the stomach. Its functions include activation of pepsinogen to pepsin and acidifying stomach contents.
2. Bile, excreted by the liver into small intestines, emulsifies fats.
3. Hormones produced in mucosa of gastrointestinal tract perform a variety of functions.

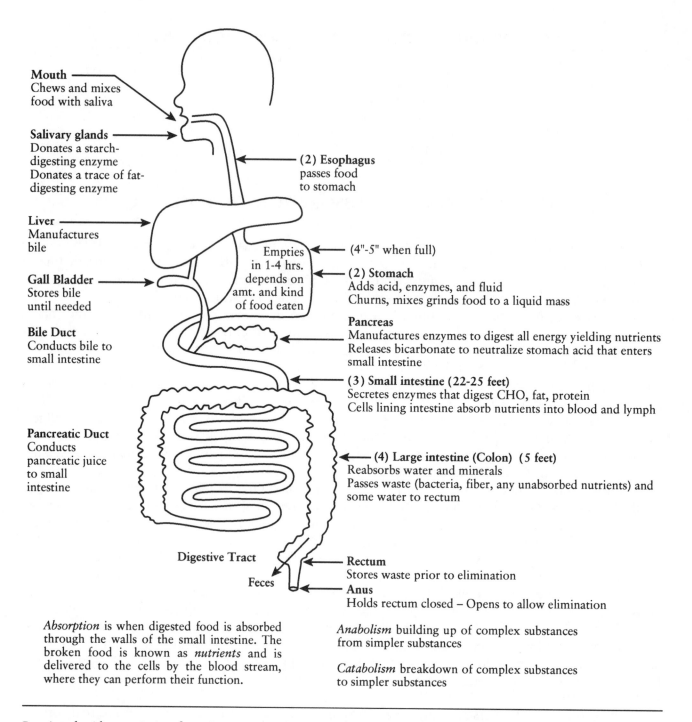

Mouth —
Chews and mixes
food with saliva

Salivary glands —
Donates a starch-
digesting enzyme
Donates a trace of fat-
digesting enzyme

(2) Esophagus
passes food
to stomach

Liver —
Manufactures
bile

(4"-5" when full)

Empties
in 1-4 hrs.
depends on
amt. and kind
of food eaten

(2) Stomach
Adds acid, enzymes, and fluid
Churns, mixes grinds food to a liquid mass

Gall Bladder —
Stores bile
until needed

Pancreas
Manufactures enzymes to digest all energy yielding nutrients
Releases bicarbonate to neutralize stomach acid that enters
small intestine

Bile Duct
Conducts bile to
small intestine

(3) Small intestine (22-25 feet)
Secretes enzymes that digest CHO, fat, protein
Cells lining intestine absorb nutrients into blood and lymph

Pancreatic Duct
Conducts
pancreatic juice
to small
intestine

(4) Large intestine (Colon) (5 feet)
Reabsorbs water and minerals
Passes waste (bacteria, fiber, any unabsorbed nutrients) and
some water to rectum

Digestive Tract

Feces

Rectum
Stores waste prior to elimination

Anus
Holds rectum closed – Opens to allow elimination

Absorption is when digested food is absorbed
through the walls of the small intestine. The
broken food is known as *nutrients* and is
delivered to the cells by the blood stream,
where they can perform their function.

Anabolism building up of complex substances
from simpler substances

Catabolism breakdown of complex substances
to simpler substances

Reprinted with permission from Dietary Managers Training Course. 1999 R. Puckett

DIGESTION: The process which food goes through before it can be used by the cells. Changes in
food are accomplished by:

1.   Mechanical action peristalsis.
2.   Chemical action is accomplished by the action of enzymes produced by various glands.

DIGESTION

1. Food taken in *mouth*. Saliva softens and lubricates food and starts the breakdown of carbohydrates to sugar.
2. Food moves down *esophagus* to stomach where muscular contractions further softens the food as it mixes with gastric juice. Proteins begin to digest in the stomach, carbohydrates continue to be digested.
3. Food is moved by gentle muscular action (peristalsis) from *stomach* to small *intestines*. Major digestion takes place here. Food is thick liquid. Digestion of protein, fats, carbohydrates are completed in small intestine. Food is now in simplest form and can be used by the cells in the body.
4. Unabsorbed food enters from *small intestine* to *large intestines*. From time food is eaten to this point, about 9 hours. Excess fluids absorbed from large intestine leaving waste which is *eliminated* as feces.

▶ ENZYMATIC DIGESTION OF CARBOHYDRATES, FATS AND PROTEINS ◀

Source of Enzyme	Enzyme	Substrate	Product

Mouth
  Salivary Glands
	Salivary amylase
	  ptyalin
		Starch (carbohydrate)	Dextrins & maltose

Stomach
  Gastric mucosa
	Gastric Proteases
	  pepsin
		Proteins	Polypeptides, proteoses, peptones

	rennin	Casein	Paracasein (insoluble)
	Gastric lipase	Emulsified fat	Fatty acids and glycerol

Small intestine
  Pancreas
	Pancreatic proteases
	  trypsin
	  chymotrypsin
	  carboxypeptidases
		Proteins and polypeptides	Smaller polypeptides and amino acids

	Pancreatic lipase
	  steapsin
		Fats	Mono & diglycerides
			  fatty acids and glycerol

	Pancreatic amylase amylopsin	Starch	Maltose

Intestinal
  Brush border
	Intestinal peptidases
	  aminopeptidase
	  dipeptidase
		Polypeptides
		Dipeptides
			Smaller polypeptides and amino acids

	Intestinal disaccharidases
	  sucrose
	  maltase
	  lactase
		Sucrose
		Maltose
		Lactose
			Glucose & fructose
			Glucose (2 molecules)
			Glucose & galactose

Key Words

1. *Peristalsis*—the wave-like muscular squeezing of the esophagus, stomach, and small intestine that pushes their content along
2. *Chyme*—the fluid resulting from the actions of the stomach upon a meal
3. *Pyloric valve*—the circular muscle of the lower stomach that regulates the flow of partly digested food into the small intestine.

4. **Bile**—a compound made by the liver, stored in the gall bladder, and released into the small intestine when needed
5. **Bicarbonate**—a common alkaline chemical: a secretion of the pancreas
6. **Mucous**—a slippery coating of the intestine tract and other body linings that protects the cells from exposure to digestive juices and other destructive agents.

References

Drewnowski, A. Sensory Properties of Fat and Fat Replacements, *Nutrition Reviews,* 50, 117–1120, 1992.

Hahn, N. Setting the nations health agenda J. Amer. Dietet. Assoc. 99, 4, 415–420. 1999

Hamilton, EVN, Whitney, EN, Sizer, FS, *Nutrition Concepts and Controversies, 5th ed.,* West Publishing Co., St. Paul, MN 1991.

Hauff, K. "Water—The Forgotten Nutrient", *Support Line, Newsletter of Dietitians in Nutrition Support,* 13:11–16, October, 1991.

Sizer, FS, Whitney EN, Hamilton/Whitney's Nutrition Concepts & Controversies 6th ed, West Publishers NY, 1994

Healthy People 2000: National Health Promotion and Disease Prevention Objectives, U.S. Dept. of Health and Human Services, Public Health Service, Washington, DC. 1990.

January 8, 1996 issue of *Time Magazine* (laypersons guide to fat substitutes)

Larson, D.E. Mayo Clinic Family Health Book 2nd ed., William Morrow & Co., Inc. NY 1996.

National Library of Medicine "Adverse Effects of Aspartame", (GPO No. 817-006=00014-1) *Current Bibliographies in Medicine,* 1991, Superintendent of Documents, U.S. Printing Office, Washington, DC 20402

Nutrition and Your Health: Dietary Guidelines for American, 3rd ed., Home and Garden Bulletin No. 232, U.S. Dept. of Agriculture and U.S. Department of Health and Human Services, Washington, DC. 1990 and 1995.

Position of the American Dietetic Assoc.: Fat Replacement, J. *Amer. Dietet. Assoc.,* 98:463, 1998.

Position of the American Dietetic Assoc.: Health implications of dietary fiber J. Amer. Dietet. Assoc. 97:1157, 1997

Position of the American Dietetic Assoc.: Use of nutritive and non-nutritive sweeteners, J. Amer. Dietet. Assoc. 98: 98: 580, 1998

Puckett, RP, Brown, SM, Shands, *Hospital at the University of Florida: Guide to Clinical Dietetics, 5th ed.,* Kendall/Hunt Publishing Co., Dubuque, IA. 1993.

Recommended Daily Allowances, 10th Ed., Food and Nutrition Board, National Academy of Science, Washington, DC. 1989.

Robinson, CH, Weigley, ES, Mueller, DH, *Basic Nutrition and Diet Therapy, 7th ed.,* Macmillan Publishing Co., New York, 1993.

Slavin, J., "Nutritional Benefits of Soy Protein and Soy Fiber", J. *Amer. Dietet. Assoc.,* 91:816–19. 1991.

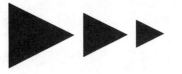

Module 2

Nutrition Through the Life Cycle

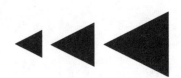

▶ PRECONCEPTIONAL NUTRITION ◀

The physical and mental health of the woman prior to conception may have a profound effect on the pregnancy outcome. In order to decrease the infant mortality rate women of childbearing age need to have adequate diets and be healthy before conception. Weight management, both under and over weight can place the fetus at risk. Infants born to women who have a body weight of less than 85 per cent of ideal body weight (IBW) are more likely to have preterm infants of low birth weight, and possible delay.

Women who have a weight of 120 percent or greater than the IBW have a greater chance of developing hypertension and gestation diabetes. Infants born to these women are more likely to suffer birth trauma, suffer from neonatal hypoglycemia, and become overweight by the 12th month of age.

Other concerns include:
▶ women with chronic dieting
▶ women who skip meals or fast
▶ women who eat a limited variety of foods
▶ women of low income
▶ women who have conceived within 12 months of previous pregnancy
▶ women with a history of problematic obesity
▶ women who are smokers, alcoholics, and/or drug addicts
▶ women who have chronic systemic diseases (diabetes mellitus)
▶ women who are HIV positive
▶ women 35 years and older

A healthy women who has practiced good nutritional habits before becoming pregnant has a very good chance of delivering a healthy, full term baby of normal weight. Good nutrition before and during pregnancy affects both present and future development of the infant.

▶ PREGNANCY AND LACTATION ◀

Prenatal care is essential. Good nutrition is essential to the health of the pregnant woman and her unborn child. If the diet is inadequate, the baby may obtain its needs at the mother's expense or suffer from mental or physical malformation.

The physician may recommend a prenatal multivitamin and/or iron supplement to meet these needs.

It is acceptable to gain 25–35 pounds during the nine months, in addition to the ideal maternal weight (first trimester, 1 to 1½ pounds a month; second trimester ½ to ¾ pounds a week; third trimester, ¾ to 1 pound per week.) A daily intake of 2000 calories should supply a steady but slow weight gain. Protein should be increased to 4–6 ounces of meat or meat substitute daily. Milk should be emphasized (2–4 cups daily), since the calcium and phosphorus provides for bone and tooth formation of the infant.

Breads and cereals furnish energy and other necessary nutrients. In case of excess weight, bread and cereal may be limited, but should not be completely omitted. Vegetables and fruits contain vitamins and minerals. Fresh fruits and green vegetables also encourage daily elimination. The Food Guide Pyramid (pg) is a good model for healthful daily eating.

Fats and sugars furnish necessary calories and energy. They may be limited if weight gain is a problem.

Discuss the use of salt, artificial sweeteners and caffeine with the physician. Most physicians suggest avoiding caffeine-containing foods and drugs whenever possible. Herbal teas should also be avoided.

If the mother elects to breastfeed her baby after its birth, she will need enough calories to furnish milk. A daily intake of approximately 3,000 calories is suggested; on the ideal intake the mother will not be gaining or losing weight.

Again, protein should be emphasized with an intake of 6–8 ounces of meat or meat substitute daily. Milk should increase to 1 quart daily.

Breads and cereals may be used as desired. Three to five servings of fruits and vegetables should be eaten daily. Strongly flavored vegetables should be limited, since the flavor will be passed into the breast milk. The laxative property of prune juice also passes into the milk.

Fats and sugars may be used as desired.

No restrictive diets should be attempted in pregnancy without a physician's knowledge and approval.

Drink 6–8, 8 ounce glasses of liquid each day, to include at least 3-, 8 ounce glasses of water. Avoid herbal teas as they may cause nausea, vomiting, and convulsions.

Pregnancy places demands for increased intake of foods to provide energy and a greater need for increased nutrients. (See RDA in Appendix W)

Nutritional Concerns: PICA

Food cravings, such as pickles, ice cream, or watermelon aren't necessarily of concern, unless they interfere with the consumption of a balanced diet. The craving for cornstarch, dirt, clay and laundry starch is known as pica and presents a problem for healthcare providers. Patients must be educated about the need to discontinue this practice since the intake of these products may reduce the intake of nutritious foods and interfere with iron absorption. Most pregnant women who practice these cravings are considered at risk of developing nutritional deficiencies. Cravings may reflect a diet that is nutrient poor, however, these cravings usually do not reflect a physiological need.

Fad Diets, Skipping Meals

The growing fetus needs a constant source of well balanced nutrients for proper growth and development. Skipping meals or following a fad diet has an adverse effect on the development of the fetus.

Nausea

Some women experience nausea, frequently referred to as "morning sickness" during the first trimester of pregnancy. **See suggested meal plans that follow.**

Constipation

If constipation occurs, an increase in high fiber food is recommended. Foods such as fresh fruits, vegetables, prunes and whole grain breads and cereals are natural laxatives. Increase the fluid intake, the majority being from water. Get plenty of rest. Exercise on the advice of the physician. If the conditions continue after an increased intake of these foods the woman will need to discuss the problem with her physician.

Other Concerns

Heartburn, bloating/cramping, muscle cramps, and frequency of urination may present problems for some women. In the case of heartburn, eating small and frequent meals that are more bland may give relief. Try to plan and eat meals in a relaxed atmosphere. Avoid large, heavy fat meals just before bedtime. Bloating/cramping may also be reduced by the elimination of greasy foods, reduction in the amount of roughage in the diet and reduction of the drinking of cold (iced) beverages. Frequency and urgency of urination can be reduced by avoiding caffeine beverages, alcohol and spices.

Major Concerns

There are some substances that can be harmful to the fetus. Healthcare personnel will need to carefully question and monitor the mother concerning the use of these substances. Pregnant women must be encouraged to eat a healthy diet and forgo the use of the following substances, or on the advise of her physician practice moderation.

▶ *Limit the intake of caffeine.* Some nutritionists suggest the complete elimination of caffeine during pregnancy, others suggest no more than 4–8 ounce cups per day and others no more than 2–8 ounce cups per day.

▶ *Quit smoking.* Smoking stunts growth, thus increasing the risk of mental retardation. The surgeon general has warned that smoking can be lethal to an otherwise normal fetus or newborn. Even inhaling "second-hand" smoke may be hazardous to a pregnant woman and her unborn child.

▶ *Do not use over-the-counter (OTC) and street drugs.* Some OTC, unprescribed drugs, excessive vitamins as they may cause serious birth defects. Street drugs, such as marijuana, crack, coke, cocaine, heroin, etc. have been found to cause nervous disorders and withdrawal symptoms for the newborn as well as other possible serious health problems to both the mother and the fetus/infant.

▶ *Do not drink alcohol during pregnancy.* Drinking excessive alcohol during pregnancy leads to fetal alcohol syndrome (FAS). FAS threatens the fetus with irreversible brain damage and mental and physical retardation. Every container of beer, wine and liquor that is sold must carry a warning label to pregnant women of the danger to their health.

Some pregnant women experience gestation diabetes, and pregnancy-induced hypertension. Each condition must be properly managed by a physician and the nutrition care team. (See Diet for gestation diabetes in Section 2, Module 3.) If a pregnant woman becomes infected by an infectious disease during pregnancy, the physician must be contacted immediately.

Modification for Pregnancy

Excessive weight gain in pregnancy may call for a low calorie or low sodium diet. The regular restrictions may be ordered or a combination of the two diets may be ordered as is outlined below. Any other dietary restrictions may be ordered by indicating the type diet desired.

► **1500 CALORIE RESTRICTED SODIUM #3 DIET** ◄
FOR OBESITY AND TOXEMIA OF PREGNANCY
CHO-155 gm, Pro–91 gm, Fat–55 gm, Sodium 1.5–2 gm, (65.2–87 mEq)

Breakfast
Fruit, 1 serving from Fruit List below
Salt-free Egg, 1 (boiled or poached—not fried)
Bread, 2 slices (may substitute 1/2 cup of any cereal cooked without salt or 3/4 cup of puffed rice, puffed wheat or shredded wheat for a slice of bread)
Margarine or unsalted butter, 1 pat (1 teaspoon)
Skim milk, 1 cup (8 ounces)
Coffee or tea, if desired—no sugar or cream. Sugar substitute may be used.
(Limit intake of coffee, tea. Keep total intake below 200 milligrams per day.)

Lunch and Dinner
Meat, fish or chicken, 1 medium serving of lean meat (3 oz.) both meals. Use fresh meat such as beef, veal, mutton, lamb, liver, chicken, turkey, rabbit, squirrel, fish. DO NOT FRY the meat or make stew or gravy with it. Do not cook meat with salt. Two eggs may be substituted for the meat.
Vegetables, 1 cup from the Vegetable list. Try to eat one raw vegetable every day. Do not add salt in cooking.
Bread, 1 slice (may substitute ½ cup of potato, rice, corn, spaghetti, macaroni, noodles, grits, dried beans, or dried peas for the slice of bread.) Do not add salt.
Margarine or unsalted butter, 1 pat (1 teaspoon)
Fruit, 1 serving from Fruit List
Skim milk, 1 cup (8 ounces)
Coffee or tea, if desired. No sugar or cream. Sugar substitute may be used
(Limit intake of coffee, tea use decaffeinated.)

Bedtime
1 cup skim milk
Fruit, 1 serving from Fruit List

▶ FRUIT LIST ◀
(Must be fresh or unsweetened)

1 Apple	1 Orange	1 Tangerine, Satsuma or Mandarin
3 medium Apricots	1 Peach	½ cup of unsweetened Fruit Juice
½ Banana	1 Pear	½ cup of unsweetened Citrus Sections
¼ cantaloupe	2 Plums	
1 fresh Fig	1 cup Strawberries	
½ Grapefruit	½ slice Watermelon	

▶ VEGETABLE LIST ◀
(1 cup, use fresh, frozen or canned without salt)

Asparagus	Eggplant	Pumpkin
Beans, green or wax	Green or red peppers	Rutabagas
Broccoli	Green peas (not frozen)	Snap beans
Brussel sprouts	Lettuce	Squash
Cabbage	Mushroom	Tomatoes
Carrots	Mustard greens	Turnips, roots and greens
Cauliflower	Okra	
Cucumber	Onions	

Rules:
1. Eat 3 meals a day following the patterns given above and using only the foods listed.
2. The milk used may be fresh skimmed milk or powdered skim milk (mix 3 tablespoons of powder to 1 cup water). Be sure you get 4 glasses of milk a day.
3. Do not fry anything. Boil, bake, roast, steam or broil meat.
4. Do not add sugar or flour to anything.
5. Do not eat pancakes, waffles, biscuits, pies, cakes, cookies, doughnuts, pastries, ice creams, puddings, jellies, candy, syrups and other sweets.
6. Cook vegetables in plain water without salt.
7. Do not use fat meat, bacon grease or oil to season vegetables.
8. Never use cooking soda with vegetables.
9. Drink 12 glasses of fluid a day. Do not drink carbonated beverages or alcoholic beverages.
10. Between meals you may have limited coffee, tea and lemonade. Use a sugar substitute if you want them sweetened. Sucaryl® calcium—the liquid or the tablet does not contain any sodium.
11. Do not eat: ham, bacon, bacon grease, salt pork, pickled meat, sausage, frankfurters, canned meats, corned beef, luncheon meats, cheese, peanut butter, bottled salad dressings and sauces, pickles, olives, canned foods with added salt, soda crackers, saltines, prepared mustard or horseradish.
12. For seasoning may use: pepper, garlic, paprika, vinegar, lemon juice, lemon extract, vanilla, cinnamon, allspice, ginger, nutmeg, mustard powder, caraway, sage, thyme, tumeric and mace.
13. Read labels carefully. Do not use anything which is made with salt, baking powder, baking soda, sodium benzoate or monosodium glutamate.

Dry Diets for Vomiting in Pregnancy (Morning Sickness)

During the first trimester of pregnancy there may be trouble with nausea. Foods which had been taken without trouble previously may not be tolerated. Fats are a common cause of upset, although butter and cream may be well tolerated in reasonable amounts. Nausea and vomiting may be minimized by giving dry foods which are high in carbohydrate and low in fat and residue.

Two diets are available. The physician may order whichever one he feels is suitable for the individual.

Dry Diet No. 1 is intended as the initial diet. It consists of small amounts of foods which are high in carbohydrate and low in fat and residue, with no fluids given by mouth. This is an inadequate diet which should be used for a short period only and supplemented by vitamin and mineral concentrates. As soon as the patient is able to retain food on this diet, Dry Diet No. 2 may be started. As soon as progress allows, the patient should be put on Dry Diet No. 2 which is the Maintenance Diet for vomiting in pregnancy.

▶ DRY DIET #1 ◀
PATTERN MEAL PLAN
Fluids Given Parenterally

7:00 A.M.
  2 soda crackers with jelly
Breakfast
  Cooked cereal (½–¾ cup)
  Butter (1 pat)
  S. C. or poached egg (1)
  Toast (1 slice)
  Jelly
10:00 AM
  2 soda crackers
  Butter (1 pat)
Lunch
  Meat (2 oz.)
  Rice, noodles, or grits (½ cup)
  Butter (1 pat)
  Plain cookies or graham crackers

Dinner
  Meat (2 oz.)
  Baked potato (1)
  Butter (1 pat)
  Toast (1 slice)
  Jelly
  Jello, plain custard, or plain pudding
  (3 oz.) Plain cake or plain cookies
3:00 P.M.
  Jello, plain custard, or plain pudding (3 oz.) Plain
      cookies or graham crackers
8:00 P.M.
  Custard or jello (3 oz.)
  Plain cookies

▶ DRY DIET #2 ◀
WET/DRY DIET
(Maintenance Diet for Vomiting in Pregnancy)

On the maintenance diet, fluids by mouth are allowed 1 hour before or 1 hour after meals. Small frequent feedings are employed, rich and greasy foods are avoided. This is a nutritionally adequate diet.

Type of Food	Food Allowed	Foods Omitted
Beverages	Milk–1 qt. daily; crushed ice, fruit juice, Popsicles; carbonated beverages; fruit juices 1 hr. before or 1 hr. after meals	Any with meals
Meat; fish; poultry	Lean meats, fish and poultry prepared without grease.	Fried meats; fried or greasy fish; fatty meats such as pork
Egg	1 daily	Fried eggs
Cheese	Cottage cheese; mild cheddar	Any strongly flavored cheese
Fruits	All fruits and juices	Fruit juice with meals
Vegetables	All except those omitted	Strongly flavored vegetables; juices with meals
Potato or substitute	Potato; sweet potato; rice, corn; grits; macaroni, noodles; spaghetti	Fried potatoes; dried peas and beans
Cereals	All cooked cereals	Ready to eat cereals since these require milk with them
Bread	All	None

Type of Food	Food Allowed	Foods Omitted
Desserts	Plain cakes; cookies; custards; puddings; jello, popsicles	Rich pastries; doughnuts; pies
Other sweets	Sugar; honey; syrup; molasses; jam; jelly; preserves; marmalade	Any in excessive amounts
Fats	Butter; margarine; salad dressings; bacon; cream–in small amounts	Excessively fat foods
Soups	Any (except those omitted 1 hour before or 1 hour after meals)	Cream soups
Miscellaneous	Salt; spices; vinegar; flavoring; extracts; seasonings	Gravies; cream sauces; peanut butter; nuts

► DRY DIET #2 ◄
PATTERN MEAL PLAN
Upon awakening–2 soda crackers with jelly

Breakfast	*Lunch*	*Supper*
Fruit–no juice (4 oz.)	Meat (3 oz.)	Meat (3 oz.)
Cereal (¾–1 cup)	Potato or substitute (½ cup)	Potato or substitute (½ cup)
Sugar (1T.)	Vegetable or salad (½ cup)	Vegetable or salad (½ cup)
Egg (1)	Dessert, as allowed	Dessert, as allowed
9:00 AM	*1:00 P.M.*	*7:00 P.M.*
Milk (8 oz.)	Milk (8 oz.)	Milk (8 oz.)
Water, as desired	Water, as desired	Water, as desired
10:00 AM	*2:00 P.M.*	*8:00 P.M.*
Toast (1 slice)	Sandwich (1)	Fruit juice (8 oz.)
Jelly	*3:00 P.M.*	Water, as desired
	Milk (8 oz.)	
	Water, as desired	
	4:00 P.M.	
	Fruit juice (4 oz.)	
	Water, as desired	

► BREASTFEEDING* ◄

The Committee on Nutrition of the American Academy of Pediatrics (AAP) issued this statement: "Breastfeeding is strongly recommended for full-term infants, except in the few instances where specific contraindication exists". When mothers choose to breastfeed their newborn, adequate nutrition is essential and especially in the proper amount of nutrients (See Appendix A—for RDAs). Extra fluids may be needed to prevent dehydration of the mother. Additional calories are needed for women who are breastfeeding more than one infant, who are below their IBW, and women who are breastfeeding while pregnant 1200 mg Ca should be consumed daily.

Some infants may be sensitive to some foods, such as spicy and gas-forming, the mother eats. If the mother observes that the infant is uncomfortable after she has ingested certain foods the mother

---

*The LaLeche League is an international organization who helps mothers with breastfeeding concerns. Check your local chapter or contact: LaLeche League International
9616 Minneapolis Avenue
Franklin Park, IL 60131
Avoid crash diets to lose weight; 1–4 pounds per month is safe.

should leave them off for a few days. She should try these foods again in a few days to determine if the infant still experiences difficulty.

The mother should avoid caffeine-containing beverages by limiting to one 8-ounce serving per day. Smoking and the use of alcohol should be avoided. Take only medicines prescribed or approved by the physician. Avoid fad diets and rapid weight loss. Avoid herbal teas as they can cause nausea, vomiting and convulsions in both the mother and infant.

There may be times when a mother should not breastfeed her infant. If she is taking any over the counter or prescription drugs, has increased the use of alcohol since the birth of the infant she will need to consult with her pediatrician who will advise her of any impending dangers to her and/or the infant. If she has a communicable disease such as tuberculosis, hepatitis or AIDs the mother should not breastfeed her infant without discussing it with her physician. In the case of mothers infected with the AIDs virus studies show that AIDs may be passed from an infected mother to her infant during pregnancy or birth or through breastfeeding (See chapter—on AIDs).

The American Academy of Pediatrics recommends breast feeding for one year. Breast feeding should be on demand and usually averages out to every three hours.

▶ INFANT ◀

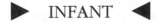

Infancy is a period of very rapid growth. During the first five months, infants gain from 5 to 8 ounces per week. Most newborns spend a good part of the day sleeping and eating. By the end of the 8th month, an infant has doubled his birth weight. From 8 months to 12 months, the weight increase is 4–5 ounces per week. By the age of 10–12 months, the birth weight has tripled. By the end of the year, the height has increased approximately 10–12 inches.

The stomach of the newborn has a capacity of one ounce; at the end of one year, 8 ounces.

During the first years, the central nervous system continues to develop so that by the age of four, the brain has reached 90% of the size of an adult. During this period of time, if a child is severely malnourished, the central nervous system will not develop adequately; a condition that cannot be corrected later in life. Therefore, the child can never reach his full mental potential.

Infant mortality in the United States has declined, but the United States still ranks thirteenth (13) among the nations of the world.

Infant Feeding (Birth–Six Months)

Breast Feeding

Breast milk provides optimum nutrition for infants and should be encouraged and supported by the medical staff. The guidelines for breast feeding infants are as follows:

1. Breast feeding should begin as soon after delivery as possible. The infant will receive colostrum for the first 2–3 days until the mother's milk comes in. Early, frequent suckling will help prevent maternal engorgement when the true milk is produced. Both breasts should be offered at each feeding alternating which is offered first (beginning with 5–10 minutes on each breast).
2. The infant will develop his/her own pattern of feeding which is generally every 2–5 hours. Some babies will breast feed every 2 hours through the day and sleep most of the night; others will feed every 3 hours throughout the day and night. Nursing time will vary from 10–30 minutes on each breast.
3. The best indication of adequate breast milk intake is by monitoring the infant's weight gain. An infant should at least regain his/her birth weight by 10–14 days. The following table reflects the average daily weight gain that may be expected in an appropriately fed infant.
4. If an infant is not gaining weight appropriately, the mother should be encouraged to feed the baby more frequently. Her diet and activity level should be checked. Supplemental bottles should only be used in special cases.

▶ EXPECTED MEAN WEIGHT GAIN FOR INFANTS ◀

Age	Males (gm/day)	Females (gm/day)
1–3 months	31.0	27.0
3–6 months	19.5	20.7
6–9 months	14.7	14.7
9–12 months	11.7	10.9
12–18 months	8.2	7.2
18–24 months	6.0	6.5
24–36 months	5.4	5.8

5. Daily supplements for the breast feeding baby:
   a. If a mother's vitamin D nutriture is inadequate or if an infant does not have ultraviolet light exposure, 400 IU/day of vitamin D may be necessary.
   b. In a completely breast fed infant receiving very little fluoridated water, 0.25 mg fluoride/day is recommended.
6. Interruption of Breast Feeding.
   If breast feeding is interrupted for medical reasons and the mother wishes to continue nursing, she must be encouraged to pump her breast at the same time each day.

Formula Feeding

The guidelines for formula feeding are as follows:

1. Although infants are born with sufficient iron reserves for the first four months, the American Academy of Pediatrics Committee on Nutrition recommends feeding an iron-fortified formula from birth to 1 year.
2. If a child is fed ready-to-feed formula or if formula is prepared with unfluoridated water, (<0.3 ppm) an infant should be supplemented with 0.25 mg of fluoride/day.
3. Bottle-fed babies should always be held in a semi-upright position while feeding. Propping a bottle can be dangerous and can lead to dental caries as well as otitis media. Eye to eye contact during feeding is important.
4. An infant should receive formula or breast milk until he/she is a year old. (Whole, low fat, or skim milk should not be fed.)
5. If infants are fed water, do not add sugar, corn syrup or honey.
6. Infants should be permitted to stop eating when they show the first signs of being full.

▶ SUGGESTED AMOUNTS OF FORMULA FOR INFANTS ◀

Body Weight (kg)	Approximate Age	Average quantity per feeding	Average # of feedings*	Total Volume in 24 hours
2.7–3.5	1 week	60–90 cc	6–8	450–670
3.8–4.8	2–4 weeks	90–150 cc	6–8	640–810
5.0–6.0	2–3 months	120–180 cc	5–6	770–1000
6.2–7.2	4–5 months	180–240 cc	5	900–1200
7.2–8.5	6 months	180–240 cc	4–5	1200

*Most infants establish their own particular feeding pattern, usually wanting to feed every 2–5 hours depending on how long the infants sleeps at night.

Physicians Order

Use Pediatric Enteral Formula Order Form. Specify type of formula and amount.

Infant Feeding (6–12 Months)

The purpose of the infant diet is to provide the infant with soft foods (mainly strained) which will meet their nutritional requirements and will be compatible with their particular stage of development. A variety of foods are included in the diet to introduce the infant to new taste experiences. The following table indicates an appropriate schedule for introducing foods into the diet.

Physician's Order

Use Pediatric Enteral Formula Order Form. Specify formula and amount. If solid food desired, order Pureed Diet; specify age.

▶ INTRODUCTION OF SOLID FOODS ◀

Age	Food Introduced Into Diet
4–6 months	Iron fortified cereal (single grain first)
5–7 months	Strained vegetables
6–8 months	Strained fruits & fruit juices (except citrus)
9 months	Strained meats
10 months	Egg yolk and citrus fruits and juices
11–12 months	Egg whites

Guidelines for feeding infants:

1. The introduction of solid foods should be delayed until at least five months of age (Check with the physician.) At this age the infant's tongue and swallowing movements become coordinated and the infant has reasonable control of head and neck. Nutritionally speaking, solid foods are not necessary until five or six months of age.
2. Strained foods are introduced one at a time with an interval of three to five days to allow for easy detection of intolerances or food allergies. Initially, new foods are offered in small amounts (one to two teaspoons) and at first can be thinned with small amounts of formula until the food is easily accepted.
3. Infants should be fed solid food with a spoon. Baby food should not be put in a bottle or infant feeder.
4. Use plain varieties of fruits, vegetables, meats, and dry cereals. They offer a greater source of nutrients than fruit desserts, vegetable dinners, or wet pack cereals.
5. Between eight and nine months of age, soft table foods such as chopped or mashed cooked fruit, soft cooked vegetables, plain crackers, or ground meats may be offered. These help to develop chewing skills and fine motor development. Avoid foods that may choke the baby. Such foods are hot dogs, grapes, popcorn, nuts, raisins, and raw carrots.
6. Junior foods are expensive and unnecessary. Use fresh or frozen (not canned) foods. Canned foods contain excess sodium and may contain traces of lead. Use salt and sugar sparingly.
7. At age eight to nine months, small amounts of formula can be put into a cup and offered at mealtime.
8. Fruit juices should never be offered from a bottle. This practice can contribute to the development of nursing bottle caries. Nap time milk bottles can also lead to nursing bottle caries due to the constant bathing of the teeth in sugary solution. Offer a cup when feeding fruit juices.
9. Avoid over and under feeding.
10. Introduce new foods as tolerated.

▶ SAMPLE FEEDING PATTERN FOR INFANTS ◀

Time	4–6 Months	7–8 Months	9–10 Months	11–12 Months
MORNING	Breast milk or Formula 180–240 cc Breast milk or Formula 120–180 cc	Breast milk or Formula 180–240 cc Breast milk or Formula 120–180 cc Dry cereal 3–4 tbsp	Breast milk or Formula 120–180 cc Str Fruit 2–4 tbsp	Breast milk or Formula 120–180 cc Fruit 4 tbsp Egg 1
	*Dry cereal 2–4 tbsp	Str Fruit 1–4 tbsp		
AFTERNOON	Breast milk or Formula 120–180 cc *Dry cereal 2–4 tbsp	Breast milk or Formula 120–180 cc Dry cereal 3–4 tbsp Str Vegetable 1–4 tbsp	Breast milk or Formula 120–180 cc Str Meat 1–2 tbsp Str Vegetable 2–4 tbsp Toast 1/2 slice	Breast milk or Formula 120–180 cc Vegetables 4 tbsp Meat 2–3 tbsp Toast 1/2 slice
EVENING	Breast milk or Formula 120–180 cc Dry cereal 2–4 tbsp Breast milk or Formula 180–240 cc	Breast milk or Formula 120–180 cc Str Vegetable 1–4 tbsp Str Fruit 1–4 tbsp Breast milk or Formula 180–240 cc	Fruit Juice 120 cc Crackers 2 Breast milk or Formula 120–180 cc Str Meat 1–2 tbsp Str Vegetable 2 tbsp Str Fruit 2–4 tbsp Dry cereal 2 tbsp Breast milk or Formula 120–180 cc	Fruit Juice 12-cc Crackers 2 Breast milk or Formula 120–180 cc Starch 2–4 tbsp Meat 2–3 tbsp Vegetable 4 tbsp Fruit 2–4 tbsp Breast milk or Formula 120–180 cc
Calories	650–750	700–800	800–900	900–1000
Protein	18–18 gm	16–18 gm	16–18 gm	20–25 gm

*Cereal is baby type cereal.

▶ INFANT DIET ◀

Type of Foods	Foods Allowed	Foods Not Allowed
Beverages	Breast milk, iron-fortified formula, water, strained juices	All other citrus juices
Meat, Poultry, Eggs, Fish & Cheese 2–3 servings (2 tbsp each)	Strained beef, chicken, ham, lamb, turkey, veal, fine cottage cheese strained or mashed, cooked egg yolk	Fish, other cheeses, egg white until 1 year
Fruits 2 or more servings (2–4 tbsp each)	Strained cooked apples, apricots, peaches, pears, pineapple, plums, prunes, alone or in combination, mashed ripe bananas	All others, raw fruits any with small seeds (citrus fruits until infant is 9–10 months)
Vegetable 2 servings (2–4 tbsp each)	Strained cooked beets, carrots, green beans, peas, spinach, squash	All others (especially strong flavored), raw vegetables
Starches, Cereals 2 or more servings (2–4 tbsp each)	Iron-fortified dry infant cereals Cheerios®	All others

Type of Foods	Foods Allowed	Foods Not Allowed
Other occasionally (2–5 tbsp each)	Mashed white potato, mashed or strained sweet potato, grits	All others
Breads occasionally	Teething biscuits, Rusk®, zwieback®, toast, saltine crackers	All others
Desserts	None	All
Fats	None	All
Miscellaneous		Excessive use of sugar, syrup or salt
Soups	None	All

Note: The nutrient composition of commercially prepared strained dinners are almost identical to the strained vegetables. The protein content of the high meat dinners is between 50–75% of the protein content of the strained meats. Therefore, these foods are not recommended.

▶ TODDLER AND PRESCHOOL 1–6 YEARS ◀

Children age one to three should be introduced to good foods and healthy eating habits. Toddlers usually can't stay still to finish a meal as they are so busy exploring the world. At ages two to three the toddler wants to feed himself usually expressing himself with "want" and "no". Sometimes their "no" is just a way of expressing their control over a given situation.

Children continue to develop new food behavior patterns as they grow older and are introduced to a variety of foods. The child from age three to five is energetic, active, and restless which leads to a high caloric intake. Snacks of high nutritive value should be offered. Children in this age group learn by imitating the people they come in contact with—family, friends, neighbors, etc. They begin to develop food habits like their family and will request those foods eaten by their peers.

Health Concerns

 Iron-deficiency anemia. Many children from low income families, those who have an ignorance of nutritious foods, and have developed poor eating habits are the most likely children to have iron-deficiency anemia. Lack of iron may cause an energy crisis, but can also affect behavior, mood, attention span, and learning ability. Iron deficiency is the most widespread nutrition problem of children.

▶ ***Obesity.*** From the age of birth to four years and seven to eleven, the incidence of obesity is high. Some overweight/fat children may have emotional problems, have a lack of physical exercise, eat excessive high fat, high calorie snacks, overeat and while others may be imitating family eating patterns. A controlled calorie intake and exercise are recommended. (See chapter on weight management)

▶ ***Dental caries.*** This is a lessening problem in most areas as water and toothpaste have been fluoridated. Regular dental check-ups are recommended.

▶ ***Allergies.*** Many childhood allergies are caused by food. Milk is the most common, followed by egg whites, citrus, chocolate, seafood, wheat and nuts. Symptoms vary and may include respiratory difficulties, skin rashes, diarrhea, nausea, and/or vomiting.

Diagnosing food allergies is difficult. Tests must be made to determine if an allergy is present. Suggested diets for allergies are included in Module 6.

Toddler Soft Diet (10–18 Months)

The soft diet is designed to meet the nutritional requirements of a child who no longer needs all his foods pureed or strained but is not yet able to tolerate a chopped diet. This diet includes soft cooked whole foods and ground meats, many of which may be finger fed. Raw vegetables and hard raw fruits are omitted.

Nutritional Adequacy

This diet should supply the RDA for all nutrients if a variety of foods from the Food Guide Pyramid is consumed in adequate amounts.

Physician's Order

Toddler Soft Diet, specify age.

▶ TODDLER SOFT DIET ◀

Type of Foods	Foods Allowed	Foods Not Allowed
Beverages Milk–4 servings (4–6 oz each)	Whole milk, iron fortified formula water, fruit juices	All other
Meat, Poultry, Eggs, Fish, Cheese 2–3 servings (¼ cup each)	Ground beef, chicken, ham, lamb, liver, pork, turkey, veal, frankfurter, luncheon meat, milk, cheese (such as American), flaked fish, eggs, tuna, creamy peanut butter	Fish with small bones; sharp cheeses
Fruits 2 or more servings (¼ cup each)	Applesauce, crushed pineapple, canned peaches, pears, fruit cocktail, peeled apricots, ripe banana, orange with tough membrane and seeds removed	All others; most raw fruits; any with small seeds
Vegetable 2 or more servings (¼ cup each)	Cooked beets, carrots, squash, green beans, peas, creamed corn, chopped spinach or greens	All other (especially strong flavored vegetables), raw vegetables
Starches 1 or more serving (¼ cup each)	Boiled or mashed white or sweet potatoes, baked french fries, macaroni, noodles, rice, spaghetti, grits	Highly seasoned rice or pasta mixture
Cereals 1 or more servings (½ cup each)	Cooked cereals, any easily digested, ready to eat cereals such as cornflakes, rice flakes, wheat flakes or Cheerios;rM	Dry, course cereals such as shredded wheat or bran, any containing nuts, hard dried fruit; excessive use of sugar coated cereals
Breads 3 or more servings (½ slice bread or 2 crackers each)	White enriched or whole wheat bread or toast, teething biscuit, saltines or graham crackers, Rusk®, zwieback®	All others
Desserts in moderation	Simple custards, puddings, gelatin, desserts, plain cakes, and cookies, smooth fruit ice, ice cream and sherbet	Any with nuts, all others (especially any highly concentrated sweetened dessert)

Type of Foods	Foods Allowed	Foods Not Allowed
Fats 3 or more servings (1 tsp each)	Margarine, butter, bacon, mild gravy	All others
Soups	All mildly seasoned and blenderized to a smooth consistency	Any highly seasoned or those that contain foods which are not allowed.
Miscellaneous	Salt (iodized), sugar, clear jelly, vanilla flavoring, cocoa, mild spices such as cinnamon	Excessive use of salt and sugar

► **SAMPLE MEAL PATTERN** ◀
Toddler Soft Diet

Breakfast	Lunch	Afternoon Snack	Dinner	HS Snack

½ c milk
1 scrambled egg
½ c orange juice
¼ c cream of
    wheat or grits
½ slice toast
½ tsp margarine
	¼ c ground chicken
	½ slice bread
	¼ c peas
	½ tsp margarine
	¼ c chopped
	    peaches
	½ c milk
		½ c apple juice
		2 saltine crackers
			¼ c ground beef
			¼ c mashed potato
			¼ c carrots
			¼ c applesauce
			½ c milk
			1 tsp margarine
				½ c milk
				1 graham cracker

Preschool Diet (18 Months–4/5 Years)

The preschool diet is designed to meet the nutritional requirements of the child aged 18 months to 4 years. This diet stresses the use of "finger foods" which serves to promote motor development and encourage the chewing process. Bite size chopped meats should be used to avoid choking.

Nutritional Adequacy

This diet should supply the RDA for all nutrients if a variety of foods from the Food Guide Pyramid is consumed in adequate amounts.

Physician's Order

Preschool Diet, specify age.

▶ PRESCHOOL DIET ◀

Type of Foods	Foods Allowed	Foods Not Allowed
Beverages Milk—4 servings (4 oz each)	Milk, water, fruit drinks, juices carbonated beverages.	Coffee, tea, excessive use of sugar and caffeinated drinks
Meat, Poultry, Eggs, **Fish & Cheese** 2–4 servings (4 oz each)	Any chopped tender meat, poultry, or fish without bones, hotdogs & luncheon meat in moderation, peanut butter, milk, cheeses eggs, hard or soft cooked, poached or fried.	Any fried or highly seasoned meat or fish, fish containing small bones, strong flavored cheeses.
Fruits 2 or more servings (¼ cup each)	Applesauce, chopped pineapple, canned peeled apricot, cherries, peaches, pears, strawberries, fruit cocktail, raw fruit suitable as finger foods such as peeled apples, pears, or peach wedges, banana, orange sections and melon.	Fruit with seeds or tough skin.
Vegetables 2 servings (¼ cup)	Well-cooked tender vegetables suitable as finger foods, asparagus tips, beet slices, carrots, green or wax beans peas, chopped spinach, squash, stewed tomatoes, creamed corn, raw carrots & celery sticks, shredded lettuce, tomato wedges, green pepper rings, (include a serving of dark green or yellow vegetable daily for a source of vitamin A)	Strongly flavored or gas-forming vegetables such as brussel sprouts cabbage, cauliflower, whole kernel kohlrabi, radishes, turnips, dried raw vegetables
Starches 1 serving (¼ cup)	White potato (no skin): baked, creamed, scalloped, mashed, boiled, french fried; sweet potato (no skins); macaroni, noodles, rice, spaghetti.	Highly seasoned rice and pasta mixtures
Breads 3 servings (½ slice each or equivalent)	White enriched, whole wheat, rye bread, toast, simple yeast buns or rolls, plain saltine or graham crackers, Rusk®, zweiback®.	Excessive use of donuts or sweet rolls, pancakes or waffles, breads with seeds or nuts
Cereals 1 serving (1/3 cup cooked or 1/2 cup ready to eat)	Refined cooked cereal, plain dry cereals.	Any dry course cereals, any containing nuts or hard dried fruit.
Desserts in moderation	Plain puddings, cakes, cookies, ice cream, gelatin, sherbet.	Any with nuts, all others (especially any highly concentrated sweet desserts).
Fats 3 or more servings (1 tsp each)	Butter, margarine, cream, oil, vegetable shortening, mayonnaise, gravy, bacon, plain salad dressing.	Excessive use of fats.
Soups (as desired)	Any made from allowed foods.	Any high seasoned or made from foods not allowed.
Miscellaneous	Salt (iodized), sugar, honey, clear jelly, syrup, cocoa, milk flavoring and extracts, pickles.	Jams, marmalade, preserves (made with skins or seeds), coconut, whole nuts, olives, popcorn, relishes, pepper, spices.

► **SAMPLE MEAL PATTERN** ◄

Preschool Diet

Breakfast	Lunch	Afternoon Snack	Dinner	HS Snack
½ c milk*	½ roast beef	½ c apple juice	2 oz chopped chicken	½ c milk*
1 poached egg	sandwich	2 saltine crackers	¼ c mashed potato	2 graham crackers
½ c orange juice	½ tsp mayonnaise		¼ c carrots	
½ c corn flakes	carrot sticks		1 slice bread	
½ slice toast	¼ c canned peaches		½ tsp margarine	
½ tsp margarine	½ c milk*		½ c milk*	
& jelly				

*2% milk (after 2nd birthday) other low fat selections may be made at the advise of the physician.

► 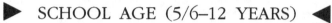 SCHOOL AGE (5/6–12 YEARS) ◄

This diet is designed to meet the nutritional requirements of the child aged 6 to 12 years, through a selective menu. All foods and beverages are included in this diet with the exception of coffee, strong tea, and highly seasoned foods. Excessive use of highly concentrated sweets and fat is discouraged.

Nutritional Adequacy

This diet should supply the RDAs for all nutrients if a variety of foods from the Food Guide Pyramid is consumed in adequate amounts. Iron-deficiency anemia may become problem. Iron and zinc and other essential minerals will be adequate when the Food Guide Pyramid is followed.

Physician's Order

Juvenile Regular Diet, specify age:

► **SAMPLE MEAL PATTERN** ◄

School Age Diet

Breakfast	Lunch	Afternoon Snack	Dinner	HS Snack
½ c orange juice	6 oz tomato soup	1 granola bar	2 oz roast beef	½ c milk*
1 scrambled egg	turkey (2 oz)	4 oz apple juice	¼ c mashed potato	2 graham crackers
½ c grits	sandwich		⅛ c gravy	
1 tsp margarine	celery and carrot		¼ c green beans	
1 slice bacon	sticks		1 roll	
1 slice toast	fresh fruit		1 tsp margarine**	
½ tsp margarine**	1 c milk*		¼ c sliced peaches	
& jelly			½ c vanilla pudding	
1 c milk*			1 c milk*	

*Whole, skim, 2%, evaporate or buttermilk

**Fats and sweets should be determined on an individual need for calories.

▶ SCHOOL CHILD (6–12 YEARS) ◀

During the next six years of a child's life, his weight and height develop at a steady pace. During these years he may gain from 30–35 pounds and grow 10–12 inches. There is a marked increase in his food consumption.

It is at this period that a child begins school and is faced with a new set of problems. He must begin the day with a well balanced breakfast to prevent late morning fatigue and slower learning processes. He also must decide whether to eat in the school cafeteria, the vending machines or pack a lunch from home.

The child still requires the same basic foods, but in greater quantities to meet his increased needs. His peer group plays a vital role in his food acceptance during this period. Empty calories, such as sodas, coffee, tea, sweets and pastries should be discouraged.

Health Concerns

▶ *Iron-deficiency anemia.* Many children from low income families, those who have an ignorance of nutritious foods, and have developed poor eating habits are the most likely children to have iron-deficiency anemia. Lack of iron may cause an energy crisis, but can also affect behavior, mood, attention span, and learning ability. Iron deficiency is the most widespread nutrition problem of children.

▶ *Obesity.* From the age of birth to four years and seven to eleven, the incidence of obesity is high. Some overweight/fat children may have emotional problems, have a lack of physical exercise, eat excessive high fat, high calorie snacks, overeat and others may be imitating family eating patterns. A controlled calorie intake and exercise are recommended. (See chapter on weight management)

▶ *Dental caries.* This is a diminishing problem in most areas as water and toothpaste have been fluoridated. Regular dental check-ups are recommended.

▶ *Allergies.* Many childhood allergies are caused by food. Milk is the most common, followed by egg whites, citrus, chocolate, seafood, wheat and nuts. Symptoms vary and may include respiratory difficulties, skin rashes, diarrhea, nausea, and/or vomiting.

Diagnosing food allergies is difficult. Tests must be made to determine if an allergy is present. Suggested diets for allergies are included in Module 6.

School Foodservice

The school foodservice has as its mission: "To improve the health and education of children by creating innovative public and private partnerships that promote food choices for a healthful diet through the media, schools, families, and the community". School foodservice must follow the guidelines as established by the USDA. Recent mandate is to reduce fat, salt, cholesterol, sugar calories; increase the fiber in the meal. Some schools offer both school breakfast, school lunch and after school snacks. The school lunch should meet 1/3 of the Recommended Daily Allowances. Some schools have implemented a service called "a-la-carte". This service mimics the fast food outlets, by establishing salad bars, potato bars and taco bars. Pizza recipes have been developed to meet the nutrient requirements of school lunch programs and are among the best accepted food on the menu. Some schools allow vending machines on the campus that sell canned drinks, juices, sugary confections, while other schools vending machines offer more nutritious foods such as fresh fruit, milk, and other more nutritious foods. (see reference—ADA Position Paper)

▶ ADOLESCENCE (13–19 YEARS) ◀

During the teenage years, the second major growth period of life occurs. With the heightened growth rate come increased needs for all nutrients—calories, protein, vitamins and minerals.

In America, teenage males are typically better nourished than teenage females. This occurs principally because boys tend to exercise more than girls, thus consuming a greater quantity of food. However, because the quality of foods selected is often low, diets of both boys and girls tend to be deficient in iron, calcium and ascorbic acid.

Breakfast should be eaten and not hurried or skipped. The nutrients that breakfast would furnish are difficult to make up during the day. A study conducted at Iowa University, showed that children who omit breakfast or have an inadequate breakfast, become more fatigued, less attentive and are not able to achieve as much as those who have an adequate intake of the nutrients. Those who ate breakfast worked, played and were sharper in thinking and action during the late morning hours.

Adolescents enjoy snack time. Most of the snacks are "empty calories". These empty calories usually take away appetite for more nutritious foods. Snacks must be considered a part of the total day's intake.

Teenagers may develop poor eating habits as they are involved in an array of after school activities. It is at this time that many teens may not eat a single meal with the family at regular meal times. A large portion of the energy intakes comes from snacks usually being eaten on the "run". Fast food becomes a favorite with pizza being the first choice.

Health Concerns

▶ Teenage sexuality and pregnancy is an increasing problem as many of the teens are at high nutritional risk. Between 1/3 to 1/2 of the pregnancies actually give birth, many of the full term infants may suffer from low-birth weight and other deficiencies. A pregnant teenager has a very high need for a well balanced diet high in all the essential nutrients. Dietitians and other healthcare providers will need to counsel these girls in good nutritional practices/choices for the protection of the unborn fetus as well as the mother.

▶ Anorexia nervosa and bulimia are eating disorders that many teenagers and young women face. (Few men have these disorders). Medical, psychiatric, and nutritional intervention is necessary for treatment. Anorexia nervosa is life threatening and is known as the "self-starvation" disorder. The symptoms include controlling food intake, usually limiting the intake to low calorie foods. The loss of weight is very pronounced since the sufferer will not allow herself to eat/gain weight. If she feels she has gained an ounce she will engage in excessive physical exercise and or take laxatives or self-induce vomiting to remove the weight. The anorexic is preoccupied with food and knows the caloric content of foods and counts calories to maintain an intake of 500-900 calories per day. This behavior presents problems such as extreme weight loss, hormonal aberrations, hair loss, impaired immune system, malnutrition, dry skin, abnormal nerve function, sleeplessness, heat and other internal organ problems and in some cases death. Many anorexia patients are admitted to healthcare institutions for psychiatric treatment. A team approach made up of psychiatrists, physicians, nurses, dietitians, family psychologist work together to treat the patient/family. The goal is to initiate a weight gain and to maintain the gain. In severe cases the patient may be force fed through a tube, for others a diet of increased calories is offered and a reward system for weight gain and maintenance may become part of the treatment. Psychological and psychiatric counseling involving the family and patient is vital. Few of the patients make a full recovery about one-half fall back into some type of eating disorder.

▶ Bulimia is binge eating, impulsive gorging in a short period of time followed by self-induced vomiting or purging by laxatives or diuretics to control weight. Bulimia is seen in older teenagers and women and some men. The eating binge is a compulsion and the binger may eat as few as 1,000 to as much as 10,000 calories at one time. The foods consumed are easy-to-eat, high fat and high carbohydrates. After the ingestion of so much food the bulimia person feels ashamed and disgusted and must find a method to rid the body of the food. Strong laxatives, vomiting, periods of fasting and/or enemas are used to purge the body of the food. Unlike persons with anorexia nervosa, bulimic persons are aware that their behavior is abnormal. Bulimia is a serious problem causing physical problems from emotional tensions. The constant bingeing-purging may cause dehydration, malnutrition, esophageal irritation, erosion and decay of teeth and glandular and metabolic disturbances. Treatment calls for a team approach of psychiatric, family counselors, nurses, dietitians. The dietary goal is to help the patient gain control over food and establish regular eating habits, maintain weight, rather than yo-yo and to develop a life-long plan to prevent relapse.***

▶ Other concerns include the use of alcohol, drugs and smoking. Each of these habits can have an affect on the nutritional health of the person.

▶ Obesity is increased during this period due to the decreased physical activity and the increased use of high fat, high carbohydrate foods that are of little nutritional value.

▶ Acne may or may not be related to food choices. Fatty foods, cola drinks, milk, nuts, sugar and chocolate have been accused as the culprits. Some scientist suggest that a low intake of zinc and increased consumption of alcohol may be the cause. Stress seems to worsen acne.

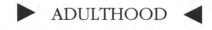

▶ **ADULTHOOD** ◀

Adulthood has been defined from 19 to 55 years and from 18 to 65 years. Early adulthood is considered from 18–30 and middle adulthood from 30–65. In the United States the life expectancy of females is 78+ years and for males it is 72+ years. The elderly may be confined to extended care facilities, others live with their children, however a large portion continue to function independently until late in life. The population of over 65 years of age is about 13+ percent and is expected to be 22 percent by 2040. The over 65 year age group uses approximately 32 percent of all healthcare services. The so called "baby boomers" are reaching 50 years old in the late 1990s. It is not uncommon now a days to find many people over the age of 100. Life span (the maximum number of years of life attainable by a member of a species) is 115 for humans.

As the body grows older changes take place such as an increase in fat, reduction in bone density, the increased frequency of arthritis and osteomalacia. The ability to perform strenuous physical activities decrease with age. Life styles change and these health changes have an affect on the food habits. Elderly patients admitted to healthcare facilities often have multiple, chronic medical problems and tend to have longer healthcare stays than younger patients.

Health Concerns

▶ Long time use of alcohol, drugs, and smoking increases the possibility of cancer and other health problems.

▶ Chronic exposure to environmental pollutants is a health hazard, especially in large industrial cities.

▶ Obesity, arthritis, osteomalacia are more common and for women osteoporosis is common.

▶ Cardiovascular diseases and cancer are the leading causes of death.

▶ There is a great deal of emphasis being placed on women's health. As women grow older pregnancy, lactation and menopause change the nutrient needs. Some contraceptives devices can create some problems with certain nutrients, especially iron and some vitamins. Women who use contraceptives should have regular check-ups and their nutritional status checked. Abortions may affect the iron status of a woman. Women who are menopausal iron needs decreases while the need for calcium increases. Physical activity is important as one ages. Thirty minutes per day of exercise is recommended. Dehydration may become a problem. Fiber becomes very important for its role in reducing constipation. Fats should be limited, the need for Vitamin D

***The American Anorexia/Bulimia Assoc., Inc. 133 Cedar Lane, Teaneck, NJ 07006 and National Anorexia Aid Society hotline (614-436-1112) provides information and services for clients and their families as well as health care personnel.

may become a problem as older adults may not drink Vitamin D fortified milk and may go for days without exposure to the sunlight.

▶ Depression and mid-life crisis.

▶ THE ELDERLY ◀

There are 26 million Americans over 65 years old one person in ten and one-third of this 26 million is over 76 years old. Many of these elderly live in poverty, have poor health and are suffering from hunger and malnutrition.

To be a healthy senior citizen, one must begin early in life in practicing good food habits. Nutrition is vital. The needs of nutrients for the elderly do not differ significantly from those of the young adult. However, due to the aging process, this group must be given special consideration.

Some elderly persons do have problems with adequate nutrition. Many of these problems relate to long standing faulty dietary habits. Other causes include the loss of teeth, poorly fitting dentures or absence of teeth, which usually results in a modification of eating habits, sometimes reducing the recommended intake of nutrients and the development of a monotonous diet.

As one grows older, most of the pleasure of eating is removed, due to the decrease of the taste and smell senses. The satisfaction of eating with loved ones or friends may also be lessened.

The physical discomfort of heartburn, belching, flatulence and indigestion is more pronounced in the older citizen. The effort to eliminate these conditions usually means the avoidance of nutritious foods.

Because of the loss of neuromuscular activity, some elderly develop an inability to handle eating utensils. Rather than to be embarrassed with spilled food, inability to cut meat or eat soup, the elderly will avoid these foods. In most cases, they will eat soft low fiber foods and then develop a tendency to become constipated.

Economics play a vital role in the nutrition of the elderly. The desire to remain independent and to live on a meager income, forces many elderly persons to choose the less expensive, readily available carbohydrate foods, rather than those that contain the needed nutrients.

Living alone, poor cooking facilities, boredom, frustration and fear reduces the desire to prepare food. The elderly person develops irregular eating hours, usually snacking on unbalanced meals.

Because of fear of illness, the elderly fall prey to the food faddist and quack who promise them eternal youth, excellent health, vigor and cure of disease.

The elderly still have the need for all the nutrients. Due to a decrease in activity, there should be a decrease in the number of calories ingested per day. If the appetite is poor, frequent small meals should be eaten. Breakfast should be eaten and the noon meal should be the largest meal of the day. If coffee and tea produce insomnia, they should be eliminated and a decaffeinated substance substituted.

It is suggested that dietary supplements not be taken unless a complete dietary history is taken and it is determined that the person is lacking the essential nutrients.

The elderly, like other age groups, need special understanding. Approximately 10% of persons over 65 suffer from some form of chronic abuse—verbal, psychological and/or physical.

Health Concerns

Loss of teeth, reduced salvia, diminished taste and smell and decreased ability to digest food are some of the changes that occur as one ages. A complete diet history must be taken and a diet formulated that will meet the needs of each patient. Dysphagia may occur. Dysphagia is a difficulty in swallowing liquids or solid foods, caused by an underlying central neurologic disorder or an isolated mechanical dysfunction. It most often is seen in patients who have had a head injury, Parkinson's disease, cancer of the head and neck, multiple sclerosis, Alzheimer's disease and cerebrovascular accidents. Many dysphagia patient who are hospitalized are malnourished, a serious consequence of dysphasia. As a result the patient may require enternal and/or parenteral nutrition (See chapter—enteral and parenteral nutrition.)

Daily millions of sufferers must decide what they will do in coping with an incurable disease. Arthritis can generate depression and stress that may develop from fear, chronic pain, stress and fatigue due to the affect on the lifestyle.

The Arthritis Foundation suggest the following:
▶ Learn about the disease.
▶ Accept that changes are necessary.
▶ Balance rest and activity.
▶ Learn to deal with fatigue.
▶ Practice joint protection.
▶ Think realistic.
▶ Beware of unproved remedies.
▶ Avoid large doses of vitamins, snake venom, steroids, and drugs with hidden ingredients.

Special adaptive feeding devices may be required. The use of these devices should be carefully monitored to determine their effectiveness and appropriateness. Osteoporosis is a condition where there is a decrease in bone mass, which can lead to fractures and possible disability. Osteoporosis is most often seen in Caucasian and Oriental females and risk factors include aging, early menopause, family history, low body weight, low calcium intake, sedentary life style, nulliparity, smoking and alcohol abuse. Calcium supplements may be indicated, as well as increased vitamin D to insure that the calcium is absorbed, increase of weight-bearing exercises such as walking, and estrogen replacement. Women will need to have a complete physical before venturing on their own to increase the intake of calcium, and exercise. The physician will determine the most appropriate supplement, the increased need for vitamin, the most appropriate type of exercise and estrogen replacement.

▶ Increased use of laxatives and decreased fluid intake may lead to dehydration and interference of nutrient absorption. Many elderly suffer from chronic constipation which may be caused by decreased/lack of physical activity, decreased intake of fiber and fluids and the intake of some medications.

▶ Change in eye sight such as cataracts that may lead to the problems in reading recipes, labels, and "seeing" unsanitary conditions, such as unclean dishes, pots and pans.

▶ Alcoholism is a major problem among the elderly, especially those living alone.

▶ Obesity is a major problem as caloric intake remains high while physical activity is reduced. The body composition changes as there is a decrease in lean body mass, subsequent reduction in total body water, and an increase in adipose (fat) tissue.

▶ Non-insulin-dependent diabetes type II (NIDDM) is a common problem and is sometimes referred to as "maturity on-set diabetes". Over three-fourth of people with this type of diabetes are overweight or obese. Most people can control the disease by diet alone. The most effective treatment is to reduce and maintain normal body weight. (see chapter on weight management/diabetes mellitus).

▶ Diverticulosis is a problem characterized by the weakening of the intestinal walls resulting in the development of "pouches" along the colon called diverticuli. A diet in high fiber has been found to be helpful. (see chapter on GI)

▶ Cancer is the second most common cause of death among the elderly in the US. The incidence and mortality rates of cancer increase with age until 84 years, when they plateau and possibly decline. Risk factors that contribute to cancer development include smoking, heredity, alcohol consumption, sunlight, radiation, some dietary habits, environmental pollutants, occupational hazards and predisposing medical conditions, (see chapter on cancer).

▶ Hypertension and atherosclerosis are two common problems among both males and females as they grow older. Salt, alcohol, smoking, body fat (excessive weight/obesity) are thought to contribute to hypertension. Some researchers also suggest that stress plays a role. Coronary heart disease is the leading cause of death in the US, especially among the elderly. (see chapter—cardiovascular disease)

▶ Alteration in sensory abilities such as smell, taste and hearing impairment may compromise nutritional status especially if the elderly do not enjoy eating and as a consequence reduce the intake of food.

▶ Pressure sores, also called decubitus ulcers and bed sores, are inflammation sores, or ulcers over a bony prominence such as the sacrum, shoulder blades, heels, elbows, back of the head and hip/pelvic area. Pressure sores occur in about one-fourth of the elderly population confined to long term care facilities. Surveying agencies have stated "hospital acquired decubitus ulcers are an indication of poor quality care". The skin breaks down and results in pressure sores due to pressure, friction, shearing and maceration. These ulcers are most often caused by prolonged immobilization and patients confined to the bed or wheelchair for extended periods of time without moving the patient (turning the patient, changing the position of the body), exercise and good skin care (such as the use of moisturizing skin rubs and special sleeping pads for bed and chair). Other factors include incontinence, altered mental state, inadequate nutrition (especially protein and vitamins, especially Vitamin C and of the mineral zinc), hydration, edema, infections, anemia, diabetes mellitus, cerebral vascular accidents, dementia, malignancies, and possibly stress and smoking. To prevent most pressure sores the removal of the pressure in most case will eliminate the sores. The diet most often prescribed is: High protein (75–100 g/per day), High vitamin C (100-200 mg per day), increased zinc (15–25 mg/day), and high calorie (2,200–3,500 calories/day), increased fluids (2,000–2,500 cc/per day). In the most severe cases nutritional supplements may be prescribed and if oral intake is inadequate enteral tube feedings may be ordered.

▶ Abnormal deterioration of the brain called senile dementia of the Alzheimer's type (SDAT) afflicts 5 percent of the population by age 65 and by age 80, over 20 percent. The progression of the disease is gradual and varies among individuals. The diagnosis is difficult but the symptoms include gradual losses of memory and reasoning, the ability to verbally communicate, progressive decline in the ability to perform activities of daily living until the person becomes totally dependent on the care giver and eventually loss of life. There is no known cure. Treatment involves providing relief and support to the patient and the family. As the dementia progresses increased supervision and controlled dining environments may be necessary to decrease confusion, distraction, agitation and resistive behavior. It may be necessary to have the care giver feed the patient. The food consistency may need to be modified, frequent small meals may be necessary for the more difficult patients that is fed by others and as the last resort enteral tube feeding may become necessary.

▶ Psychological and socioeconomic factors play a role in the nutritional status of this age group. Factors such as reduced income, inability to shop, food prejudices, food fads, inadequate cooking facilities and lack of the desire to prepare meals, eating alone, limited nutrition knowledge, the feeling of loss of independence and depression may increase the possibility of malnutrition. The interdisciplinary team needs to complete a diet history, screening/assessment of the elderly patient and develop an individualized care plan to meet the needs of the patient. Careful consideration must be given to the medication taken by the patient and the possibility of nutrient-food interaction. If appropriate the pharmacist should be consulted. A complete psychological and socioeconomic evaluation can be completed with input from the social worker and dietitian. If special feeding tools are needed the occupational therapist should be consulted. The patient and the family should be involved in the care plan for the patient. Other concerns that may play a role in good nutrition status include reduced mobility, constipation, lack of adequate intake of fluids, especially water; depression, skin problems and ingestion of too many medications that may lead to drug interactions

▶ Faddism and quackery, nutrient and food interaction are also considered to be problems faced by the elderly. (see following section on these topics).

▶ FADDISM AND QUACKERY ◀

Americans are extremely diet conscious. They desire to be thin, beautiful, with long shining hair and clear, soft skin without the effort required to accomplish this desire. Quackery and charlatans prey on the gullibility, superstitions and susceptibility of these people with misleading, misinformation and fear. Americans spend approximately 10 billion dollars annually on nutritional supplements, wraps, exercise gear, other devices, books, and other "cures". Every year one out of four Americans will use quack medicine treatment.

Many of the fad diets present health problems as most often they do not follow appropriate nutritional guidelines. Some diets are severely restrictive such as the Rice diet, to severely imbalanced such as the Air force diet, thereby creating an imbalance in the body's nutriture. Fortunately most diets are so restrictive that people will adhere to them for only several days to a week.

Many people fall prey to herbal remedies, other old old wives tales such as honey and vinegar to "cure" arthritis, others to the unknown such as laetrile to cure cancer, Vitamin E to delay aging. The very low calorie diet (VLCD) has caused a great deal of concern among nutritionist and physicians. (see chapter on weight control)

Another fad is the omission of food because it is thought to be harmful. An example would be omitting enriched foods because of the danger of "chemical" poisoning.

The largest group of faddists are those that put emphasis on "natural" foods as being the only safe food to consume. Honey has been claimed to have unique nutritional benefits—UNTRUE Honey has the same nutritional properties as ordinary sugar

The food quack is hard to distinguish. However, one should become suspicious when one hears talk about "wonder foods", "miracle foods", "health foods", or "organically grown", "nature's own food", "food cures", "secret formula", "proven", "foreign", "breakthrough" and "good and bad foods".

The food quack appeals to the emotion—to the psyche; he makes exaggerated claims for his product, youth, glamour, cure of disease, beauty. He will sell anything, but he is out to sell books, food products, gimmicks. Many quacks are in the form of "door bell doctors", who convince housewives they are depriving their family of health and well being. They sell cookware, vitamins, food supplements and cures for all ills. The food quack also gives lectures to people who have been invited to attend a "special invitation only" meeting.

Drug and Nutrient Interaction

Some drugs interfere with nutrients in the food. Nutrients may increase or decrease the potency of some drugs. It is important that the interdisciplinary team develop a working knowledge in this area.

The effect of nutrients on drug therapy depends in part on the timing of the meal and the level of certain nutrients in the diet such as milk, fiber, alcohol and protein foods. A drug may hinder absorption of a nutrient in the gastrointestinal tract, or it may interfere with the action of the nutrient after it is absorbed. Certain foods or dietary patterns may destroy a drug's effectiveness. Some drug-nutrient interactions cause nausea, altered taste, decreased appetite, stomach distress, dizziness, malabsorption, dehydration, and hypertension. The most susceptible people are very young children, the elderly, alcoholics and the chronically ill. (see chapter on drug and nutrient interaction)

Physical Fitness and Sports Medicine

Exercise should be part of everyone's life. Studies show that children do not get enough exercise and adults have been labeled "couch potatoes". Many studies confirm that children, teenagers and adults are physically unfit. Their intake is high in calories, sweets, and fats and the intake exceeds the output causing a nation of overweight, obese people. Before an inactive, over 35 year old, overweight or physically handicapped person begins an exercise program they should see a physician who will perform a physical and identify the best exercise program for the individual. The program should be initiated gradually with 5–10 minutes to start, building up to 30 minutes to one hour at each session. A warm-up period of 3–5 minutes should precede any intense exercise and a gradual cool-down period at the termination of the exercise.

Some physicians will recommend aerobic exercise, especially for persons over 35. Aerobic exercise include walking, running, jogging, swimming, and bicycling. Whatever form of exercise is chosen it should be enjoyable, continuous, convenient, and affordable. There are no special foods or supplements needed by the person who exercises regularly.

Competitive athletes constantly desire to improve their performance and endurance and require additional calories due to the expenditure of energy. The caloric requirement for competitive athletes varies from 3,000–6,000 kcal during intense periods of activity. During the "off-season" these athletes will need to reduce their caloric intake to meet a more sedentary life style.

During training the athlete will need to secure 50–55 percent of calories from carbohydrates such as breads, pasta, rice, potatoes, cereal and other starchy foods. The amount of carbohydrates needed by the athlete will depend on the intensity and duration of the exercise and the degree of training to perform the exercise.

The protein intake will need to be from 1.0–1.5 grams per kg of weight. Increased fluid intake is vital as athletes are constantly facing dehydration due to loss of water in sweat, and respiration. Loss of as little as 2 percent of body can impair performance. It has been recommended that athletes drink 16 ounces of water 2 hours before competition and another 16 ounces 15 minutes before the competition. Sodium and chloride are the main electrolytes loss through perspiration. Some athletes take salt pills to replenish their supply. This is not recommended as they can irritate the stomach and cause nausea. Some athletes drink commercially prepared electrolytes. Most athletes don't need the salt pills but can replenish the salt through eating salty foods and using extra salt at meals. Citrus foods should be increased.

Athletes have a need for increased calcium and iron in the diet. Calcium supplements and or estrogen replacement for females may be indicated. Some athletes develop sports anemia which is usually seen in the early stages of training. The iron status of girls and teens should be monitored as they have a tendency to develop iron deficiency. The need for additional vitamins is unclear. Studies continue to be conducted. Most active people will meet the RDAs for vitamins if they consume a diet that is sufficient to meet their energy needs.

When engaging in vigorous exercise in which perspiration is high, drink an extra pint of water 2 hours before the competition or workout and 3–6 ounces every 10–20 minutes during exercise.

Many athletes who compete in endurance events (continuous uninterrupted activity for 11/2 hours or more) will carbohydrate load before the event. The body can deplete the glycogen during an endurance event and the athlete may feel fatigue and exhaustion during the competition.

Carbohydrate overloading regime is:

▶ The week prior to the competition the athlete will begin to taper off on exercise and the day before the event will be at complete rest.

▶ Increase the carbohydrate intake for seven days preceding the event.

▶ Increase the amount of carbohydrates from 350g per/day with an increase to 525–555g per/day for three days before the event.

Carbohydrate overloading is not recommended for children, teens and for persons engaged in short intense activities and is recommended for endurance athletes no more than four times per year.

Precompetition meals should be eaten 3–4 hours before the event. The meal should be high in complex carbohydrates, low in fat, moderately low in protein. Pasta, rice, vegetables, fruits, bread and other grains should contribute between 300–800 kcal.

Ergogenic Products

Ergogenic products are supposed to have special enhancing powers. Many quacks and charlatans peddle these wares to athletes. Some of the products (steroids, steroid-drug substitutes, protein supplements, muscle building powder etc.) are gimmicks and vary in their effect from useless to dangerous. Most athletes believe the many products will help them improve their performance. Caffeine is used by some athletes who believe it helps the performance while others say it has no effect.

Steroids, an illegal drug, is forbidden in sports competition, however, they are used by many athletes to promote the development of muscle mass. There are serious side effects from the use of these drugs that include liver and heart damage, mood swings, growth stunting, and appearance of muscular characteristics in women.

Some of the other ergogenic products are bee pollen, ginseng, gelatin, herbal steroids, lecithin, kelp, wheat germ, vitamin supplements, herbs made into pills that promote improved athletic performance, and spirulina that is used as a supplement and can be potentially dangerous.

▶ CULTURAL, RELIGIOUS, LIFESTYLES AND FOOD LORE ◀

We eat because our bodies need the nutrients to sustain life. The body gives off signals when it is hungry or thirsty. We eat the kinds of food we do because of custom, folk food lore, geography, climate, religion, lifestyles, culture, emotions, availability and sociability.

Everyone's eating pattern is affected by:

▶ *Geography.* The place where we live has a profound influence on the foods we eat and are familiar with. Regional food patterns still exist. The foods we are familiar with provide us with a feeling of comfort, pleasure and safety.

▶ *Economic factors.* Inadequate and low income does not allow for a great variety and quantity of foods. People with more income may also have poor food choices due to types of foods eaten/chosen. Neither group may practice or have access to good nutritional practices.

▶ *Psychological factors.* Food is often used as a means of rewards and punishment. We reward ourselves when we have completed a special project with gooey chocolate candy bar/cake, or express our happiness with birthday, anniversary parties, dine at fine restaurants with the one we love, eat when we are sad, lonely and depressed to give us comfort and security. We overeat sometimes because of our perceived failure, such as a loss of job, poor marks on a report card, unpopularity. Elderly people may not eat because of loneliness and depression. Some people use food as a punishment. Children may be scolded during meal times for their poor performance in sports or grades and they associate food with failure and unhappiness. Others withhold food especially desserts if the child didn't eat all the food placed on the plate. Food is sometimes used as a bribe for good behavior with favorite foods such as ice cream, candy, cookies. Some of the psychological factors of food intake can lead to obesity.

▶ *Family traditions.* Positive and negative attitudes about foods are learned in the home. Children will copy the habits of the parent. Children will learn to eat and appreciate a variety of foods if the parents prepare and serve a variety of food items. Children can learn cooking skills and nutrition information when they assist in meal preparation.

▶ *Folk food lore.* Some societies still practice food lore. They may believe that these lore have a cause and effect on health or outcome of a situation. For example, believe that eating fish and drinking milk at the same meal with make one ill, while other customs may include eating certain foods during pregnancy will produce a specific sex child. Most of the customs practiced have no scientific basis, but are superstitions that may have been practiced or handed down for generations.

Ethnic and religion play major roles in food selections. The following influences are not all inconclusive.

Religious Food Patterns

A number of religions have food restrictions as part of the religious code. Many are based on rabbinical dietary laws and the Old Testament of the Bible

Jewish: The degree to which these rules are followed in the United States depends on whether the individual is an Orthodox, Conservative, or Reform Jew. Orthodox Jews adhere to the biblical and rabbinical dietary laws called Rules of Kashruth and follow them under all conditions. Conservative Jews are less stringent, and Reform Jews give little emphasis to the dietary law.

According to Orthodox rules, pork, shellfish, and scavenger fish are prohibited. Animals and poultry are slaughtered according to ritual. This method of slaughter minimizes pain for the animal and maximizes blood drainage. The meat is soaked in cold water, salted to remove the blood, drained, and rinsed three times. This meat is considered *kosher*. Meat from the flesh of all quadruped with cloven hoofs that chew cud, such as cattle, sheep, goat, and deer, are acceptable but only the forequarter (rib section forward) is used. Meat from pork is prohibited.

Dairy products may not be eaten at the same meal with meat or meat products. Milk, sour cream, and cottage cheese are used in dairy meals. Usually 2 meals per day are dairy meals. Six hours must elapse after a meal before dairy foods may be eaten; half an hour must elapse after eating a dairy food before meat may be eaten.

Fish with fins and scales, eggs, fruits, bread, and vegetables may be eaten with the dairy, as well as the meat meals. Shellfish is prohibited. If these food items are to be served with meat, no milk, butter, or other dairy product may be used in the food preparation. Separate utensils and dishes are used for the preparation and service of the meat and dairy meals. No food preparation takes place on the Sabbath, which is Saturday. For special religious holidays, special foods are prepared; food items also are used symbolically. On Yom Kipper, no food or drink is taken for 24 hours.

Symbols used to indicate rabbinical supervision and kosher foods include:

▶ U—Union of Orthodox Jewish Congregations of America, used for canned, boxed, and batter products.

▶ VH or VHI—Vaad Haroborium of Massachusetts

▶ K—Organized Kashrus Laboratories, K (the letter) indicates rabbinical supervision by the individual company, not always approved by Orthodox rabbis.

Muslims: Muslims abstain from eating pork and the use of alcoholic beverages. Meat is slaughtered in a prescribed manner and in the name of Allah. Some Muslims will choose to eat kosher meat, substitute fish, slaughter their own, or eliminate meat from the diet. Young pigeons are allowed. Birds that are permitted to fly around and search for their own food are not allowed. Chicken is allowed if raised under controlled conditions. Fish must weigh at least 10 pounds. Milk is used extensively. Aged cheese is prohibited.

Because alcohol and pork products are forbidden, any flavorings that contain alcohol (such as extracts) or any cosmetics or drugs that contain alcohol and/or pork products are never used.

Foods may not be fried, white sugar is not used, and nuts are not allowed. Only 1 meal a day is eaten and there is no between-meal snacking.

During Ramadan, Muslims fast for a month. During this month, the practice is to abstain from food, water, and tobacco from dawn until after dark.

Hindus: As a basic rule, Hindus cannot eat any animal food. Most Hindus are prohibited from eating onions and garlic. Beef is a supreme taboo. Widows cannot eat any animal food. Drinking alcohol is a major sin. The Hindu religion is characterized by a caste system. No Hindu can eat with anyone who does not belong to the same caste. Each caste system practices different food regulations. The Brahmins (highest caste) are strict vegetarians; the lower caste may eat meat if meat is killed in the prescribed manner; the "untouchables" (lowest caste) can eat anything obtained in virtually any manner.

Others:

▶ *Buddhists* are essentially vegetarians and most will not eat the flesh of any animal.

▶ *Latter-day Saints* (Mormons) do not drink coffee, tea, or alcohol.

Traditional vegetarian groups, such as the Seventh-day Adventists and Trappist monks, generally differ little from non-vegetarians in their attitudes toward healthcare. In contrast, members of various groups (eg. macrobiotics, Zen Buddhist, Hare Krishnas, raw food eaters, some yogics) often hold negative attitudes toward orthodox or "Western" healthcare services and rely on homeopaths or lay healers for all but the most serious illnesses.

Regional Food Habits

Regional food habits have almost faded from the American scene due to the ease of travel, advertising, and the availability of food items. However, some foods and food habits still exist. The most common ones are:

▶ South—grits, cornbread, greens, okra, sweet potatoes, biscuits, fried chicken
▶ Southwest—Mexican dishes
▶ New England—clam chowder, baked beans, lobster
▶ Pennsylvania Dutch—scrapple, shoofly pie, German style sausage
▶ New Orleans—Creole and French cuisine
▶ Midwest—dairy products, Idaho potatoes
▶ West—salmon, fruits, vegetables, fresh foods, anything new

Cultural Food Patterns

America is a melting pot of races, culture, and traditions. In some areas, culture plays a large role in the food selection of the people. The most common cultural habits are:

▶ Native American
▶ African American
▶ Puerto Rican
▶ Mexican American
▶ Oriental
▶ Meditteranean

Native American: There is no true Native American diet as it varies from tribe to tribe. Corn, squash, tomato, peppers, and pumpkins continue to be widely used. Game, such as turkey, deer, bear, elk, fish, makes up the major protein source. Some studies point out that Native Americans are often lactose-intolerant.

African American: African Americans adopt many of the food customs of the South. Both Caucasians and African Americans in the South enjoy the same foods that are common to the region. African Americans do not consume a great deal of milk or milk products. There is a prevalence of lactose-intolerance in this population. Many African Americans consume:

▶ Large quantities of sweets (cakes, pies, candy, soft drinks)
▶ Large amounts of fat as fried foods are usually preferred (fish, poultry, pork).
▶ Vegetables cooked for long periods of time in ham, bacon, or salt pork. The liquid from the vegetables is eaten. Potatoes, onions, tomatoes, hot peppers, okra, sweet potatoes, green leafy vegs are preferred.
High blood pressure, obesity, and dental caries are common nutritional problems.

Puerto Rican: The basic Puerto Rican diet contains all the essential nutrients. The staple diet includes rices, chick peas, red beans, black beans, and other legumes. A combination of rice and beans may be eaten once a day and served with a highly seasoned tomato dish called *sofrito* (tomatoes, peppers, onion, garlic, spices, herbs, anato seeds, and lard). Starchy vegetables called *viandas* (plantains, green bananas, cassava, and white sweet potatoes) are used frequently. They are boiled and served with oil and oil vinegar, and in some cases may be fried. Chicken, pork, and dried cod fish are the basic meats. Beverages consist of *malta* (caramel, malt extract, and sugar), which is popular with pregnant women and *café con leché* (very strong coffee, warm milk, and sugar). Many fruits are grown in Puerto Rico and are readily available at road stands, as well as supermarkets. Few green leafy vegetables are eaten.

Mexican American: The Mexican American diet has had a great influence on the Southwest and has been popularized in several fast food chains and restaurants in America. The basic diet includes corn, pinto or calico beans, rice, chili pepper, tomatoes, onions, avocados, sour cream, garlic, and spices.

Beans are usually eaten with the evening meal. Refried beans are a staple. Stewed tomatoes, avocados, sour cream, tomato paste, and lard are greatly utilized. *Masa,* the staple of the diet, is dried corn that has been soaked in lime water, washed, and pounded to a jellylike consistency. *Masa* is baked on a hot griddle and used to make tortillas and tacos. Various bean mixtures, ground meat, cheese, onion, lettuce, and tomato sauce are served with these products. *Tamales* are another dish made with corn dough and ground beef, wrapped in a corn-husk, and steamed. *Chili con carne* consists of beans, meat, garlic, tomatoes, chili peppers, and other spices. Potatoes, pumpkins, greens, carrots, bananas, melons, and peaches are the most commonly used fruits and vegetables. Potatoes are usually served 3 times per day. Sweets, sweet rolls, candy, and sugar are consumed in high amounts. Wheat products are beginning to replace some of the corn products, thus reducing the calcium intake. May exclude green leafy vegetables and yellow vegetables. Chocolate and strong coffee drinks are served at least once a day.

Oriental: Oriental food habits may be Chinese, Japanese, Vietnamese, Korean, and Filipino. Rice, wheat, soybean, tofu, sprouts, poultry, pork, eggs, and fish are commonly used in combination with vegetables and noodles. Cheese is rarely used and only in small quantities. Almost every part of an animal is used. Blood pudding is eaten frequently by the Chinese. Vegetables are cooked for short periods of time, and the cooking liquid is served with the vegetables. Fruits are considered a delicacy in China. A large variety of fruits are used in Japan. Soy sauce, which is high in sodium, is widely used. Soybean, sesame, lard, and peanut oils are used for cooking. Tea is the most popular beverage. Soft drinks and beer are also highly consumed. Lactose intolerance may be common. The Filipino diet is similar to Japanese and Chinese. Rice is the main carbohydrate. Fish, meat, eggs, legumes, and nuts are protein sources. Milk and milk products are limited due to lactose-intolerance.

Meditteranean: This diet includes the increased use of olive oil instead of butter or shortening, high use of vegetables, seafood, seasonings, grain breads, seeds, including lentils and beans, goat cheese, fruits, especially grapes and figs, drank wine diluted half and half with water, egg plants, lemons, garlic and herbs, such as dill, mint, and parsley; lamb, yogurt, tomatoes, cucumbers, honey. This diet is approximately 42% fat. Diets vary from Greece, Italy and even within regions of each country.

Physician's Order

When a diet is requested for religious, cultural, or regional reasons, write a nutrition consult for the registered dietitian (RD) to plan the diet. Notice of 24 hours, preferably 48 hours is requested.

Food Lore

In many societies food has been used traditionally as well as symbolic. Most beliefs are not founded in scientific principles. Many people hold superstitutions and fear about some foods, especially at times of high stress such as death, aging, and illness.

Some cults determine that when certain foods are eaten a successful pregnancy and delivery will be assured.

Most food lores begin in childhood and may never be overcome. The healthcare provider should NEVER voice overt criticisms concerning one's beliefs but counsel the client to eat a well balanced diet incorporating a variety of foods.

General References/Bibliography

Chicago Dietetic Association and South Suburban Dietetic Association, *Manual of Clinical Dietetics,* American Dietetic Association, Chicago, 1992.

Food and Nutrition Board, Subcommittee on the Tenth Edition of the RDA's. *Recommended Dietary Allowances,* (10th ed.), National Academy Press, Washington, DC, 1989.

Hamilton, E.M.N., Whitney, E.N., Sienkiewicz, F.S., *Nutrition: Concepts and Controversies,* (5th ed), West Publishing Co., St. Paul, MN, 1991.

Hommerson, S., *Practical Guide to Nutritional Care for Dietitians and other Health Care professional,* AB Hospital, University of Alabama, Birmingham, 1992.

Pemberton, C.M., Moxness, K.E., German, M.J., Nelson, J.K., Gastineau, C.F., Rochester, Methodist Hospital and Saint Mary's Hospital, *Mayo Clinic Diet Manual: A Handbook of Dietary Practices,* (6th ed), B. C. Decker, Inc. Toronto, 1988.

Puckett, R.P., Brown, S.M., *Shands Hospital at the University of Florida Guide to Clinical Dietetics,* (5th ed), Kendall/Hunt Publishing Co., Dubuque, Iowa, 1993.

Robinson, C.H., Weigley, E.S. Mueller, D.H., *Basic Nutrition and Diet Therapy,* (7th ed), Macmillan Publishing Co., New York, 1993.

Sizer, F., Whitney, E., Hamiltons and Whiteney's *Nutrition Concepts and Controversies,* (6th ed), West Publishing Co., Minneapolis/St. Paul, 1994.

USDA and USDHHS, *Nutrition and Your Health: Dietary Guidelines for Americans* (2nd ed), Revised November, 1990 and (3rd ed) Revised 1996. 1990 edition—home and Gardens Bulletin 232, USDA/USDHHS, Washington, DC, August 1985.

Specific Topic Bibliography

Abrams, W.B., Berkow, R. Fletcher, A.J. Abrass, I.B. Besdine, R.W. Butler, R.N., Rowe, J.W., Solomon, D.H., *The Merck Manual of Geriatrics,* Merck Sharp & Dohne Research Laboratories, Rathway, NJ, 1990.

American Academy of Pediatrics, Committee on Nutrition, *Pedatric Nutrition Handbook,* 2nd ed, American Academy of Pediatrics, Elk Grove Village, IL.

American Dietetic Association, *Understanding Food Patterns in the USA,* Chicago, American Dietetic Association, 1969.

Atkins, F.M., Food allergies and behavior: Definitions, mechanism, and a review of the evidence, *Nutrition Review Supplement,* May 1986.

Bagby, B.H., Aging: Global trends and national perspectives, *J. Home Econ.,* 81:48–53, Spring 1991.

Chaudhuri, N.C., *Hinduism,* Oxford University Press, New York, pp. 192–201, 1979.

Chicago Dietetic Association and South Suburban Dietetic Association, *Manual of Clinical Dietetics,* American Dietetic Association, Chicago, pp. 27–32, 1988.

Craig, L., *Nutrition and Aging,* Ross Laboratories, Columbus, Ohio, 1991.

Dobler, M.L., Food Allergies, *J. Amer. Dietet. A.,* 91:1–5, 1991.

Dwyer, J., Fitzgerald, J., Teenagers' diets. Hazards, virtues problems, solutions, *Nutr. & the M.D.,* 172/14/961–3 November, 1991.

Food and Nutrition Services, Shands Hospital at the University of Florida, *Guide to Normal Nutrition and Diet Modification,* (3rd ed), Gamesville, Florida, pp. 217–200, 1983.

Gray, P.J., Goodwin, J., *Aging: In The Surgeon General's Report on Nutrition and Health,* U.S. Public Health Service, U.S. Department of Health and Human Services, Washington, DC, 1988, Chap. 16, pp 595–617.

Havala, S., Dwyer, J., Position of the American Dietetic Association. Vegetarian diets, *Journal of the American Dietetic Association,* 88(3), pp. 351–355, 1988.

Hendricks, K.M., Walker, W.A., *Manual of Pediatric Nutrition,* (2nd ed), B.C. Decker, Inc., Toronto, pp 170–173, 1990.

Higgins, C. Warshaw H.S. Jewish food practices, customs and holidays, Ethnic & Regional Food Practices (series) Chicago and Alexandria, VA: American Dietetic Assoc. and American Diabetes Assoc. 1989.

Hoffman, C.J. Coleman, E. An eating plan update on Recommended Dietary Practices for Endurance Athletes, *J. Am. Dietet. A.,* 91: 325–30, 1991.

Holm, K., Walker, J., Osteoporosis Treatment and prevention upate, *Geriatric Nursing,* May/June, 1990.

Hui, Y.H., *Principles and Issues in Nutrition,* Wadsworth Health Sciences Division, monterey, California, pp. 606–623, 1985.

Infant feeding and allergy, *Nutr. & M.D.,* 16 3–4, September 1990.

Institute of medicine Subcommittee on Nutritional Status and Weight Gain During Pregnancy, *Summary Nutrition During Pregnancy,* National Academy Press, Washington, DC, 1990.

Kris-Etherton, P.M., Nutrition and athletic performance, *Nutr. Today,* 25:35–37, September/October 1990.

Lappe. F.M., *Diet for a Small Planet,* Ballatine Books, New York, 1982.

Lawrence, R.A., *Breastfeeding: A Guide for the Medical Profession,* St. Louis: Mosby, 1989.

Logemann, J.A., *Dysphagic: A Review for Health Professionals,* Milani Foods, Melrose Park, IL, pp. 6–17, 1991.

Masana, L and coauthors. The Mediterranean type diet; Is there a need for further modifications? American Journal of Clinical Nutrition 53 (1991): 886–889.

McIntosh, W.A., et al. The relationship between beliefs about nutrition and dietary practices of the elderly, *J. Am. Dietet. A.,* 90:671–76, 1990.

Mead Johnson Enteral Nutritional, *Preventing Pressure Sores,* Study Guide, Bristol-Meyers Squibb Co., Evansville, IN, 1989.

Meador, R., Montalbano, B., Practical application of kosher foodservice in a nonkosher residential health care facility, *Journal of Nutrition for the Elderly,* 2(1), pp. 61–69, 1982.

Miller, S.A., Health Claims: an ethical conflict?, *Food Technol.,* 452/14/96130-39, May 1991.

Muhammad, E., *How to Live to Eat,* Chicago, Perkin, J.E., *Food Allergies and Adverse Reactions,* Aspen Publishers, Inc., Gaithersburg, MD, 1990.

Position Paper of the American Dietetic Association: School-based nutrition programs and services, *J. Am. Dietet. A.,* 95:367–69, 1995.

Sitzmann, J.V., Nutritional support of the dysphagic patient: Methods, risk and complication of therapy, *Journal of Parenteral and Enteral Nutrition,* 14(1), pp. 60–63, 1990.

Srisuphon, W., Bracken, B.M., Caffeine consumption during pregnancy and associated with late spontaneous abortion, *Am J. of Obstetrics and Gynecology,* 154, 14–20, 1986.

Stjernfeldt, M. et al. Maternal smoking during pregnancy and the risk of childhood cancer. *Lancet,* 1, 1350–1352, 1986.

Weigley, E.S., Changing patterns in offering solids to infants, *Pediatr. Nursing,* 16, 439–41, 452, 1990.

Worthington-Roberts, B., Williams, S.R. *Nutrition in Pregnancy and Lactation,* (4th ed), Times Mirror/Mosby College Publishing, St. Louis, MO, 1989.

Zheng, JJ., Rosenberg, I.H., What is the Nutritional status of the elderly? *Geriatrics,* 44(6), 1989.

Zuckerman, B. et al., Effects of maternal marijuana and cocaine use on fetal growth, *New England J. of Med.,* 320, 762–768, 1989.

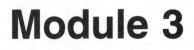
Module 3

Healthcare Food and Nutrition Services

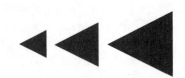

▶ INTERDISCIPLINARY TEAM APPROACH TO PATIENT CARE ◀

Nutrition care provided to the patient and family is best provided by an interdisciplinary team. The team may be composed of physicians, dietitians, nurses, social workers, pharmacist, and rehabilitative professionals. A nutrition team composed of registered dietitians (RDs), dietetic technicians, dietary managers, patient representatives, and other food and nutritional employees provide both direct and indirect nutritional care to the patient. The goal of this team is to provide optimal nutrition to the patient with input from the patient and family concerning the care. Nutrition is an essential part of the total care of the patient and should be provided by persons with the expertise to provide the care.

The RD is the team leader. The RD has the educational background necessary to provide the following services:

▶ Screen patients to determine their nutritional status.

▶ Assess and reassess the nutritional status of patients.

▶ Develop, implement, monitor, and evaluate nutritional care plans.

▶ Involve patients and families in the development of care plans.

▶ Teach and counsel patients and families concerning nutrition, diet plans, nutrient and drug interactions.

▶ Participate as a member of the interdisciplinary team.

▶ Provide educational programs to other professionals including students.

▶ Maintain competency through the participation in professional activities, continuing education, literature review, research, etc.

▶ Communicate with team members concerning the progress, needs, perceptions, and treatment of the individual patient.

▶ Develop educational materials including materials for the organization's diet manual.

▶ Serve as the liaison to the food service through the translation of diet orders into food and menus.

▶ Record pertinent data in the patient's medical record.

▶ Provide discharge materials to referring agencies, physicians, or community agencies.

▶ Serve as a change agent for improvement of performance with measurable outcomes.

▶ Provide cost effective services.

The dietetic technician works in conjunction with the RD to provide screening, leveling of patients for service, data collection, planning specialized menus to meet the needs of patients, providing direct contact with patients and families to obtain diet histories, nutrient intake, and instructing patients on modified diets. Diet technicians may also plan menus, supervise food service personnel, assist patients with menu selection, record pertinent data in the medical record, supervise dietary managers, and/or clerical staff. They may also be responsible for calorie counts, enteral nutrition formula room activities and other duties specific to the individual organization.

Other members of the nutrition team may be responsible for the manufacturing of enteral/tube feedings, passing nourishments, assisting with menu selection, ordering food and supplies from a central warehouse, and for preparing and delivering meal trays. Regardless of the role of each individual team member the nutrition team has as its primary goal to translate the art and science of nutrition into food and feeding the patient a balance diet.

Each team member has its specific role. In conjunction with the physician the RD prescribes the ***diet order after*** reviewing the screening and assessment information. The RD translates the diet order into menus and food. An ***initial diet order*** should be prescribed for new patients and written in the patients' medical record. The order is then transmitted to the Food and Nutrition Services department who records the information in a kardex or computer order system. The information should include complete information such as: patient's full name (first and last name), room number, and all pertinent details concerning diet. For pediatric patients, the age should be provided. When a diet is to be held the order is ***Hold diet.*** A hold diet order is for patients having tests, minor surgery, laboratory or radiological tests and/or other minor treatments. Hold diet orders are used to restrict food for a period of less than a day. A **NPO diet order** is used for patients who will have food restricted for 24 hours or longer. If a patient is on NPO for more than 72 hours a nutritional assessment should be made on the patient.

      Diet histories, diet recall and food diaries are considered as a component of the dietary assessment and are used in conjunction with other assessments to provide a nutritional profile of the patient. A *diet history* (see below) may be taken by a RD, dietetic technician and/or a certified dietary manager. A diet history is information gathered from the patient/family member to assist the nutrition team to determine the possibility of malnutrition. The history contains information on food likes, dislikes, meal patterns, food frequency record, alcohol consumption, smoking habits and medication record. A *diet recall* is the recollection of what the patient ate in the last 24 hours, including snacks. A *food diary* is a written record of specific foods and nutrients consumed over 3–7 days. The record is maintained by the patient/family. It records the portion sizes of all food and beverages consumed during the period. The intake record information is recorded in the diary, entered into a computer software program for a nutrient analysis profile. A *nutrient analysis* is a mathematical calculation of the nutrients consumed in a given period of time, usually three days. This analysis provides data to the nutrition and interdisciplinary teams as to food patterns, deficiencies in various nutrients, and alcohol consumption of the patient. This data can be used for recommending the diet order.

► FOOD AND NUTRITION SERVICE DIET HISTORY FORM ◄

To be filled out by a member of the Nutritional Care team during the initial visit. Data will be available to the interdisciplinary team.

Name ————————————————— Date: ————————————

Room Number: ————————————— Attending physician: ——————————

Occupation: ——————————————— Diet Order: ——————————————

1. Do you live alone? Y — N — If no, with whom do you live? ————————————

2. Who does the majority of grocery shopping and cooking in your household? ————————————————————————————————

3. If you eat most of your meals away from home, where do you eat, and how often? ————————————————————————————————

4. Do you order food out, such as pizza, pick up food on the way home? Y — N — If yes, what types of foods, how often? ————————————————————

5. Type of diet followed at home. ————————————————————————

6. Is your appetite good? Y — N — poor? Y — N —

7. Have there been any recent changes in your life style that would affect your appetite? Y — N — What? ————————————————————————

8. Do you have any food allergies? Y — N — What? ————————————————
   Any food intolerance? Y — N — What? ————————————————————
   Any food dislikes? ————————————————————————————————
   Any foods you prefer? ————————————————————————————

9. Are there any foods you avoid due to religious, cultural or philosophical reasons? Y — N — If yes, describe ————————————————————————

10. Do you wear glasses? Y — N — Hearing aid? Y — N — Dentures? Y — N — Do you have a problem with chewing? Y — N — Swallowing? Y — N — Do you need your foods chopped? Y — N — pureed? Y — N — special feeding tools? Y — N — feed self? Y — N — need assistance with feeding? Y — N —

11. Do you smoke? Y — N — cigarettes per day? ———— cigars? Y — N — number per day ———— chew tobacco? Y — N — dip snuff? Y — N —

12. Do you drink alcoholic beverages? Y __ N __ How much? _____
    How often? _____ What type? beer __ wine __ mixed drinks __ liquor __

13. Do you drink caffeine containing beverages? Which ones and how much per day?
    coffee? _____ tea? _____ regular canned sodas? _____ diet sodas? _____

14. How much water do you drink per day? _____ milk? _____juice? _____
    other beverages? _____

15. Do you exercise regularly? Y __ N __ How often? _____
    Type of exercise _____

16. Do you take any vitamin, mineral, herbs or other types of nutritional supplements? Y __ N __
    What type? _____ How often? _____

17. Are you on a reduction diet? _____ Who prescribed it? _____
    Have you ever been on a fad diet to lose weight? Y __ N __

Other pertinent information: _____

_____

_____

_____

_____

_____

_____

_____

_____

_____

_____

                                History taken by: _____
                                Date: _____

_____

© Copyright Ruby P. Puckett MA, RD, LD, used with permission.

▶ NUTRITIONAL SCREENING ◀

Nutritional screening should be completed within 24 hours of admission for patients who are at high risk. To provide appropriate nutrition care for all patients screening levels are suggested. Level 1 patients are those patients who are not in need of nutrition intervention at this time. Patients in this category include those with less than a 24-hour stay and patients with no related nutritional requests. In most instances Level II screening is accomplished by the dietetic technician. Level II patients include patients who have food allergies, food intolerances, special nutrition/food request, patients who need assistance with menus, patients with chewing/swallowing problems and or have self-feeding difficulty, and patients who have an unintentional weight loss/gain in one month and or six months. Level III patients will be seen by the registered dietitian. Level III patients are considered to be at high nutritional risk. Patients in this category include a diagnosis of malnutrition, failure to thrive, kwashiorkor/marasmus and severe malabsorption problems. Other parameters include unintentional weight loss of greater than 10% of the usual body weight (UBW) in the last one month as well as the last six months; poor visceral protein (albumin of less than 2.7–3.0 g/dl), medical problems that include diarrhea, vomiting, constipation, poor appetite with minimal food intake for five days before admission, chemotherapy, surgery in the last 3 months, dysphagia, pressure sores, and patients who are on eternal or parental nutrition feedings.

Nutrition Risk Screening

(To be completed within 24 hours of admission)
Chart Review: *(To be completed by Certified dietary manager or diet technician)*
▶ Height and weight
▶ Allergies
▶ Medications (especially drugs that may interfere with nutrients)
▶ Diagnosis
▶ Physician and service
▶ Diet Order
▶ Pertinent history and physical data
▶ Lab values (if available)
        albumin
        triglycerides
        cholesterol

    Direct Patient Contact: *(To be accomplished by patient nutrition representative, certified dietary manager, diet technician registered or registered dietitian)*
▶ Meal rounds
- acceptance of meals/appetite
▶ Patient interviews
- modified diet
- weight history
- chewing/swallowing problems

Nutrition Screening and Assessment Tools*

The Nutrition Screening Initiative (NSI) was developed in the early 1990s as a cooperative effort of the American Academy of Family Physicians, the American Dietetic Association, and the National Council on the Aging, Inc.

The NSI developed two levels of screening. The NSI level 1 Screen is used by non-professionals to identify the risk of malnutrition and includes:

Height and weight to determine body mass index
Specific questions about eating habits, living arrangements, and functional habits
The NSI Level II Screen, for professional use, includes the following *anthropometric data:*
BMI
Mid-arm circumference
Triceps skinfold
Mid-arm *muscle* circumference
Laboratory values:
Serum albumin (risk = >3.5g/dL)
Serum cholesterol (risk = <160 mg/dL)
Serum cholesterol (risk = 240 mg/dL)
Other data:
Drug-use history
Clinical history
Eating habits
Living environment and income
Functional status
Mental and cognitive status

---

*The NSI materials summarized and used by permission of the Nutrition Screening Initiative, 2626 Pennsylvania Avenue NW, Suite 301, Washington, DC 20037

► FOOD AND NUTRITION SCREENING FORM© ◀

Name: _____ Room number: _____ Age: _____

Male: _____ Female: _____ Child: _____ Adult: _____ Elderly: _____

Diagnosis: _____

Diet order: _____ Physician: _____

CLINICAL DATA:

Medical history prior to admission: (last 1–3 months)

Decubitus ulcer? _____ Radiation therapy? _____ Chemotherapy? _____

Surgery? _____ Acute illness greater than 3 days? _____ Height? _____

Weight? _____ Loss 3/months? _____ Gain 3/months? _____ UBW? _____

IBW? _____ Condition of mouth, lips, tongue, gums? _____

BIOCHEMICAL DATA:

Serum Albumin? _____ Transferrin? _____ Nitrogen balance? _____

FOOD AND NUTRITIONAL HISTORY PRIOR TO ADMISSION:

Diarrhea? _____ Constipation? _____ Nausea/Vomiting? _____

Heartburn? _____ Bloating? _____ Cramping? _____

Appetite? Loss? _____ Increased? _____ Chewing/swallowing problems? _____

NPO or limited intake greater than 3 days? _____ Home TPEN? _____

Diabetic? _____ NIDD? _____ Number of calories? _____

Any other diet modification? Y __ N __ What? _____

Bulimia? Y __ N __ Anorexia nervosa? Y __ N __

MEDICATIONS AND HERBS _____

_____

Vitamins? _____ Minerals? _____

Other supplements? _____

SCREENED:

_____ Patient screened at Level I—no nutritional intervention required at this time.

Provide basic food service (selective menu, etc)

_____ Patient screened at Level II—requires assistance of Nutritional care team, no malnutrition but may be at low risk.

Provide basic food service, (may need assistance with menu, education, may re-screen within 7 days)

_____ Patient screened at Level III—requires RD intervention. Moderately malnourished.

Provide basic food service, follow-up in 3–5 days. Document in patient's medical history.

_____ Patient screened, severe malnutrition, referred to the TPEN team and RD. Referred to out-patient nutrition clinic, referring physician and/or community agency.

Document outcome in medical history. Forward data to appropriate person/agency.

Screened by: _____ Date: _____ Time: _____

► **GOAL OF NUTRITION SCREENING** ◄

To Identify High-Risk Patients who may be Prone to Poor Nutritional Status

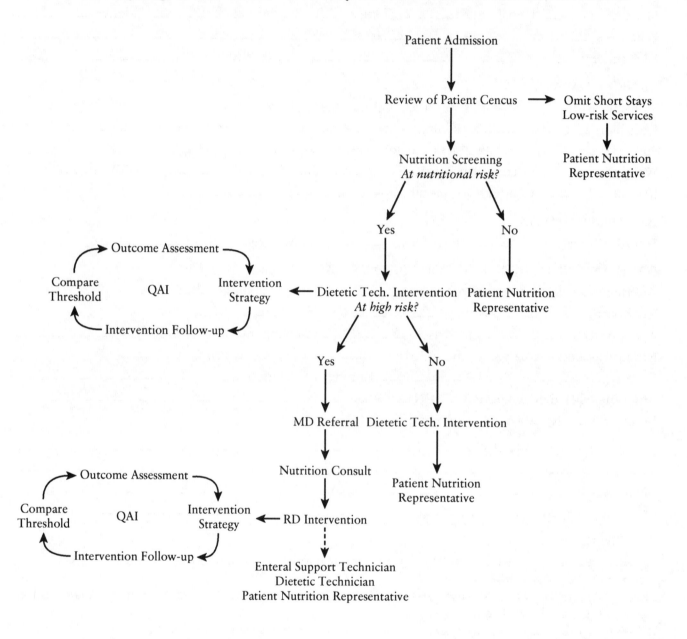

Recent evidence has shown a high incidence of malnutrition in hospitals, adversely affecting patient recovery time and survival rate. Nutritional assessment has become a vital component in the prevention and treatment of hospital malnutrition. Assessment parameters have been established to identify individuals at risk, to provide guidelines for appropriate intervention and to evaluate the effectiveness of therapy. Because not all patients require a comprehensive nutritional assessment, routine screening of the patient population should be performed to identify patients with or at risk of developing malnutrition.

► DETERMINATION OF NUTRITIONAL STATUS ◄

Nutritional status may be determined through the synthesis of four indices:

1. clinical data
2. dietary assessment
3. anthropometric measurements
4. biochemical data

Clinical Data

The patient's medical, family and social history, physical exam, and admitting diagnosis should be evaluated. Physical signs of malnutrition are often found in the medical history. Clinical features frequently correlated with poor nutritional status follow below.

► THE CLINICAL NUTRITION EXAM ◄

Clinical Findings	Consider Deficiency	Comment
Hair/Nails		
Hair easily pluckable, sparse, straight, hypopigmentation,	Protein	
Dull, spoon-shaped nails	Chronic iron	
Brittle, ridged, lined nails	Non-specific	
Skin		
Petechiae, purpura, corkscrew hairs	Ascorbic acid	Symptoms of scurvy can occur within 40 days of deficient intake
Pigmentation, desquamation	Niacin (pellagra)	Sun-exposed areas, symmetric
Follicular keratosis	Vitamin A	Keratin plugs in follicles
Dry, scaling	Non-specific	
Subcutaneous fat loss	Calories	Minimal fat reserves if triceps skinfold 1/4" between fingers
Eyes		
Dull, dry conjunctiva	Vitamin A	
Blepharitis	B-complex	
Ophthalmoplegia	Thiamin	Wernicke's syndrome: prompt treatment necessary
Perioral		
Angular fissures, scars	B-complex, iron	Also with ill-fitting dentures
Cheilosis	Pyridoxine, niacin, riboflavin, iron	

The Clinical Nutrition Exam—Continued

Clinical Findings	Consider Deficiency	Comment
Oral		
Ageusia, dysgeusia	Zinc, vitamin A	Also associated with altered sense of smell
Glossitis, depapillation	Niacin, riboflavin, B;i1;i2, folate, iron	
Swollen, bleeding gums	Ascorbic acid	
Glands		
Parotid enlargement	Protein	
Sicca syndrome	Ascorbic acid	
Thyroid enlargement	Iodine	
Heart		
Small heart, decreased output		
Enlargement, tachycardia, high-output failure	Protein Thiamin	"Wet beriberi"
Sudden failure, death	Ascorbic acid	
Abdomen		
Hepatomegaly (fatty)	Protein	
Muscles, Extremities		
Muscle, wastage evident in temporal area, dorsum of hand between thumb and index finger, calf muscles	Protein, calorie	
Pain in calves, weak thighs	Thiamin	
Edema	Protein, thiamin	
Bones, Joints		
Epiphyseal thickening, deformities	Vitamin D (rickets)	
Bone pain (adult)	Osteomalacia	No sun, steatorrhea, repeated pregnancies with poor calcium intake
Bone pain (child)	Ascorbic acid	Subperiosteal hemorrhage
Neurologic		
Arthralgia	Ascorbic acid	
Ophthalmoplegia, footdrop	Thiamin	Wernicke's encephalopathy
Confabulation, disorientation	Thiamin	Korsakoff's psychosis
Decreased position, vibratory sense, ataxia	B_{12}	Subacute combined cord degeneration
Weakness, paresthesia of legs	B_{12}, thiamin, pyridoxine, pantothenic acids	Nutritional polyneuropathy, especially with alcoholism
Other		
Delayed healing and tissue repair (eg, wound, infarct, abscess)	Ascorbic acid, zinc, protein calories	

▶ DETERMINING DEGREE OF MALNUTRITION ◀

	Mild	Moderate	Severe
Fat Reserves			
triceps skinfold	40 to 50th percentile	30 to 39th percentile	less than 30th percentile
Somatic Protein			
Arm muscle area, sq. cm	40 to 50th percentile	30 to 39th percentile	less than 30th percentile
Wt. as % ideal	80 to 90%	70 to 79%	less than 70%
Wt. as % usual	85 to 90%	70 to 84%	less than 75%
Creatinine Height	60 to 80%	40 to 59%	less than 40%
Visceral Protein			
Albumin, grams per 100 ml	2.8 to 3.4	2.1 to 2.7	less than 2.1
Transferrin, mg per 100 ml	150 to 200	100 to 149	less than 100
Immune Competence			
Total lymphocyte count	1200 to 2000	800 to 1199	less than 800
Cell-mediated immunity (reactivity to skin tests)	Reactive	Reactive	Anergic

Used by permission. Ann Grant and Susan DeHoog, from Nutritional Assessment and Support, 1991. Published by Grant/Dehoog. 1991.

Evaluation of Weight

The term *ideal body weight* is difficult to define and to be *accurate* in defining weight. Insurance companies charts are also rarely utilized since the charts are based on people from age 25–29 years old and then applied to everyone. The bases for these charts are from persons who purchased insurance in the last 12 years. A *healthy weight* is a more appropriate term. A healthy weight is a balance between lean and fat tissues. However, for a quick reference the following formulas may be used, with the knowledge that they are only an estimate.

Frisancho developed weight standards as percentiles according to frame size and by age group which are based on extensive data merged from the NHANES I and NHANES II studies. These studies were a cross-sectional sample of over 43,000 subjects age 1 to 74. These standards are perhaps the most representative data available on adult, non-institutionalized population.

The Hamwi method for determining ideal body weight is:

Females:	Males:
100 lbs for first 5 feet	106 lbs for first 5 feet
Additional 5 lbs for each inch over 5 feet	Additoinal 6 lbs for each inch over 5 feet

Add 10 percent for large frame, subtract 10 percent for small frame

Peiffer et al suggest for adjustments for paraplegia—subtract 10–15 pounds from the IBW and adjustments for quadriplegia—subtract 15–20 pounds from the IBW.

The Guidelines for Long Term Care Tag number 325 states: "Parameters of nutritional status which are unacceptable include unplanned weight loss as well as other indices such as peripheral edema, cachexia, and laboratory test indicating malnutrition.

Weight: Since ideal body weight charts have not yet been validated for institutionalized elderly, weight loss (or gain) is a guide in determining nutritional status. An analysis of weight loss or gain should be examined in the light of the individual's former life style as well as current diagnosis."

Body Mass Index (BMI) is an indicator of body fat content. An index greater than 27.2 in men and 26.9 in women means a need for weight reduction.

$BMI = \dfrac{wt, kg}{ht^2, meters}$ Example: client 66 inches (168 cm or 1.68 m) 154 pounds (70 kg) $BMI = \dfrac{70}{2.82} = 24.8$

Suggested parameters for evaluating significance or unplanned and undesired weight loss are:

Interval	Significant loss	Severe loss
1 month	5%	Greater than 5%
3 months	7.5%	Greater than 7.5%
6 months	10%	Greater than 10%

The following formula determines percentage of loss

$$\text{\% of body weight loss} = \frac{\text{usual weight} - \text{actual weight} \times 100}{\text{usual weight}}$$

overweight = 10–20% above accepted standard
obese = 20% or more above standard
morbidity obese = 100 pounds or 100% above accepted standard

In evaluating weight loss, consider the resident's usual weight through adult life, the assessment of potential for weight loss, and care plan for weight management. Also, was the resident on a calorie restricted diet, or if newly admitted and obese, and on a normal diet, are fewer calories provided than prior to admission? Was the resident edematous when initially weighted, and with treatment no longer has edema? Has the resident refused food?

Anthropometric Assessment

Anthropometry is the science that deals with measurements of size, weight, and proportions of the human body. Triceps skinfold, subscapular skinfold, sometimes skinfolds such as the elbowbreath, midarm and wrist circumference are also used. For children head and chest circumferences are frequently used. Comparison of the anthropometric measurement can be compared to standard measurements to determine the percentile of growth for age and sex, as well as possible nutritional deficiency, fatness and leanness, water retention. Growth charts for children are found in Appendix.

Mid-Arm Circumferences (MAC). Mid-arm circumference is used to derive the mid-arm muscle circumference (MAMC), which provides a sensitive estimate of skeletal muscle mass. Comparison of measurements to established standards is used to evaluate severity and type of malnutrition.
    Procedure:

1. Place tape around arm at midpoint. Be sure tape fits snugly but does not constrict arm. See figure.
2. Record measurement in centimeters.
3. Calculate MAMC as follows:
   MAMC cm = MAC cm − (0.314 × TSF mm)

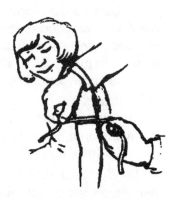

**Determination of
mid-arm circumference**

▶ STANDARDS OF ANTHROPOMETRY ◀			
	Standard	**90%**	**< 90–60%**	**< 60%**
Female				
TSF (mm)	16.5	14.9	14.8–9.9	9.8 or less
MAC (cm)	28.5	25.7	25.6–17.6	17.5 or less
MAMC (cm)	23.2	20.9	20.8–13.9	13.8 or less
Male				
TSF (mm)	12.5	11.3	11.2–7.5	7.4 or less
MAC (cm)	29.3	26.3	26.2–17.6	17.5 or less
MAMC (mm)	25.3	22.8	22.7–15.2	15.1 or less

▶ STANDARDS FOR TRICEPS SKINFOLD AND ◀ MID-ARM CIRCUMFERENCE OF THE ELDERLY

Triceps Skinfold Percentiles (µMM)[a]

Age (years)	Males			Females		
	95%	50%	5%	95%	50%	5%
65	27.0	13.8	8.6	33.0	21.6	13.5
70	26.1	12.9	7.7	32.0	20.6	12.5
75	25.2	12.0	6.8	31.0	19.6	11.5
80	24.3	11.2	6.0	30.0	18.6	10.5
85	23.4	10.3	5.1	29.0	17.6	9.5
90	22.6	9.4	4.2	28.0	16.6	8.5

[a]Reprinted with permission of Ross Laboratories, Columbus, OH 043216, from *Nutritional Assessment of the Elderly Through Anthropometry*, pp. 24 and 26, © 1984 Ross Laboratories (6).

▶ STANDARDS FOR TRICEPS SKINFOLD AND ◀ MID-ARM CIRCUMFERENCE OF THE ELDERLY

Mid-Arm Circumference Percentiles (cm)[b]

Age (years)	Males			Females		
	95%	50%	5%	95%	50%	5%
65	37.8	31.9	26.7	37.0	30.5	25.3
70	37.2	31.3	26.0	36.6	30.2	24.9
75	36.6	30.7	25.4	36.3	29.8	24.6
80	36.0	30.1	24.8	35.9	29.5	24.2
85	35.3	29.4	24.2	35.6	29.1	23.9
90	34.7	28.8	23.5	35.2	28.9	23.5

[b]Reprinted with permission of Ross Laboratories, Columbus, OH 43216, from *Nutritional Assessment of the Elderly Through Anthropometry*, pp. 24 and 26, © 1984 Ross Laboratories (6)

▶ STANDARDS FOR MID-ARM MUSCLE AREA OF THE ELDERLY[a] ◀

$$\text{Mid-arm muscle area (cm}^2) = \frac{\text{Mid-arm circumference (cm)} - (3.14) \times \frac{(\text{triceps skinfold (mm)})^2}{10}}{12.56}$$

Mid-Arm Muscle Area Percentiles (cm²)[c]

Age (years)	Males			Females		
	95%	50%	5%	95%	50%	5%
65	77.1	59.4	43.2	66.4	44.5	33.5
70	75.3	57.7	41.4	65.9	44.1	33.0
75	73.5	55.9	39.6	65.5	43.6	32.6
80	71.7	54.1	37.8	65.1	43.2	32.2
85	69.9	52.3	36.0	64.7	42.8	31.8
90	68.2	50.5	34.3	64.2	42.4	31.3

[c]Reprinted with permission of Ross Laboratories, Columbus, OH 43216, from *Nutritional Assessment of the Elderly Through Anthropometry*, pp. 32 and 33, © 1984 Ross Laboratories (6)

Biochemical Assessment*

Biochemical data is most often used in extended nutritional assessment, however some lab values may be available for use in initial screening.

Serum Proteins. Serum albumin and serum transferrin provide biochemical indices of visceral protein status. Catabolism causes the blood concentrations of these proteins to decrease.

Serum albumin is a plasma protein which is synthesized in the liver. It is considered a reliable measure of the visceral protein compartment. However, due to its relatively long half-life (16–18 days) changes in serum albumin are not seen until protein depletion has already occurred. Still, it is a relatively inexpensive and easy test to perform and has been found to have a strong correlation with changes in mid-arm muscle circumference in adult hospital patients with malnutrition. Decreased serum albumin levels may reflect impaired synthesis, decreased protein intake or excessive loss, impaired absorption, or overhydration.

Serum transferring also originates in the liver. As another measure of the body's visceral protein compartment, it is a more sensitive indicator than albumin due to its shorter half-life (8–10 days). Therefore, a change in transferrin during catabolism will precede that of albumin. Serum transferring is indirectly derived using the total iron binding capacity (TIBC) value:

$$serum\ transferring = (TIBC \times 0.8) - 43$$

The use of serum albumin and transferring as indicators of nutritional status is limited in the following conditions: liver disease, nephrotic syndrome, congestive heart failure and excessive blood loss. Transferrin levels are usually indirectly calculated and carry a high margin of error.

Other plasma proteins currently being researched such as pre-albumin and retinol-binding protein show promise of being sensitive biochemical indices of visceral protein depletion.

▶ VISCERAL PROTEIN COMPARTMENT ◀

Serum Proteins	Normal	Moderately Depleted	Severely Depleted
ALBUMIN, g/dl	3.5–5.0	2.5–3.4	< 2.5
TRANSFERRIN, mg/dl	180–250	160–179	< 160

Cell-Mediated Immunity. Cell-mediated immunity is greatly compromised in malnutrition. The inability of the host to defend itself against infection is another indication of visceral protein depletion. The two most common parameters used in evaluation of cellular immunity include the total lymphocyte count (TLC) and skin antigen testing. Lymphocytes play a major role in the body's defense system with low levels being consistent with malnutrition and impaired defense mechanisms. Immune function will often be restored after nutritional repletion and is a good prognostic sign of recovery.

$$TLC = WBC\ (10^3/mm^3) \times lymph\ (\%) \times 10$$

Skin antigen testing also demonstrates immune competency and can be used when evaluating the overall nutritional status of the patient.

The use of skin antigen testing and TLC is limited when sepsis or multiple trauma is present and during chemotherapy.

*See Appendix V

▶ IMMUNE COMPETENCY ◀

Indices	Normal	Moderately Depleted	Severely Depleted
TOTAL LYMPHOCYTE COUNT (mm^3)	1500–3000	800–1500	less than 800
SKIN TEST (mm)	greater than 10	5–10	less than 5

Creatinine Height Index. Creatinine is a product of muscle metabolism, urinary levels are dependant on the extent of skeletal muscle metabolism especially during times of protein depletion. The creatinine height index (CHI) provides a measure of lean body mass. Actual urinary creatinine excreted (24 hour collection) is compared to ideal excretion relative to height (cm). Creatinine excretion is decreased in renal disease, therefore, renal function must be normal for test to be reliable.

$$CHI = \frac{\text{actual urinary creatinine} \times 100}{\text{ideal urinary creatinine}}$$

▶ ADULT IDEAL URINARY CREATININE VALUES ◀

Male		Female	
Height (cm)	Ideal Creatinine	Height (cm)	Ideal Creatinine
157.5	1288	147.3	830
160.5	1325	149.9	851
162.6	1359	152.4	875
165.1	1386	154.9	900
167.6	1426	157.5	925
170.2	1467	160.0	949
172.7	1513	162.6	977
175.3	1555	165.1	1006
177.8	1596	167.6	1044
180.3	1642	170.2	1076
182.9	1691	182.7	1109
185.4	1739	175.3	1141
188.0	1785	177.8	1174
190.5	1831	180.3	1206
193.0	1891	182.9	1240

Nitrogen Balance. Nitrogen (N_2) balance may be used to assess the efficacy of nutritional therapy; a positive balance indicates an anabolic state, a negative balance indicates catabolism. This value is determined by a 24 hour urinary urea nitrogen (UNN) collection and simultaneous 24 hour nitrogen intake (p.o. and/or parenteral).

This formula will not accurately reflect N_2 balance if patient has severe vomiting, diarrhea or fistula drainage unless N_2 losses from these causes are quantitated.

$$N_2 \text{ balance} = \text{nitrogen intake} - (uuN + 4^*)$$

---

*constant factor accounting for insensible N_2 losses (stool, skin)

▶ EVALUATION OF NUTRITIONAL STATUS ◀

Malnutrition can be defined as decreased nutritional status due to improper intake or absorption of nutrients necessary to meet body needs. There are three classifications of malnutrition: marasmus, kwashiorkor and protein-calorie malnutrition (maramus-kwashiorkor).

Marasmus results from a chronic deficiency of calories and is characterized by depleted somatic protein and fat stores. Visceral protein compartments are within normal limits. The patient is cachectic and thin and has suffered weight loss due to wasting of lean body mass.

Kwashiorkor is caused by chronic protein depletion and clinically presents with decreased visceral protein stores and depressed immune competence. Frequently, the patient is at or above ideal body weight with excessive somatic protein and fat stores.

Protein-calorie malnutrition is associated with a decrease in fat stores as well as somatic and visceral protein compartments.

▶ INDICES OF MALNUTRITION ◀

Classification	Weight	TSF	MAC	MAMC	Albumin	TLC	Transferrin	CHI	Skin Antigen Test
Marasmus	X	X	X	X	N	N	N	X	N
Kwashiorkor	N	N	N	N	X	X	X	N	X
Protein-Calorie Malnutrition	X	X	X	X	X	X	X	X	X

X = below normal limits
N = normal

Proper treatment of malnutrition requires evaluation of the patient's energy and protein needs. Calorie needs can be calculated using the individual's basal energy expenditure (BEE) which represents minimal calories needed per day. Protein needs vary depending on the patients level of stress. To promote optimal utilization of nitrogen, a calorie to nitrogen ratio of 150:1 to 200:1 is recommended.

▶ DETERMINATION OF CALORIE AND PROTEIN REQUIREMENTS ◀

KILOCALORIES:

Basal	Men 66 + (13.7 X wt, kg) + (5 X ht, cm) − (6.8 X age)
Energy	Women 655 + (9.6 X wt, kg) + (1.7 X ht, cm) − (4.7 X age)
Expenditure	
For Anabolism	BE X 1.5
For Maintenance	BEE X 1.2

PROTEIN:

Protein requirements X actual or ideal body weight, kg

Protein	normal:	0.8–1.0
Requirement	moderately stressed:	1.0–1.5
(grams)	stressed:	1.5–2.0
	severely stressed:	2.0–4.0
	(burns, major trauma)	

An alternate method for assessing calorie requirements may be found under Diabetes Mellitus. This method is based on activity level and may be more appropriate for ambulatory out-patients than hospitalized patients.

Physician's Order

Nutritional Assessment*

▶ NUTRITIONAL STATUS OF CHILDREN ◀

The overall nutritional status of children in the United States is relatively good. However, the nutritional status of hospitalized children is often below standard. A survey of hospitalized children in a pediatric referral center found 33% of patients with some degree of malnutrition. Nearly half were chronically malnourished with height-for-age less than 95 percent of the standard. Further studies have supported this finding.

Most protein-calorie malnutrition in the United States occurs secondary to other diseases. Problems such as malignancies, infections, organ failure, and malabsorption may result in deterioration of nutritional status. Subsequent nutritional depletion has been associated with a greater risk of infection, poor wound healing, increased surgical mortality, increased mortality of children with localized cancers, and increased length of hospital stay.

All hospitalized children should be screened to determine who will require a more complete nutritional evaluation. Routine screening should include: height, weight, weight/length ratio, head circumference, physical exam, medical history, and diet history.

A more in-depth evaluation is required for children with these conditions or diseases:

1. Height: weight ratio < 5% on NCHS Growth Charts.
2. Recent weight loss > 10% of previous weight.
3. Growth failure for one month if less than 6 months of age; 3 months in children 6–12 months of age; 5 months in children greater than 1 year of age.
4. Height: weight ratio >95% on NCHS Growth Charts.
5. Diseases/conditions predisposing to nutritional depletion:
   a. malabsorption syndromes, GI disorders
   b. burns
   c. cancer
   d. cystic fibrosis
   e. congenital heart disease
   f. other chronic illness
   g. acute illness when prolonged, especially when it requires intensive care
   h. prematurity
   i. renal disease
6. Disease/conditions requiring nutritional management:
   a. diabetes
   b. inborn errors of metabolism
   c. food allergies
   d. rampant caries
   e. nasogastric or gastrostomy feedings
   f. parenteral nutrition and transistion feedings

---

*#5006 Pocket Resource for Nutrition Assessment may be ordered from CD-HCF/ADA, 216 W. Jackson Blvd., Chicago, IL. 60606-6995 Tel. 800/877-1600 Ex 5000, FAX 312-899-4899 (1997-$16.95) Excellent-gives assistance for assessments in all types of healthcare settings anthropometeric, nutrient requirements; enteral & parenteral feeding assessment guide

7. Vitamin or mineral deficiencies.
8. Pregnancy (adolescents).
9. Low socioeconomic status (which affects adequacy of food supply).
10. Physical or mental handicaps affecting feeding such as:
    a. delayed weaning (>2 years of age)
    b. inability or unwillingness to eat
    c. limited variety of foods
    d. inappropriate food consistency for age
11. Guidance/education for special diets:
    a. low sodium
    b. vegetarian
    c. ketogenic, etc.

Determination of Nutritional Status of Children

Clinical Data

A physical exam and medical history should include present illness, past medical history, and family history of disease. Special emphasis should be placed on the perinatal period, surgical procedures, allergies, chronic medical problems, and medications. Clinical examinations of hair, face, eyes, lips, tongue, gums, teeth, glands, and skin by a trained observer may reveal signs of malnutrition.

Dietary History

The dietary history should include type of diet (strained foods/junior foods/regular) or type of infant formula with average amounts consumed.

An evaluation of adequacy or appropriateness of the diet should be determined. The patient/parent(s) should be questioned about dietary modifications or vitamin supplementation. If significant weight loss or poor growth is present, an estimation of caloric, protein, vitamin and mineral intake is especially pertinent. The availability of food and formula as well as mother-child interaction should be assessed.

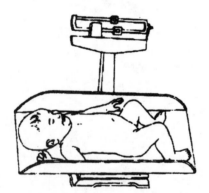

Weighing an infant*

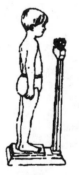

Weighing a child*

Anthropometrics for Infants and Children

A physical examination, medical history and a diet history should be completed for infants and children who are patients. The care giver should be interviewed to collect nutrition related data. The interdisciplinary team will need to be involved; the nutrition team will need to determine the type of formula/diet and the amounts consumed.

*Courtesy Ross Laboratories

Height, weight and head circumference measurements are tools that will assist the nutrition team in the assessment process. The actual measurements can then be compared to standardized growth charts.

Evaluation of Nutrition Status

Infants and children may be evaluated as failure to thrive when compared to growth charts, the parameters for concern about growth include:

▶ no growth for 1 month in <6 month of age
▶ no growth for 3 months in >6 months of age
▶ no growth for 5 months in >1 year of age

Weight

In weighing an infant, a balance-beam scale with non-detachable weights should be used. The scale should be correctly calibrated. Infants and young children should be weighed lying down, clothes removed. If the infant is weighted with clothes/diapers the weight must be subtracted from the total weight for accuracy. Children who are above 2 years old, who will stand alone and be co-operative, a platform beam scale can be used. The child should be weighted in light-weight undergarments. Probability of obesity in children:

▶ Both parents obese 80%
▶ One parent obese 40%
▶ Neither parent obese 7%

Height/Length

Infants should be measured for length/height on an examining table, using a length measuring device with a fixed headboard and a moveable foot board perpendicular to the table surface. Children 2–3 years can be measured while standing. A measuring tape may be attached to a vertical, flat surface, such as a wall. A guide for a right angle headboard is also needed. An older child may be measured on the beam scale that contains a measuring device with a headboard.

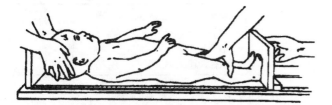

Measuring recumbent length*

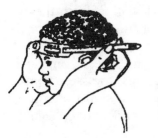

Measuring head

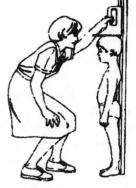

Measuring stature (standing height*)

---

*Courtesy Ross Laboratories

Head Circumference

Head circumference should be routinely measured on an infant/child until three years of age. A flexible, nonstretchable measuring tape is used. The lower edge of the tape should be positioned just above the eyebrows, above the ears, and around the occipital prominence at the back of the head. Pull the tape tight to compress the hair, read and record and compare against charts for age and sex.

Limitations of Growth Measurements

1. Normal growth patterns do not always reflect the smooth curve indicated on growth charts.
2. Several points should be plotted over time to determine an individual's normal pattern of growth.
3. Growth standards are to be used for screening tools and not exclusively for diagnosis.
4. Growth charts reflect growths patterns of normal healthy children. Charts have not been established for altered growth patterns of children with certain genetic anomalies or chronic illnesses.
5. Approximate gestational age should be determined for premature infants soon after birth. Classification as either "small for gestational age" (SGA) or "appropriate for gestational age" (AGA) should be made. If children are plotted on the standard NCHS charts, the plots should be corrected for appropriate gestational age until they are at least two years old. Growth of infants who are small for gestational age may never reach normal growth curves. SGA infants usually growth along their own curves at less than the 5th percentile.

Height and weight can also be used to determine the severity of nutritional deficits. Acute malnourished status is determined by dividing the patient's weight by the 50th percentile weight for age. Chronic malnourished status is reflected by dividing length or height by the 50th percentile length for age (see table below).

▶ ACUTE/CHRONIC MALNUTRITION ◀

Stage	Acute Malnutrition (wt/50th % wt for age)	Chronic Malnutrition (length/50th % length for age)
Stage 0	greater than 90%	greater than 95%
Stage 1	80–90%	90–95%
Stage 2	70–79%	85–89%
Stage 3	less than 70%	less than 85%

The above table provides standards by which the past nutritional history and the present nutritional status can be evaluated. Each stage represents approximately one deviation from the median of the population. Stage 1 patients are normal, but nutritionally at risk; if further insults or deficiencies occur they are likely to develop protein-calorie malnutrition.

Other anthropometric measurements include triceps skinfold thickness to assess somatic fat stores, and arm circumference and determination of midarm muscle circumference to assess somatic protein stores. Such techniques are useful in evaluating the patient's overall status and energy reserves of fat and protein. They must be interpreted relative to hydration state and only collectively give an adequate evaluation.

Laboratory Assessment

To determine visceral protein stores and micronutrient nutriture, laboratory assessment is usually necessary. Albumin and transferrin are good indicators of visceral protein stores. Iron nutriture can be assessed by hemoglobin/hematocrit, red blood cell indices and smear as well as zinc protoporphyrin (ZPP), transferrin ferritin and serum iron. Total lymphocyte counts have not been related to immune status in children. Skin testing for delayed hypersensitivity should probably be done if immune status is questionable.

▶ STANDARDS OF CARE ◀

Standards of care are developed to assure that patients receive optimal nutrition. Standards of care may be developed as a component of *critical pathways.* Critical pathways are plans of care developed by an interdisciplinary team which delineates responsibility of each care provider and times (days) they are to provide specific care. All care is collaborated and in most cases reduces length of stay and overall cost. Standards of care may also be developed generically and then individualized to meet the needs of each patient. For example, all patients would receive the diet ordered by the physician/RD, but not all patients would need/receive a complete nutritional assessment. Standards of care may also be developed after a complete assessment has been completed and the care plan has been developed to determine the level of care to be provided. Standards of care may also be developed by service (e.g. cardiology, orthopedics, etc.) or by ICD-9-CM Codes 260-263 (see Code definitions below), by feeding modalities and/or disease (e.g. diabetes). Regardless of the method utilized to develop the plan, the plan must RUMBA, that is it must be:

Realistic
Understandable
Measurable
Behavioral
Achievable

The plan needs to address a specific problem, documented for the action taken, outcomes and future plans.

International Classification of Diseases, Ninth Edition, Clinical Modification (ICD-9-CM)

Under the existing diagnosis-related group (DRG) payment system malnutrition is considered a comorbidity or complicating condition. Using the ICD-9-CM codes has the potential of changing a person's diagnosis (DRG) and increasing the reimbursement a hospital receives.

Developing care plans based on ICD-9-CM codes will also insure that the nutrition team is screening for potential malnutrition.

ICD-9-CM Code 260:
Kwashiorkor

Severe hypoalbuminemia (<25g/L), transferrin and immune response depressed, edema, change in hair color and skin pigmentation, may appear well nourished.

ICD-9-CM Code 261:
Nutritional Marasmus

Depletion of lean body mass, severe energy deficiency, body weight, triceps skinfold and/or midarm muscle circumference below standards, albumin and serum transferring are normal.

ICD-9-CM Code 262:
Other Severe Protein-Energy Malnutrition
Combination of both protein-energy malnutrition and visceral protein depletion, weight for age less than 60% of standard, nutritional edema

ICD-9-CM code 263.0, 263.1, 263.8
Moderate Forms of Protein-Energy Malnutrition
Milder forms of malnutrition. There may be a weight loss, lowered albumin and transferrin. The following shows a simple format for an individualized Nutrition Standard of Care Plan.

▶ NUTRITION STANDARD OF CARE© ◀

Patient Name: _____ Diagnosis: _____

Date: _____ Assessment complete? Y _____ N _____ Level of care: _____

Documented in Medical History? Y _____ N _____

Objective of Care: (should include plan, how to monitor and evaluate outcomes)

_____

_____

_____

_____

Problem:	Assessment:	Action Taken:	Measurable Outcomes:	Future Plans:

Plan developed by *(List all team members)*

_____

_____

_____

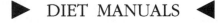

► NUTRITION CARE PLAN ◄

Before a **nutrition care plan** can be developed, data will need to be collected. This data will include both objective as well as subjective information. The data may be obtained from the patient when a diet history is taken, from the family, from the information in the medical history, laboratory and radiological information, other team members, and any other clinical findings that are applicable.

Data gathered from the assessment should be analyzed, and the need for additional nutrition intervention determined. Once it has been determined that additional intervention is needed, the **nutrition care plan** should be developed to assist the patient to improve his well being.

The plan should include at least the following data:

► Name of patient.

► Problems or needs as identified from the data collection.

► Short and long term goals that are attainable and realistic and stated in behavioral/measurable terms, and include specific time limits. Goals should be specific and address each problem separately and prioritized from the most important to the least and or in conjunction with overlapping problems.

► Methods or approaches used to attain these goals. The methods to be used in reaching the goals must be understood and accepted by the patient and family. The methods must be realistic, affordable, agreed to and the outcome measurable.

► Goals accomplished. Once the initial goal has been accomplished it will need to be communicated to all team members and new short- and or long-range goals will need to be developed/implemented. It will be important to provide positive feedback on results to the patient, family and team members.

► Department(s) responsible for the goal. Since the care plan may be developed as an interdisciplinary approach to the care, each representative department will need to have input into the goals and be given the responsibility for insuring they are accomplished.

► Long range goals, with methodologies to be used in reaching these goals. The long term goal is the ultimate level of function.

► Discharge plan includes education of patient/family, willingness of the patient and family to adhere to the diet regime, need for assistance, referral to community/admitting physician, and or return visits to the registered dietitian at the healthcare discharging facility or to a clinic.

► DIET MANUALS ◄

"Diet manuals should be available on each patient unit. Diet manuals should be developed collaboratively with interdisciplinary team input and approved by the Medical staff. The manual should be reviewed and revised at least every three years and reflect the standards for nutrition care established by the Recommended Dietary Allowances (1989) of the Food and Nutrition Board, National Research Council, of the National Academy of Science, and other publications. The manual serves as the basis for all prescriptions or orders for food and nutrition products including eternal and parenteral nutrition."***

► MENUS ◄

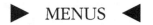

Menus are an often overlooked component of the nutritional screening process. Menu should be planned using the Food Pyramid Guide, meet the recommended daily allowance (RDA's) and modified to meet the nutritional needs of the patient. The resulting meal that is served should be consis-

---

***as quoted in 2000 JCAHO Standards of the Care of the Patient, Nutrition Care TX4.7.

tent with the planned menu and care plan in the amounts, types, and consistency. Menus should be adjusted to meet the caloric and nutrient-intake of each patient. Menus should be calculated to determine if the menu meets the RDA's for all nutrients. When a problem exists the menu should be changed and/or the deficiency for any one day documented and filed for future reference.

When surveying agencies such as OBRA, JCAHO, and state survey/certification for long term care facilities survey a facility they will make a determination concerning the nutritional adequacy of menus. They will be determining if the meals served meet the recommended daily allowances (RDA's) as well as reviewing if the meals served are consistent with the planned menu and care plan in the amounts, types and consistency of food served.

Patients on modified diets should be monitored to determine if they are eating and/or their intake meets the RDA's. In some instances a nutritional supplement may be needed and should be included as part of the care plan.

▶ REASSESSMENT ◀
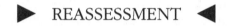

Reassessment and evaluation of the care plan by the interdisciplinary team is made at regular intervals throughout the healthcare stay. Each discipline discusses the patient's progress response to care, significant changes in condition and or diagnosis. The team makes collaborative decisions to determine if the goals and needs of the patient are being met. If changes are needed they are made before the patient is discharged. Special attention needs to be paid to the patients who were screened at Level II and especially Level III.

▶ EDUCATION, DISCHARGE PLANNING ◀

The interdisciplinary team should collaboratively develop a comprehensive education program for patient and family. The instruction will need to consider the psycho-social, spiritual, cultural values, age, learning needs, abilities, emotional barriers, desire and motivation to learn, physical and cognitive limitations, language barriers and the economics of the care choices. The teams' goal for education is to reduce the redundancy of instructions. The goal of the team should be to improve the health and well being of patient through well planned and delivered programs and materials. Patients should be provided information concerning community resources and how to obtain additional/further treatment. Return appointments, medication prescription and/or additional medical devices, diet modification, food/nutrient interaction, training in use of medical devises (crutches, walker, feeding pumps, etc.) home health, hospice or other care is a part of the discharge planning. Educating the patient for discharge should begin the day the patient is admitted to the facility. The patient and family must be involved in the after healthcare stay care. Patient and family should be evaluated on their ability to understand and follow the after discharge plan.

▶ DOCUMENTATION IN THE PATIENT'S MEDICAL HISTORY ◀

The patient's medical history is a confidential and legal document. It is a communication tool between the team members, ensures continuity of care through the notation of treatment modalities and the patient's reaction to them. The entries should be concise summaries of facts and objective observations. Documentation is timely, the information is meaningful, brief, concise, avoids professional jargon, the data is chronological, and isn't redundant and opinionated. The histories, screening, assessment, reassessment, care plans, progress notes, education and the outcome of the nutritional intervention should be documented in the patient's medical history. Other documentation includes periodic assessment of the patient's nutrient intake and tolerance to the diet modification including the effect of the patient's appetite and food habits, food intake, any substitutions made for cultural, religious, or personal preference and if the food intake meets the RDA's. Description of the nutritional education and counseling to patient/family members including subsequent knowledge of diet information presented and description of referrals made to other healthcare agencies or institutions, including diet information forwarded upon discharge should be noted.

Charting may be by exception, running narrative, computerized, SOAP (subjective, objective, assessment, plan). PIE (PROBLEMS) can be same as "S" and "O" information INTERVENTION brief discussion, calculations, recommendations with specific intervention. EVALUATION how/when/how frequently the interdisciplinary team will monitor success of intervention. PAG (PROBLEMS, APPROACHES and GOALS) and/or checklist. When verbal orders are given, the order should be noted in the patient's history as a verbal order and tabbed for the physicians signature at a later time. (usually within 24 hours) The nutrition care team may chart on medical records approved colored paper that denotes the discipline, coded charting forms, in the progress notes and/or in an area assigned by the medical records committee and approved by the chief of staff or in the medical staff bylaws.

All notations in the medical history should be signed by the person making the note, along with their credentials (i.e. RD), and the date of the entry. The color of ink utilized should meet the guidelines of the facility.

▶ **NUTRITION CARE DOCUMENTATION**© ◀

Nutrition Order: _____

SCREENING:

Completed by: RD _____ DT _____ Patient Repr _____ Team _____ Others: _____
Level 1 _____ Level 2 _____ Level 3 _____
Intervention: No further screening needed? Y ___ N ___

ASSESSMENT: Intervention needed due to:

Albumin below (3.0 g/dl) _____ Weight loss unplanned, 1 month _____ 6 months _____
Anthropometrics: _____ failure to thrive _____ malnutrition _____
Modified diet: _____ TPEN _____ age _____ transferrin, mg/dl _____
Disabilities: chewing _____ visual _____ hearing _____ speech _____
emotional barriers: _____ cognitive limitations _____ physical limitations: _____
motivation/desire to learn: _____ other _____
Needs: cultural _____ religious _____ ethnic _____

REASSESSMENT to be completed by (date) _____

CARE PLAN:

GOAL(S)_____

Involved: Patient: Y ___ N ___ Family: Y ___ N ___ Team: Y ___ N ___
Patient/family understands plan: Y ___ N ___ Will follow plan: Y ___ N ___
Critical pathway: Y ___ N ___
Food is brought in from other sources: Y ___ N ___ What source? _____
Modified diet _____ Diet orders consistent with diets in approved
diet manual? Y ___ N ___ Diet individualized for age Y ___ N ___

Nutrition Care Documentation—Continued

EDUCATION:

Food/Nutrient interaction: (list drugs)

Name of modified diet instructions: _____

Individualized and age specific to meet specific needs of patient/family: Y ___ N ___

Effectiveness of education: Patient/family: understands instructions and uses information to incorporate dietary changes: Y ___ N ___ verbalizes the special instructions: Y ___ N ___ constructs a sample menu: Y ___ N ___ list foods to include or omit: Y ___ N ___ Comments: _____

DISCHARGING PLANNING:

RD phone number included: Y ___ N ___ recommends follow-up appointment with RD: Y ___ N ___

recommends contacting community sources: Y ___ N ___

Nutrition care plan forwarded to: _____

Discharge supplies provided: _____

_____ RD

Date _____

▶ DRUG AND NUTRIENT INTERACTION ◀

Nutrient and drug interaction is another component of nutritional assessment of the patient. Nutrient interactions are of clinical significance for patients in long term care facilities, on high dosage drug therapy, or multiple drug regimes and among those patients who are of poor nutritional status or who are ingesting diets marginal in nutrients and energy. The elderly, the chronically ill, growing children, pregnant and lactating women, and tube fed patients are frequently among the most susceptible to a drug-nutrient interaction.

Some prescription drugs as well as some over-the-counter (OTC) drugs can cause a drug/nutrient reaction. The misuse of OTC drugs is seen in a variety of people regardless of age, occupation, socioeconomic, education level. When a diet history is being taken the RD/dietetic technician should inquiry about the use of laxatives, as dependence on laxatives can lead to malnutrition. The use of antacids, aspirins, vitamin supplements, herbal teas and other herbal compounds may cause problems such as iron deficiency, stomach ulcers, and inhibit the absorption of phosphorus. The use of OTC should be noted in the patient's medical history.

Points of Interaction

Medications can potentially alter the nutritional status of a patient in several ways. Alterations in taste and smell perception or the inducement of nausea and vomiting can adversely affect appetite and so reduce food intake. Nutrient absorption, metabolism, utilization, and excretion may also be affected. Table 1 lists the mechanisms by which drugs affect nutritional status.

▶ **TABLE 1. EFFECTS OF DRUGS ON** ◀
NUTRITIONAL STATUS AND NUTRIENTS

Alteration of Food Intake
    suppression/stimulation of appetite
    altered sense of taste, smell
    decreased salivary secretion
    inducement of nausea and vomiting
Alteration of Nutrient Absorption
    changes in gastrointestinal transit time
    changes in gastrointestinal pH
    changes in gastrointestinal motility
    interference with bile acid activity
    inactivation of absorptive enzymes
    damage of gut mucosa
Alteration of Nutrient's Metabolism and Utilization
    complexation of nutrient by drug
    decreased synthesis of nutrients
Alteration of Nutrient's Excretion
    electrolyte imbalances
    increased nutrient requirement

Concurrently, nutritional status and diet can have a marked effect on the efficiency of a drug regime. A patient's visceral and somatic protein profile, body weight, surface area, and fluid and electrolyte balance affect the amount of "free" versus "bound" drug. Diet can alter the pharmacokinetics of drug therapy primarily by affecting drug absorption through a variety of mechanisms (Table 2). Generally, drugs are absorbed more slowly and total drug absorption is reduced in the presence of food. (It is important to distinguish between the types of drugs where a decreased rate of absorption is clinically significant and clinical situations where drug-diet interactions may occur but are of little significance. As a general rule, a decreased rate of absorption is of significance when drug therapy consists of a single dose requiring rapid onset of activity such as analgesics or antiasthmatics, as opposed to drugs given in a multiple dose regime to achieve a constant blood level, as with antibiotics. A decrease in drug absorption is equivalent to a decrease in dosage; also, delayed absorption, even though complete, may preclude reaching effective blood levels or giving prompt relief, and possibly unduly prolong the action of the drug causing a "hangover" effect.

Proper timing of dosage in relation to food ingestion may lessen untoward side effects as well as promote optimum absorption. Specific instructions should be given when food intake is a consideration. Table 3 lists drugs according to optimum time for taking in relation to food ingestion.

The consumption of alcoholic beverages should be considered in regard to interactions with drugs as it is a standard nutrient component for many adults and the major nutrient component for alcoholics. Time-release or sustained-action drugs depend upon erosion or moisture permeability of special coatings which are generally soluble in organic solvents including alcohol. The concurrent ingestion of this type of medication and alcoholic beverages may significantly increase the release rate.

▶ **TABLE 2. EFFECTS OF DIET ON DRUG BIOAVAILABILITY** ◀

Lowers gastric pH
Alters gastrointestinal secretions
Alters gastrointestinal motility and transmit time
Alters pH of glomerular filtrate
Complexation of drug by nutrient

▶ TABLE 3. DRUG: MEAL TIMETABLE ◀

Drugs to be Taken on an Empty Stomach
    oral antibiotics
    penicillamine
    prophylactic coronary vasodilators
Drugs to be Taken 1/2 Hour Prior to Meal
    anticholinergics prescribed for GI disorders
    anorexiants
Drugs to be Taken with Meals to Lessen GI Upsets
    iron preparations
    theophylline and its salts
    corticosteriods
    tuberculosis drugs
    antiinflamatory agents
    urinary antiinfectives
    potassium supplements
Drugs to be Taken 30–45 Minutes after Meals
    antacids

If the dosage form contains the equivalent of several doses then releasing the total quantity at once may prove hazardous. Alcohol can also stimulate the metabolic breakdown of a drug through hepatic microsomal enzyme induction thus reducing the pharmacologic activity of a drug. Patients should be instructed to avoid alcoholic beverages when taking drugs listed in Table 4.

Some foods contain active substances that may cause changes in a drug's distribution, metabolism, and excretion, or antagonize the pharmacologic activity of some drugs. The most notorious food component is tyramine which, in combination with monoamine oxidase inhibitors, may cause dangerous increases in blood pressure. (See Restricted Tyramine Diet). Other pharmacologically active food components include caffeine, tartrazine, oxalates, monosodium glutamate, and licorice.

Some foods can change the way medications work in the body, just as medications may change how the body uses food. How foods and medications work "with" or "against" each other in the body is called a food (nutrient) and drug reaction.

People who should be concerned about food and drug interaction are those who:
▶ take medications for a long period of time.
▶ have poor eating habits.
▶ are tube fed.
▶ use at least the following drugs: Tetracycline, Warfarin, and certain anti-depressants.

▶ TABLE 4. DRUGS INCOMPATIBLE WITH ALCOHOL INGESTION ◀

antihistamines
antibiotics (nitrofurantoin)
anticonvulsants
anticoagulants (warfarin derivatives)
antihypertensives
sedatives, hypnotics
narcotic analgesics
tranquilizers
hypoglycemics
(insulin, sulfonylureas)

There are a number of ways a patient can avoid a possible food and drug interaction and stay healthy. They are:

▶ Eat a variety of foods following the Food Guide Pyramid.

▶ Discuss with a registered dietitian or physician before making big changes in lifestyle or eating patterns.

▶ Discuss with the registered dietitian or pharmacist the medication that is being taken and possible interaction. The RD or pharmacists should probe to determine if the patient is consuming alcohol or large amounts of certain foods and other beverages.

Good eating habits and taking medications correctly can work well together to improve or maintain health.

Alternative Therapies/Medicine

Alternative Therapies/medicine are becoming more common in modern western medicine. Some of these therapies are valid others may not be. Alternative medicine include a wide variety of unconventional therapies, that may or may not be administered by physicians. Categories of alternative medicine include:

▶ Aromatherapy: The inhaling, bathing or massaging of oils from plants and herbs into the skin.

▶ Folk remedies

▶ Yoga

▶ Macrobiotics and other lifestyle diets

▶ Megavitamin therapy

▶ Spiritual healing

▶ Relaxation therapy

▶ Hypnosis

▶ Energy healing

▶ Herbal medicine: The use of plants or plant based substances to treat a wide range of illnesses and enhance physical functions.

▶ Homeopathy: Stimulating the body's defenses with tiny doses of substances that would cause disease symptoms in larger amounts.

When screening and assessing a patient they should be asked if they use any type of alternative therapies/medicine. This should be documented in the patient's medical record.

The following tables list the most common herb therapies, their safety and side effects.

▶ COMMON HERB THERAPIES ◀

Herb	Active Ingredient	Health Claim/Use	Dosage	Notes Safety/ Side Effects
Aloe (or Aloes) *Aloe ferox Aloe barbadensis*	Anthracene derivatives	Laxative in acute constipation. Do not use for chronic constipation. No evidence for other internal effects	Daily dose is 0.05-0.2 g dry extract. Lethal dose is 1 g/day for several days.	May cause cramps or diarrhea Do not take over long period of time (may cause electrolyte imbalance). Do not use if pregnant or have a GI illness. May alter GI absorption of some drugs.
Aloe vera gel *Aloe barbadensis*	Polysaccharides	Use externally for treatment of burns and wounds. Cosmetics (astringent, emollient)	Use until healed to prevent scarring.	Allergy, though rare, may occur in susceptible individuals. Processing and storage may affect retention of activity.
Cayenne *Capsicum annuum*	Capsaicin	Cream acts as a local counterirritant for pain relief. Used for arthritis, herpes zoster, toothache, diabetic neuropathy, and muscular skeletal pain. Internally, acts as gastric stimulant and carminative. Evidence for decreasing platelet aggregation or decreasing cholesterol in humans is lacking.	3-5 times daily; massaged into the skin until no residue remains	Strong irritant. **Avoid contact with eyes.** Wash hands thoroughly after applying cream.
Echinacea *E. angustifolia Echinacea purpurea*	Polysaccharides, flavonoids, alkamides, and essential oils	Prophylaxis and treatment of upper respiratory tract infection and flu through enhancement of immune function	Do not take continuously. Stop when no longer sick. Take during exposure to virus. 250 mg extract 1 tsp once or twice/day	None expected although allergic reaction possible Efficacy of oral capsules and teas questionable AIDS patients should avoid

Common Herb Therapies—Continued

Herb	Active Ingredient	Health Claim/Use	Dosage	Notes Safety/Side Effects
Echinacea (continued)		Topically may provide antioxidant protection against UVA and UVB rays.		
Ephedra *Ephedra sinica* **(Ma Huang)**	Ephedrine and other alkaloids	Decongestant, bronchial asthma CNS stimulant Though it may decrease appetite, not recommended for weight loss	8 mg serving No more than 24 mg/day Do not use longer than 7 days.	May increase blood pressure, heart rate, heart palpitations Causes dry mouth Caffeine increases effect Should not be taken by patients with heart disease, high blood pressure, thyroid disease, or diabetes Avoid if using antihypertensive or antidepressant drugs.
Ginkgo Biloba *Ginkgo Biloba extract (Egb)*	Analytically controlled to contain 24% flavenoid glycosides quercetins) and 6% terpene lactones	Antioxidant, increases circulation Inhibition of platelet activating factor Cerebral insufficiency (particularly in geriatric patients): —concentration —memory —vertigo —confusion —dizziness —depression —tinnitus —headache —Alzheimer's disease Intermittent claudication in peripheral arterial insufficiency	40–80 mg three times daily Must be taken consistently for 12 weeks to be effective	Safety well established. Minimal side effects include headache, GI problems, and dizziness. Patients with bleeding disorders should not use. Avoid if pregnant or nursing. Overdose may cause irritability, restlessness, diarrhea, and vomiting. Fruit pulp and raw seeds toxic. Contact with pulp may cause dermatitis. Use standardized ginkgo biloba extract (GBE). **Use caution** if already taking anticoagulants.

continued

Common Herb Therapies—Continued

Herb	Active Ingredient	Health Claim/Use	Dosage	Notes Safety/Side Effects
Ginseng *Panax ginseng (Asia)* *Panax quinquefolius (America)*	Triterpenoid saponins (ginsenosides, panaxosides)	Tonic or adaptogenic; in Korea and China used as a relaxant or stimulant To reduce risk of various human cancers Regulates plasma glucose in Type II diabetics Use as an ergogenic aid in healthy men and women (not supported by clinical research)	15–20 grains of powdered herb Need for standardized doses of each type of ginseng	Generally safe. Mild side effects include headache, insomnia, anxiety, skin rashes, diarrhea. Caffeine may increase effects. Rare: Severe effects (asthma attacks, increased blood pressure, heart palpitations, menstrual changes) Avoid if pregnant or nursing. Quality root expensive. Concentration of ginsenosides varies among brands and preparations. There are numerous varieties of ginseng: • Oriental ginseng (Panax ginseng) is native to the Orient, primarily China and Korea. Today almost all Oriental ginseng is cultivated. • White ginseng is the name given to the natural unprocessed ginseng root. • Red ginseng is ginseng that has been processed thus turning a red color. There is no chemical difference between the two varieties.

Common Herb Therapies—Continued

Herb	Active Ingredient	Health Claim/Use	Dosage	Notes Safety/Side Effects
Ginseng (continued)				• American ginseng (Panax quinquefolius) grows wild, but is considered an endangered species due to widespread harvesting. Almost all American ginseng is now cultivated. • Siberian ginseng (eleutherococcus senticocus) is often labeled as ginseng but is not a true ginseng. It has some of the same properties but is relatively inexpensive compared to real ginseng. • Wild Red American ginseng is not ginseng at all.
Saw Palmetto *Serenoa repens*	Liposterolic extract containing 85%-95% fatty acids and sterols (betasitosterol)	As an antiandrogen for benign prostatic hyperplasia. May increase urinary flow, reduce residual urine, and decrease frequency of urination.	160 mg twice daily	No side effects reported If symptomatic, see doctor to rule out prostate cancer.
St. John's Wort *Hypericum perforatum*	Hypericin xanthones and flavenoids 0.3% hypercin	Mild to moderate depression, but not severe depression (suicidal, psychotic, or severe sadness)	300 mg three times daily Must take consistently for 4 weeks	GI irritation, most common complaint, may be lessened with food in some patients. Do not use other psychoactive medications.

continued

Common Herb Therapies—Continued

Herb	Active Ingredient	Health Claim/Use	Dosage	Notes Safety/Side Effects
St. John's Wort (continued)		May also have antiviral, antibacterial, and wound-healing activity.		Photosensitivity characterized by dermatitis and inflammation of mucous membranes at high levels of intake or prolonged use Prescription drug in Germany for depression
Valerian Root *Valeriana officinalis*	Valepotriates, volatile essential oils	Sedative and sleep aid Reduces nervous tension, stress, anxiety, and restlessness May reduce sleep latency and improve sleep quality	Follow directions with smallest possible dose.	Mild headache or upset stomach. Too much may cause severe headache, nausea, morning grogginess, blurry vision. Do not use if taking sedatives or anxiolytics. Mechanism of action similar to the benzodiazepines, but **nonaddictive** and ability to drive or operate machinery not affected.

Used with permission: *Clinical and Nutrient Guidelines: Part of the Drug-Nutrient Intervention System.* © ROCHE DIETITIANS, LLC; 1997. 708/442-0123.

▶ COMMON SUPPLEMENT/FOOD/HERB THERAPIES ◀

Supplement Food	Active Ingredient	Health Claim/Use	Dosage	Notes Safety/Side Effects
Black Cohash *Cimicifuga racemoosa*	Triterpenoid glycosides, isoflavones, and aglycones	Suppressed LH (but not FSH) secretion in patients receiving 8 mg/d for 8 weeks. Binds to estrogen receptors in rat uteri. One study indicated relief of hot flashes and improved mood.	Follow directions starting with smallest dose.	Large doses cause dizziness, nausea, headaches, stiffness, and trembling. Patients should not use if taking blood pressure medication or if they have heart problems.

Common Supplement/Food/Herb Therapies—Continued

Supplement Food	Active Ingredient	Health Claim/Use	Dosage	Notes Safety/Side Effects
Black Cohash (continuedi)		Eases menopause symptoms		
Chinese Angelica *Angelica sinensis (Dong quai)*	Coumarin derivatives	No clinical backup for assertions that it relieves hot flashes and vaginal dryness	Follow directions starting with smallest dose.	Efficacy and safety inconclusive Contains photoreactive substances, so avoid overexposure to sunlight.
Licorice Root *Glycerrbiza glabra*	Beta-sitosterol	May be a weak estrogen, but no studies confirm estrogenic effects in humans.	Follow directions starting with smallest dose.	Large amounts taken over a long period of time can lead to high blood pressure and edema. Patients with kidney disease or glaucoma should avoid use. Do not take with blood pressure medication.
Phytoestrogens *Soy and soy products, corn, green beans, lemon and orange peels, nuts and seeds, brown rice, flaxseed oil*	Isoflavones (genistein) phytosterols, saponins, lignins	Compounds have very mild estrogenic effect. May improve vaginal dryness. Effect on hot flashes inconsistent.	Follow directions starting with smallest dose.	No known toxicity or side effects
Strawberry *Fragaria*	Boron	Boron may increase level of circulating estrogen.	Follow directions starting with smallest dose.	No known toxicities May cause allergic reaction
Wild Yam Root *Dioscorea villosa*	Diosgenin	Diosgenin has no hormonal activity and is not converted into either estrogen or progesterone in the body. No clinical trials to assess efficacy have been published.	Follow directions starting with smallest dose.	No known toxicity; however, Japanese use an extract (dioscin) as a fish poison.

▶ COMMON HORMONE THERAPIES ◀

Hormone	Health Claim/Use	Dosage	Notes Safety/Side Effects
DHEA	Converted in the body to testosterone and estrogens	25–50 mg Check blood level before treating.	Amount of estrogen and testosterone that the body makes from DHEA varies among individuals. Precursor to testosterone and estrogen Side effects may include acne, hair growth, low energy, irritability, insomnia, headache, menstrual irregularity, increased ocular pressure, tachycardia, increased heart rate, and palpitations. Untested in long-term clinical trials Available OTC. The National Institute of Aging (NIA) does not recommend taking supplements of DHEA.
Melatonin	Regulation of the sleep-wake schedule, (eg, jet lag). May increase sleep efficiency and decrease sleep onset in persons with insomnia. Claims to protect cells from free radical damage, boost immunity, and prevent cancer. Declines with age. Only works when deficient.	Varies greatly. (See *Table 10.*)	Possible adverse side effects include inhibition of fertility, suppression of male sex drive, hypothermia, and retinal damage. High doses may cause excess sleepiness, confusion, and headache the next morning. Long-term effects unknown. Many claims unsubstantiated in human studies. Available OTC. The NIA does not recommend taking supplements of Melatonin.
Testosterone	Claims to maintain muscle mass; reduce total cholesterol, increase energy and libido Check blood level before starting treatment.	Check blood level before treating.	OTC strength and purity not regulated Can result in enlargement of prostate gland, harmful cholesterol levels, psychological problems, infertility, and acne Speeds production of RBC, which may thicken the blood and increase risk of strokes Testosterone is available only by prescription (patch, pill, injection).

► **MELATONIN THERAPIES** ◄

Melatonin Supplement vs Natural Production of Melatonin		Melatonin Supplementation Should Be Restricted in High-risk Group	
Supplement Dosage (mg)	Equivalent to Amount Produced by the Body During:	Restrict	Potential Problem
0.75	25 days	Persons taking steroids and thyroids	Melatonin may counteract effect of these drugs.
2.0	65 days	Pregnant women	Untested unknown risks.
3.0	100 days	Women wanting to conceive	Doses greater than 10 mg may prevent ovulation.
5.0	166 days	Nursing mothers	Melatonin transmitted through breast milk.
10.0	333 days	People with severe mental illness	Symptoms may be exacerbated.
		People with severe allergies, autoimmune disease, or immune system cancers (lymphoma and leukemia)	Melatonin may stimulate the immune system, thereby exaggerating allergies, autoimmune response, and immune cells.
		Normal children of all ages	Already have high levels of melatonin.

Used with permission: *Clinical and Nutrient Guidelines: Part of the Drug-Nutrient Intervention System.* © ROCHE DIETITIANS, LLC; 1997. 708/442-0123.

Caffeine

The use of caffeine containing medicines such as cold, headache remedies and weight loss pill and caffeine containing beverage is constantly increasing. Most Americans consume some form of caffeine daily. Caffeine is found in coffee, tea, soft drinks and more that a 1,000 OTC drugs, prescription drugs, candy and desserts. Caffeine is a mild stimulant that increases respiration rate, heart rate, blood pressure, headaches, sleeplessness and can act as a diuretic. Children are especially sensitive to caffeine.

On going studies are being conducted on the effect of caffeine and various diseases such as birth defects, cancer, fibrocystic breast disease, hypertension and anxiety. Due to conflicting results of the studies on the effects of caffeine it is suggested that a prudent approach to the ingestion of caffeine would be 2–8 ounce cups of coffee per day. It is a wise idea for pregnant and lactating women to limit their intake of caffeine beverages and OTC drugs. Infants (6mo–3yr) should only be given caffeine beverage and or OTC drugs on the advise of the physician. Children from the age of 3–12 years should be carefully monitored for caffeine intake. Adolescent and young adults consume a large number of caffeine containing beverages. The intake should be monitored since over indulgence may cause sweating, tenseness, inability to concentrate, insomnia and interfere with the ingestion of nutritious foods such as milk and juices.

Alcohol

Alcohol is used by persons from the age of 12 upward. Alcoholism is a chronic disease, often progressive and fatal, with genetic, psychosocial and environmental fact influencing its development. It accounts for a number of problems on college campuses. Beer and wine are the preferred beverage of the younger generation. Beer and wine contain very small amount of nutrients, while distilled alcohol furnishes none. All alcoholic beverages furnish energy, 1 gram of alcohol yields 7.1 kilocalories. Alcohol is rapidly absorbed on an empty stomach. Alcohol does not require digestion and is absorbed intact from the gastrointestinal track. It is water soluble and immediately disperses throughout the body fluids. Heavy use of alcohol may decrease the appetite, and users may substitute alcohol for food, decreasing the food intake which may lead to nutritional deficiency, especially of some vitamins. Alcohol alters one or more of the body's functions and is medically defined as a depressant drug. Persons who ingest more than 2 drinks per day or 6 drinks per week are considered to be at risk of long term effect such as seriously impaired liver functioning, increased risk of heart disease, brain and nervous system disorders. Other disorders include, noninsulin dependent diabetes (NIDD), ulcers of the stomach and intestines, skin rashes and sores, impaired immune system, bone deterioration and osteoporosis and disorders of most of the remaining organs in the body. The woman who drinks during pregnancy is giving that same drink to the fetus, a body that is defenseless against the effect. Babies born to alcoholic mothers may develop fetal alcohol syndrome (see chapter of nutrition through the life style—pregnancy). Alcoholism is not only a medical problem it is a societal problem, costing billions of dollars in medical cost, automobile accidents, lost wages, break-up of the family, criminal cost, and possible physical abuse. There are a number of drugs that should not be taken if one is or planning to ingest alcohol. The effect may be serious. When securing a diet history, food recall, and/or food diary and the medication list the dietitian or dietetic technician should carefully evaluate the daily intake of alcohol and work closely with other team members to provide education and assistance to the patient who has a tendency of abusing alcohol. Most pharmacists will provide information concerning the effect of alcohol on drugs. Most prescription drugs carry an auxiliary label warning that the medication should not be taken with alcohol. Many over the counter (OTC) drugs have a high alcohol content and should not be taken if other drugs are being used. All OTC drug labels should be read for possible reaction.

▶ CAFFEINE CONTENT OF SELECTED NON-PRESCRIPTION DRUGS ◀

Description (mg)	Brand Names	Caffeine Content (mg)
Stimulants	Caffedrine®, No-Doz®, Vivarin® 100 to 200	100 to 200
Pain relievers	Anacin®, Cope®, Excedrin®, Goody's Headache Powder®, Midol®, Vanquish®, B.C. Powder® 35 to 130	35 to 130
Aspirin	All	0
Diuretics	Aqua-Ban®, Permathene®, H₂0 Off®, Pre-Mens Forts® 100 to 200	100 to 200
Cold remedies	Cenegisic®, Coryban-D®, Dristan®, Dristan A-F®, Neo-Synephrine®, Triaminicin® 15 to 32	15 to 32
Weight control	Dexatrim®, Dietac®, Prolamine®	200 to 280 200 to 280

Note: Generic medications may contain caffeine. Read labels or check with pharmacist.

Drugs Incompatible with Alcohol

Avoid the use of alcohol with these drugs. For more specific information, consult the RD, LD or the Pharmacist.

▶ Ampicillin (Polycillin®, Omnipen®, Amcill®, Totacillian®, Principen®)
▶ Cephalosporins
▶ Chloramphenicol (Chloromycetin®)
▶ Verapamil (Isoptin®, Calan®)
▶ Clonidon (Catapres®)
▶ Nitroglycerin (Nitro-Bid®, Nitroglyn®)
▶ Methyldopa (Aldomet®)
▶ Prazosin (Minipress®)
▶ Antidiabetics
▶ Warfarin (Coumadin®)
▶ Allopurinol (Zyloprim®)
▶ Indomethacin (Indocin®)
▶ Naproxen (Anaprox®)
▶ Cimetidine (Tagamet®)
▶ Chloral hydrate (Noctec®)
▶ Haloperidol (Haldol®)
▶ Thioridazine (Mellaril®)
▶ Tricyclics
▶ Acetaminophen with codeine
▶ Codeine
▶ Hydromorphone (Dilaudid®)
▶ Propoxyphene (Darvocet®, Wygesic®)
▶ Meperidine (Demerol®)
▶ Morphine
▶ Oxycodone and acetaminophen (Roxicet®, Tylox®)
▶ Oxycodone and aspirin (Percodan®)
▶ Pentazocine (Talwin®)
▶ Hydrocodone and acetaminophen (Vicodin®)
▶ Adrenocorticoids
▶ Aminophylline/theophylline (Theo-Dur®, Thiophyl®, Elixophyllin®, Elixicon®, Slo-Phyllin®, Quibron®, Theolair™)
▶ Dyphyllline (Lufyllin®)
▶ Chlordiazepoxide and amitriptyline (Limbitrol®)
▶ Diphenhydramine (Benadryl®)
▶ Diphenoxylate and atropine (Lomotil®)

Grapefruit Juice

The interrind of grapefruit contains flavonoids that interacts with some drugs. Naringenin, one of the flavonoids, appears to interfere with liver enzymes that facilitate the metabolism of certain drugs including calcium channel blockers. Drugs associated with increased bioavailability when taken with grapefruit juice include:

▶ Plendil®
▶ Verapamil® (Calan)
▶ Procardia® (Nifedipine)
▶ Seldane® (Terfenadine)
▶ Sandimmane® (Cyclosporin)
▶ Claritin® (antihistamine)
▶ Halicon® (Triazolam),
▶ Versed® (Midazolam)

Tobacco

The use of tobacco is a major health problem causing thousands of people to suffer from cancer, cardiovascular, digestive and respiratory problems. Smoking is the single largest preventable cause of premature death and disability in the US. One out of five deaths in the US each year is associated with cigarette smoking. Approximately 400,000 annually die prematurely from the effects of smoking, millions more live with damage to lungs and heart. Smoking contributes to the development of atherosclerosis, and certain cancers. Smoking and lung cancer is common. Snuff dipping is known to cause cancer of the lips, mouth, esophagus, throat and stomach. Smoking seems to curb hunger and one of the major fears of quitting is "gaining" weight. Persons who smoke need approximately twice as much Vitamin C as non smokers. Healthcare facilities have strict smoking policies and in most cases a patient may only use tobacco upon the written order of the physician. "Second-hand" smoke from the use of tobacco also has serious health risk for people, especially for pregnant and lactating women and children.

Drug Abuse—Illicit Drugs

Recent studies show a marked increase in the use of illicit drugs. It appears that children as young as 10 years are using marijuana with the overwhelming starting age is 12–13 or the eight grade level. Marijuana is overwhelming drug of choice among these children with inhalants as a second choice. By the time these children become teenagers they have used LSD and PCP, which are powerful hallucinogens that can cause prolonged psychotic reactions. Rohypnol, a growing favorite, is a sedative that is stronger than Valium produces a feeling of euphoria. Heroin and cocaine appear to be readily available. Eight out of ten current adult users started using drugs as teens. The increased use of drugs has been attributed to the lack of concern by the government, schools and in some instances by parents. In a study of 12–17 year olds conducted for Columbia Center on Addiction and Substance Abuse, 76 percent said that the entertainment industry encourages illegal drug use. This is seen in the popular culture of "rock music" and popular rock "stars" who regularly glamorized marijuana use in songs and concerts. Marijuana is a harmful drug that disrupts short-term memory and hormonal levels. Marijuana alters brain function and harms the lungs and during a high motor skills are diminished. Marijuana is the first step to the use of other drugs. A teen (12–17 years old) who smokes marijuana is 85 times more likely to use cocaine than one who does not. The side effects of cocaine users is intense euphoria, restlessness, irritability, insomnia, loss of appetite and weight loss and possible eating disorders. Other nutrition related problems with the abuse of drugs include:
▶ money available for food is spent on drugs
▶ some drugs temporary depress appetite
▶ drugs change lifestyle including regular hours for meals
▶ the high possibility of being infected with HIV and hepatitis
▶ due to illness from infectious diseases the need for nutrients is increased
The use of illegal drugs is also linked to increased behavior problems, crime, depression, costly rehabilitation, and in some cases death.

Prescription Drugs

Physicians prescribe drugs to improve the medical condition of the patient. When the medication is taken incorrectly it may be harmful. In securing the diet history of the patient, reviewing the medical history and the medication record it is important to work in conjunction with the pharmacist and nurse to assist the patient to understand:
▶ how the drug works and when it will start to work
▶ what dose to take and when to take it
▶ what to do if a dose is missed
▶ side effects to be expected

► NUTRITION SUPPORT: ENTERAL AND ◄ PARENTERAL NUTRITION

Enteral formulas are available in three main categories
► polymeric
► predigested
► modular

Polymeric formulas are complete nutritionally lactose free and are casein or soy isolated based. Predigested formulas are minimal or no digestion required for absorption. Carbohydrate source is usually glucose oligosaccharides; protein is short-chained peptides and/or free amino acids. Modular formulas are made up of modular components.

Enteral formulas fall into the following basic categories. They include:***

► ***Standard oral supplement***—complete, balance nutrition, comes in a variety of flavors, lactose free, low residue, meets American Heart Association guidelines (polymeric)

► ***Standard oral supplement with added fiber***—comes in a variety of flavors, increased fiber, lactose free (polymeric)

► ***High nitrogen oral supplement***—comes in a variety of flavors, protein approximately 45 g/L, meets 100% of vitamins and minerals (polymeric)

► ***High calorie, high nitrogen oral supplement***—comes in several flavors, approximately 63 g protein/L

► ***Fortified pudding***—complete balance nutrition, 250 cal/5 oz serving, variety of flavors, approximately 7 g protein/5 oz

► ***Surgical oral liquids***—variety of flavors low lactose, low fat and fiber

► ***Isotonic liquid nutrition tube feedings***—lactose free, low residue, 1 cal/cc, approximately 45 g protein/L, also with fiber, fiber supplemented with ultratrace minerals, carnitine and taurine

► ***Elemental formulas, tube feedings***—low residue, lactose free, high nitrogen, and nutritionally complete, partially hydrolyzed protein

► ***Specialized formulas*** designed to meet the needs of patients with specialized diseases such as:

- abnormal glucose tolerance
- metabolically stressed
- pulmonary problems
- renal disease
- critical care, trauma
- gastrointestinal dysfunction
- HIV/AIDs
- radiation enteritis
- severe diarrhea
- intractable vomiting

These formulas are usually polymeric. Modular formulas are carbohydrate supplements that are either liquid or powder, used to increase carbohydrate calories. Protein supplements are powdered supplements used to increase protein and calories. Fat supplements are made up of medium chain tri-glycerides and or essential fatty acids. It is used to increase fat calories and for patients with malabsorption, patients undergoing high-dose chemotherapy, radiation, and bone marrow transplantation, patients with moderate to severe pancreatitis, patients who have undergone major surgery, and patients with moderate to high stress.

Tube feedings can also be used in transitional feedings when parenteral support is being tapered.

***Material furnished by Ross Products Division, Abbott Laboratories, Terry Gizesky, Representative, Gainesville, Florida

The ideal tube feeding formula* should possess the following characteristics:

1. suitable protein-kilocalorie ratio
2. balanced nutrients composition including electrolyte composition, high quality protein and well utilized supplementary sources of nutrients
3. low osmolality
4. low cost
5. bacteriologic safe
6. lactose free (due to possible lactose intolerance)
7. convenient and easy to administer

(*Blenderize tube feedings are discouraged due to the potential risk of microbial contamination from excessive manipulation of the formula. Raw eggs should never be used in a formula due to the possibility of *Salmonella* contamination.)

Enteral Delivery Routes

Patients who are unable to take in enough food to promote positive nitrogen balance are nutritionally supported via feeding tubes. The final selection of the enteral route sites include: physiology of the gastrointestinal tract, risk of aspiration, anticipated length of enteral support, whether surgical placement of a feeding tube is an option and the age and medical condition of the patient.

Tubes may enter through a variety of sites, some require a surgical procedure and a radiology test to determine if the tube is in place. The most common route is the *nasogastric* placement. The tube is inserted through the nose down to the stomach. This type of feeding tube is for patients who will be on the feeding less than 6 weeks. It is used for individuals who cannot or will not consume adequate nutrient intake. Do not use this site if the patient is at increased risk for aspiration. This procedure doesn't require surgery.

Nasoduodenal or *nasojejunal* feedings are prescribed for patients whose disease involves the stomach and for patients who have gastroparesis. The tube passes the nasal route to the duodenum or jejunum. These routes are preferred for patients who are at increased risk for aspiration. This type of feeding does not require surgery.

Gastrostomy feeding tubes are surgically or percutaneously placed into the stomach. This type of feeding tube is used for patients who will be on enteral/parental feedings for a prolong period of time. They are used when the nasal route is not feasible and when no esophageal reflux is present.

Jejunostomy feedings tubes are surgically placed into the jejunum. This type of feeding tube is indicated when there is an obstruction, fistula or stricture at a higher level of the gastrointestinal tract. When hyperosmolar solutions are entered quickly into the jejunum, a condition known as "dumping syndrome" occurs. This may be corrected by initially reducing the concentration of the formula (usually by adding more water), the rate of the feeding and using low osmolality formulas.

Esophagostomy/cervical pharyngostomy feeding tubes are surgically required as the nasal access is not available. This type of tube feeding sites are used for patients who have cancer that resulted in surgery to the head and neck area or surgical repair of the maxillofacial area.

Delivery Methods for Tube Feeding

Tube feedings are administered via continuous infusion using an appropriate pump, intermittent gravity drip or bolus gravity. The choice of the delivery method is made in accordance with the patient's tolerance, type and location of the feeding tube and the formula being administered. Continuous feedings are preferable for the critically ill, for patients who haven't eaten for 3 or more days and when duodenal and jejunal sites are used. Intermittent feedings are generally 5-8 times per day to simulate meal patterns. Each feeding usually consist of no more than 250 ml of formula delivered in 30 or more minutes. Other schedules may be desired such as 12-16 or more hours with the amount of feeding controlled by the setting on the pump.

Bolus feedings do not require a pump for delivery of the feeding. The feeding is poured directly into the tube feeding site with the aid of a syringe or gravity drip method. In this method larger volumes are given over a shorter period of time. Once the feeding is completed, the tube is usually flushed with clean (in some cases sterile) water.

Cautions

The hang time for a tube feeding is an on going debate. Some facilities use 8 hours other 12 and others 24 hours. This decision must be made by each individual facility in conjunction with the infection control service and approved by the medical staff. Warmer weather, type of tube feeding, handling oft the formula, all play a role in the desired hang time. The manufacturer of the product/bags/tubes/and pump should be contacted for their suggestion on hang time.

Other cautions include:

▶ Wash hands **before** handling formula and the administration and **after** *completing the task.*
▶ **Do not** add fresh formula to a formula that is already hanging.
▶ Wash the can top (preferably the entire can) of formula before opening it.
▶ When additional materials (such as oil, carbohydrate, protein, vitamin/minerals) are added to the canned formula a semi-sterile area should be available for adding the materials. The staff member adding the materials should be trained in correct measuring and mixing techniques, and safe and sanitary procedures for proper food handling. Make certain that **hands, equipment,** and **work area is** meticulously clean and the hang time meets the policies approved by the infection control committee/medical staff and regulatory agencies.
▶ Rinse the administration containers and tubing with water before adding fresh formula.
▶ The administration of medications through enteral feeding tubes should be avoided if possible due to risk of tube occlusion and incompatibility of medications with TF formulas.

Osmolality

The osmolality of a formula is a measure of the concentration of a solute per kilogram of solvent. Osmolality is a measure of solute per liter of solution. Normal serum osmolality is 280-295 mOSm/kg. The osmolality of a formula is an important factor in patient tolerance of the formula. Since carbohydrates are digested most rapidly, they have the greatest influence on osmolality. Glucose and sucrose have a higher osmolality than complex carbohydrates; free amino acids have a higher osmolality than intact protein; fat has little effect; a high level of electrolytes increase the osmolality of the formula. A formula that is hyperosmolar may cause rapid fluid and electrolyte shifts, especially if they flow into the small intestine. This can cause diarrhea, electrolyte imbalances, and dehydration.

Enteral feedings may be administered through a nasagastric tube, nasduodenal tube, neither of which requires surgery and may be safer to use than those put into place through a surgical procedure (GI). Gastrostomy and jejunostomy feeding tubes have been surgically inserted into the gastrointestinal tract when the upper GI tract is obstructed, when the condition of the patient does not permit naso insertion and/or when the feeding is expected to be prolong.

Feedings may be bolus, gravity drip or syringe, slow continuous feeding and/or infusion controlled by a pump.

There are complications of tube feedings. They include:

▶ diarrhea
▶ nausea/vomiting
▶ constipation
▶ hyperglycemia
▶ dehydration
▶ electrolyte imbalance
▶ tube displacement
▶ clogged tube
▶ aspiration

A nutritional analysis of enteral formulas has not been included in this work as manufacturers frequently change the composition of the formula and are constantly developing new products. There are a number of companies who produce formulas and maintain up-to-date product information on their respective formulas as well as their competitors. It is suggested that you contact one of these companies for comparison data.

Formulary

Many healthcare institutions have established Nutrition Committees, who establish and monitor the use of enteral products in the facility. This committee may suggest that the facility establish a formulary. A *formulary* is an approved listing of formulas that are to be used by the facility. The formulary may be based on such characteristics as:

▶ calories per ml
▶ sodium mEq/100 ml
▶ potassium mEq/100 ml
▶ carbohydrates, protein grams/100 ml, fat grams/100 ml
▶ osmolality, mOsm/kg water
▶ milliliter needed to meet the RDA's
▶ taste
▶ cost
▶ representative service, knowledge

Patients have the right to forgo or withdraw life sustaining treatment. The US Supreme has ruled that patients have rights in avoiding unwanted medical treatment. It also implied that the right includes "a constitutionally protected liberty interest of being free of unwanted artificial nutrition and hydration. (US Supreme Court, Cruzan *vs Missouri Department of Health, 1990* WL84074.) Healthcare facilities have procedures in place that are referred to as advance directives, living wills, power of attorney, or surrogacy appointment that honors a patient concerning treatment including the withholding of nutrition. The American Dietetic Association has issued a position paper on "Issues in Feeding the Terminally Ill Adult" (copies may be ordered from the American Dietetic Association, 216 West Jackson Blvd, Chicago, IL 60606-6995.)

Parenteral Therapy

Parenteral therapy (TPN, PPN, Hyperalimentation) refers to the infusion of nutrients via an intravenous route for the purpose of maintaining and/or improving the nutritional status, weight, and healing ability of the patient. Parenteral nutrition is used to provide sufficient caloric and nitrogen to meet patient daily requirement.

TPN is indicated for:

▶ Diagnosis indicates the need for gastrointestinal rest; the patient is unable to adequately eat orally or by enterel feedings, such as paralytic ileus, or Crohns Disease with obstruction.
▶ Incidents where oral or enteral feeding are contraindicated, such as patients with acute pancreatitis or high enterocutaneous fistula.
▶ Patient intake is insufficient to maintain an anabolic state and other means have not been successful, such as, in patients with severe burns, malnutrition, shortbowel syndrome, cancer, radiationenteritis, bowel ischemia.
▶ Patients who are in a malnourished state or are at risk because of anticipated procedures.

Parenteral Therapy Prescription

The dietitian and the pharmacist are consulted for the calculation, design, recommendations, and compounding of solutions. Standard solutions and standard electrolyte patterns should be available. Special central and peripheral base solutions and electrolyte formulas should be made available to meet specific patient requirements for whom standard solutions/electrolyte patterns are not acceptable.

The solutions should be labeled to specific contents. All hyperalimentation solutions should be prepared under laminar flow hoods in accordance with the facility standard operating procedures. All discontinued solutions should be returned to pharmacy and stored under refrigeration.

The standard peripheral solution usually contains:**

500 ml of 8.5% Aminosyn
500 ml of 10% Dextrose
170 non protein calories and 41 grams of protein per liter

Standard central parenteral solution**

500 ml of 8.5% Aminosyn
500 ml of 50% Dextrose
850 non protein calories and 41 grams of protein per liter

Standard electrolyte pattern (in total concentration per liter)** Available commercially as a single additive and can be added as needed to the PN solution except for calcium and phosphorous

Na 35 mEq
K 42.7mEq

In GRANT's *Handbook of Total Parenteral Nutrition,* the average electrolyte requirements are higher than those listed.Follow your organization's policy.*

Cl 51 mEq
Mg. 8 mEq
Ca 5 mEq
PO4 15 mEq
Ac 41.0 mEq

Additives are frequently prescribed for TPN include multivitamins, folic acid, regular insulin, trace minerals, heparin, and H2 antagonist (Tagament, Zantac, and Pepcid). All other additives prescribed should be added only after careful evaluation of compatibility with the TPN mixture.

Administration of the solution(s) should follow the standard operating procedure for the facility. The pharmacist and dietitian should be responsible for making recommendations for administration based upon patient responses to therapy, estimated caloric and protein requirements.

Monitoring of the Nutrition Care

Ongoing monitoring of the patient response to parenteral therapy is a collaborative effort of the interdisciplinary team. Monitoring of therapy includes:
▶ identification of patients who are receiving adequate nutrition intake
▶ evaluation of patient's response to parenteral therapy

**The standard solutions are suggestions. They may or may not be compatible with your standard operating procedures. Before any solution is mixed the contents should be verified by the dietitian and pharmacist.
*Calculation is based on calorie and protein content of the concentration and volume. There are a number of metabolic complications of TPN. Monitoring is essential.

▶ assessment of biological, hematological and other pertinent diagnostic data including clinical signs of nutrient deficiencies and excesses

▶ evaluation of patient's consumption of oral intake and transitional feedings

The attending physician must be altered by the team to patient's who are experiencing a suboptimal response or potential adverse events to the therapy.

If the gut works, parenteral nutrition therapy should not be ordered, but the less expensive enteral therapy. Transition from parenteral therapy to enteral should be made as fast as it is medically safe.

▶ JCAHO AND ENTERAL TUBEFEEDING SAFETY ◀

There is an ongoing concern by accreditation agencies concerning the safe handling of food, water, and especially enteral tube feedings. As a result in August, 1999 Update 3 in the **Comprehensive Accreditation Manual for Hospital** for Standard TX.4 Care of Patients-Nutrition Care and Standard IC, Survellance, Prevention and Control of Infections there were "revised" intent, examples of evidence of performance, and examples of implementation concerning safe handling for food and enteral tube feedings. The evidence of performance for TX.4, TX.4.3, TX.4.4 and TX.4.6 "documentation of HACCP for food and enteral tube feedings' and evidence of performance for TX.4.7 "documentation of HACCP for food, enteral nutrition and water." Examples of implementation TX.4.3 "Responsibilities are assigned for all activities involved in safe and accurate provision of food and nutrition products."

The organization uses the Hazard Analysis Critical Control Point (HACCP) process to manage food and enteral tube feeding safety. The organization uses performance improvement techniques that emphasize the interdepartmental influence an *open* enteral tube feeding systems and food safety.

TX.4.5 and TX.4.7 further discuss monitoring interdisciplinary committee review, survey, inconsistencies noted and corrections addressed.

In the JCAHO Infection Control Standards (IC 20 & IC 21) it states "a hospital follows the processes outlined to reduce contamination of food products for patients receiving enteral products. Sterile water is suggested for all formula use including flushing the tube.

Other Health Care Services

Patients may use a variety of healthcare services. The most familiar services include hospitals, extended care facilities, residential living, out patient clinics and day surgery. Other services are also available and may save money and stress on the family. These services include: **home health, home delivered meals, hospice and adult day care centers.** Many patients who utilize the services of home health are on modified diets including enteral and parenteral nutrition. Others have chronic diseases that affect their nutritional status. Home health agencies offer a variety of services such as nursing, home health aids, physical, occupational and speech therapy, social services and in some agencies nutrition services by a consulting dietitian. Home delivered meals are delivered to the home of patients by volunteers through the Meals on Wheels program. These meals consist of a hot meal delivered before noon and frequently a cold meal for supper. Hospice care is for the terminally ill patient. The patient may be confined to a facility or may be at home as long as possible or is feasible. The goal of hospice is to provide continuity of care while meeting the needs/preferences of the patient and family. Pain alleviation is an important factor in these cases. Patients rights and advance directives are honored. Adult day care centers are available for family members who are the care givers of a patient. These centers are used as needed by the care giver and may include as little as one day per week/month to five days a week. The patient is "dropped off" at the center and picked up at a specified time by the care giver. The patient is furnished meals, given his medication, activities, and bed rest as needed. This type of care frequently reduces the stress on the care giver.

References

Beaglow, W.S., Fetal alcohol syndrome: A review, *Journal of the American Dietetic Association,* 79, p. 274, 1981.

Charles, E.J. Charting by Exception: A Solution to the Challegene of 1996 JCAHO's Nutrition Care Standards Journal of American Dietetic Assoc. Supplement vol. 97 no 2 5131–138

Comprehensive Accreditation Manual for Hospitals, Joint Commission on the Accreditation of Healthcare Organizations, Chicago, IL, update 3 Aug. 1999

Determine Your Nutritional Health, The Nutritional Screening Initiative, a project of the American Family Physicians, the American Dietetic Association and the National Council on the Aging, Inc., funded in part by a grant from Ross Division, Abbott Laboratories, Washington, DC.

Florida Alcohol and Drug Abuse Association, Resource Center, 1030 Lafayette St., Suite 100, Tallahassee, FL 3201

Frisancho, R.A., *Anthropometric Standards for the Assessment of Growth and Nutritional status,* The University of Michigan Press, Ann Arbor, Michigan, 1990.

Grant, A., DeHoog, S. *Nutritional Assessment and Support,* (4th ed), Anne Grant Publisher, Seattle, Washington.

Grant, JP Hand book of Total Parenteral Nutrition. Philadelphia, PA. WB Saunders 1992.

Healthy People 2000: National Health Promotion and Disease Prevention Objectives, U.S. Department of Health and Human Services, Washington, DC, 1990.

Hommerson, S. (Ed) *Practical Guide to Nutritional Care for Dietitians and other health Professionals,* University of Alabama, Birmingham, 1992.

Hunt, D.R., Maslovitz, A., Rowlands, B.J., Brooks, B.A., A simple nutrition screening procedure for hospital patients, *Journal of the American Dietetic Association,* 85(3), pp. 332–335, 1985.

Larson, D.E. Mayo Clinic Family Health Book 2nd ed. William Morrow & Co. Inc. N.Y. 1996

Leiber, C.S., The influence of alcohol on nutritional status, *Nutritional Review,* 46, pp. 241–254, 1988

Mohs, M.E., Watson, R.R., Leonard-Green, T., Nutritional effects of marijuana, heroin, cocaine, and nicotine, *Journal of the American Dietetic Association,* 90(9), pp. 1261–1267, 1990.

Murray, J.A., Healy, M.D., Drug-mineral interactions: A new responsibility for the hospital Dietitian, *Journal of the American Dietetic Association,* pp. 66–70, 73, 1991.

National Academy of Science, *Recommended Dietary Allowances* (10th ed), National Academy Press, Washington, 1989.

Niedert, K.C. editor Nutrition Care of the Older Adult American Dietetic Assoc., Chicago, IL. 1998

Nutritional Assessment of the Elderly through Anthropometry, Ross Products Division, Abbott Laboratories, Columbus, Ohio, 1984.

Physicians Desk Reference Medical Economics Co. Oradell N.J 1999

Physicians Desk Reference, (49th ed), Medical Economics Company, Oradell, New Jersey, 1998 published annually.

Pressman, AF, Buffs. The Complete Idiot's Guide to Alternative Medicine Alpha Books NY 1999

Puckett, R.P., Brown, S.M. *Shands Hospital at the University Guide to Clinical Dietetics* (5th ed), Kendall Hunt, Dubuque, Iowa, 1993.

Robinson, C.H., Weigley, E.S., and Mueller, D.H., *Basic Nutrition and Diet Therapy,* (7th ed), MacMillan Publishing Co., New York, 1993.

Roche Dietitians Clinical and Nutrient Guidelines: LLC 1997

Sizer, F., Whitney, E., *Hamilton and Whitney's Nutrition Concepts and Controversies,* (6th ed)., West Publishing Co., Minneapolis/St. Paul, 1994.

State Operations Manual, Provider Certification, Department of Health and human Services, Health Care Financing Administration, (PB 95-950009), national Technical Information Service, US. Department of Commerce, Springfield, Va. 1995.

Time Life the Drug and Medicine Advisor Time-Life NY 1997

The American Dietetic Association Paper, Issues in feeding the terminally ill adult, *Dietitians in Nutrition Support,* 11(2), pp. 2-9, 1989.

Watson, R, Caffeine: Is it dangerous to health?, *American Journal of Health Promotion,* Spring 1988, pp 13-22.

Weinsier, R.L., Heimburger, D.C., Butterworth, C.E., *Handbook of Clinical Nutrition,* (2nd ed), C.V. Mosby Co., St. Louis, Missouri.

What you should know about . . . *Caffeine,* International Food Information Council, Washington, DC, 1991.

Suggested Herb References

The American Pharmaceutical Assoc. Practical Guide to Natural Medicines (ISBN 0-688-16151-0) 728 pages $35-can order on line www.amazon.com

Herbal PDR

Handbook of Complementary and Alternative Medicines http://www.springnet.com click on "Herbal Medicines"

American Botanical Council-handout: Common Herbs: An Introductory Guide to Herbal Healthcare P.O Box 201660, Austin, TX 78720-1660

Food and Drug Sites

http://www.kian.net/interact/interact.htm
http://www.foodsafety.org/sf/sf162.htm
http://www.physsportmed.com/issues/may_96/food_drg.htm
http://www.channel2000.com/news/health/stories/news-health-981118-182628.html
http://bewell.com/heathy/eating/1996/foodrug/foodrug.shtml
http://www.wvu.edu/~uacdd/nutrition/foodmed/interact.htm
http://www.wvy.edu/~uacdd/nutrition/foodmed/suggest.htm
http://www.wvu.edu/~uacdd/nutrition/foodmed/how.htm
http://www.wvu.edu/~uacdd/nutrition/foodmed/test.htm
http://pharminfo.com/pubs/msb/gfj_effect.html
http://www.ksi.com/dump/news/cc/foodncl.htm
http://www.pharmasave.com/healthnotes/2/6/druginteraction.html
http://www.openhand.org/nutrition/posnut9/mdn.table2.html
http://vm.cfsan.fda.gov/~lrd/fdinter.html

Food-Medication Interactions, P.O. Box 659, Pottstown, PA 19464. Or call 610-970-7143. They now offer a windows software program too ($189.95). $18.95 plus shipping and handling of $4.00

Drug/Nutrient Interactions

Nutrition Screening Initiative's (NSI) new publication "The Role of Nutrition in Chronic Disease" has numerous references and 10 tables of potential drug/nutrient interactions for drugs used to treat commonchronic disease states that occur in those age 65 and older. This publication can be ordered through the NSI by calling (202) 625-1662 or writing to them at 1010 Wisconsin Ave. NW Suite 800, Washington DC 20007. This document can also be ordered through ADA at 1-800-877-1600 ext.5000

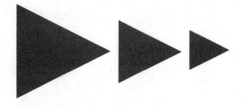

SECTION 2

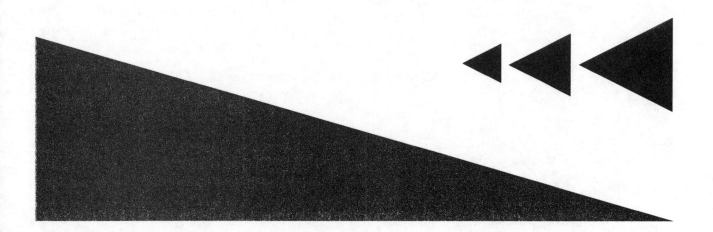

▶ INTRODUCTION TO SECTION 2 ◀

Diet modification is based on the modification of basic nutrients, consistency or texture, calorie distribution and seasoning from a normal or regular diet. The purpose of diet modification is to maintain or restore the nutritional status of an individual (patient).

When a diet modification is ordered the nutrition team will need to consider the psychological, physiological, economic, cultural, ethnic, social and religious behaviors/needs of the patient as they develop care plans and educational materials for the patient. When an individual becomes ill they may exhibit behaviors that don't fit their normal patterns. Some persons may express fear, anger, stress, anxiety and a marked difference in personality/behavior. Other patients may express strong preferences for comfort foods, childhood favorites, or they may reject all food and/or will eat only foods from their own household. Others may refuse to make any changes in their lifestyle and refuse all counseling/education. Taste may be modified due to the illness or medication. In these instances the nutrition team will need to educate the person in techniques on "how" to change food preparation.

Included in this section is a meal pattern for each of the modified diets. These meal patterns can be used as a guide in menu planning for the organization or as guidelines for developing educational materials. When meal patterns are used appropriately they can provide patients adequate nutrients, with correct portion sizes, and help to insure patients are receiving optimal nutrition.

Utilizing the tools from Section 1 the nutrition care team can identify and meet the needs of the patients. The nutritional care plan will need to be based on accurate, sound, scientific research for the specific disease entity. The care plan will need to involve the patient/family and be individualized for each patient.

The following diet modification and meal patterns contain the latest research the authors were able to obtain. Due to the identified problem of egg safety due to Salmonella Enteritidis (SE) and the number of outbreaks that invalued approximately 30,000 illnesses, 3,000 hospitalization and 79 deaths (1985-1988), we have eliminated all soft cooked eggs in the menu. Eggs need to be thoroughly cooked before consumption. (President's Council on Food Safety 2000.) These diet modifications may not be the ones used in your organization, however, they may be changed to meet your individual needs.

If additional information is needed see the references at the end of each diet for a more comprehensive review.

▶ REGULAR DIET ◀

Description

The regular diet is designed to maintain or attain optimal nutritional status. This diet is based on the basic food group plan and provides a selection of commonly known and well prepared foods. It may be used by individuals who do not require specific nutrient alterations for pre-existing disorders. Individual requirements for specific nutrients may very based on sex, age, height, weight, and activity level.

THERE ARE NO RESTRICTIONS ON THE REGULAR DIET.

It should be noted that the Surgeon General, the American Heart Association, and the Dietary Guidelines for Americans, have made recommendations for a more optimal diet. These recommendations include:

▶ 30% of less of calories from fat.
▶ 55–60% of calories from carbohydrates—with emphasis on complex carbohydrates.
▶ 10–20% of calories from protein.
▶ 300 mg or less of cholesterol per day.
▶ Salt intake should not exceed 6 grams of Sodium chloride (table salt) daily or slightly more than one teaspoon of salt. Sodium in processed and/or cured foods should be considered.
▶ Intake of fiber should be 25–30 grams daily from foods, not supplements.
▶ Avoidance of foods high is sugar.
▶ More emphasis should be placed on exercise and weight maintenance.

Adequacy

This diet is adequate for all nutrients according to the 1989 National Research Council's Recommended Dietary Allowances.

To meet the Recommended Dietary Allowances for protein, vitamins and minerals set by the Food and Nutrition Board of the National Research Council, the daily pattern should include the following *minimum* servings of foods:

▶ DAILY FOOD GUIDE—REGULAR DIET ◀

Food Group	Recommended Minimum Number of Servings				
	Child	Teenager	Adult	Pregnant Woman	Lactating Woman
MILK 1 c. Milk, Yogurt *or* calcium equivalent: 2 c. Cottage Cheese 1½ oz. Cheddar Cheese 1¾ c. Ice Cream 1 c. Pudding	3	4	2	4	4
MEAT 2 oz. Cooked Lean Meat, Fish, Poultry *or* Protein equivalent: 2 Eggs 2 oz. Cheddar Cheese ½ c. Cottage Cheese 1 c. Dried Beans, Peas 4 T. Peanut Butter	2	2	2	3	2

Food Group	Recommended Minimum Number of Servings				
	Child	Teenager	Adult	Pregnant Woman	Lactating Woman
VEGETABLE, FRUIT Vitamin A ½ c. Cooked Vegetable or 1 c. Juice 1 c. Raw Vegetable (deep yellow or dark green) Vitamin C 1 med. Fruit or ½ c. Juice (citrus, tomatoes, strawberries, cantaloupe, papaya, mango)	4	5	5	5	5
BREAD-CEREAL-GRAIN Whole Grain, Fortified, Enriched: 1 Slice Bread ½ English Muffin or Hamburger Bun 1 oz. Ready to Eat Cereal ½ c. Cooked Cereal, Pasta, Grits, Rice	4	6	6	6	6

ALL FOODS ARE ALLOWED

Food Groups	Choose ↑ More Often	Choose ↓ Less Often	Major Nutrient Contribution
Milk and Milk products (2–4 servings/day)	Lowfat or skim milk Lowfat cheeses Lowfat yogurt	Whole milk Whole milk cheeses Whole milk yogurt Ice Cream	Calories, calcium, protein, phosphorus, vitamins A & D, riboflavin
Meat, Poultry, Fish and Meat Substitutes (2–3 servings/day, total 5–7 oz./day)	Lean meats, fish, shellfish, poultry without skin Lowfat cheeses (such as cottage and part skimmed mozzarella) peanut butter, soybeans, tofu, dry beans and peas	Fried or fatty meats, fish, fried poultry or poultry with skin High fat cheeses (such as cheddar and processed cheeses) Eggs–*limit to three per week* Nuts	Calories, protein, iron, zinc, copper, B-complex vitamin
Fruit (2–4 servings/day)	Unsweetened fruits or juices, fresh fruit. Include one citrus fruit/juice or one tomato/juice daily	Sweetened fruits/juices Coconut Avocado	Calories, dietary fiber, vitamins A & C
Vegetables, including Starchy Vegetables (3–5 servings/day)	Fresh, frozen, or canned potatoes - baked or boiled Include one dark green or deep yellow vegetable daily	Deep-fat fried vegetables, chips Pickled vegetables Highly salted vegetables or juices	Calories, vitamins A & C, dietary fiber, potassium, zinc, cobalt, folic acid
Bread, Cereal, Rice, and Pasta (6–11 servings/day)	Whole grain breads or cereals. Enriched breads or cereals, muffins, bagels, tortillas, pasta, rice, grits, or noodles	Snack chips or crackers, sweetened cereals, pancakes, doughnuts, biscuits	Calories, B-complex vitamins, magnesium, copper, iron, dietary fiber

Food Groups	Choose ↑ More Often	Choose ↓ Less Often	Major Nutrient Contribution
Fats and Oils (4–5 tsp./day)	Corn, cottonseed, olive, sesame, soybean, safflower, peanut, canola oils, margarine (made from above oils) mayonnaise or salad dressing (made from above oils)	Avocado, butter, lard, margarine made hydrogenated, or saturated fats, coconuts or palm oil, hydrogenated vegetable shortening, olives, bacon, meat fat/drippings, gravy, sauces	Vitamin A, calories, essential fatty acids
Soups	Lightly salted soups with fat skimmed Cream-style soups (with lowfat milk) Reduced sodium soups	Commercially prepared soups and mixes	Fluid, calories (may contain a variety of vitamins, minerals, and protein, dependent upon type)
Desserts	Desserts that have been sweetened lightly and/or contain only moderate fat, such as puddings made from skim milk, angel food cake, fruit based deserts	Desserts high in sugar and/or fats, such as candy, pastries, cakes, pies, whole milk puddings, cookies	Calories (fats, carbohydrates)
Beverages (6 or more servings/day)	Water, unsweetened soft drinks Decaffeinated drinks	Sweetened beverages Caffeine containing beverages Alcoholic beverages	Fluids, Calories (unless sugar substitute used)
Miscellaneous	Herbs, spices, flavoring	Salt and salt/spice combinations	Sodium

Sample Menu

Breakfast	Lunch	Supper
½ c. Orange Juice	Hamburger:	3 oz. Chicken Breast
¾ c. Cornflakes	3 oz. Lean Beef	Mashed Potatoes
2 Slices Whole Wheat Toast-Jelly	Bun, Lettuce, Tomato	Broccoli
1 tsp. Margarine	1 Corn on the Cob	Tossed Salad with Dressing
1 c. 2% Milk	1 Apple	Dinner Roll–1 tsp. Margarine
Coffee–Sugar	1 tsp. Mayonnaise	Gelatin with Fruit
	1 tsp. Margarine	1 c. 2% Milk
	Coffee, Tea	Coffee, Tea

References

American Dietetic Association: Manual of Clinical Dietetics. Chicago: 1988.

Dallas–Fort Worth Hospital Council: Dallas–Fort Worth Hospital Council Diet Manual. Irving: 1992.

Florida Dietetic Association: Diet Manual, Manual of Clinical Dietetics, 1990.

Mahan, K. and Arlin, M.: Krause's Food, Nutrition and Diet Therapy. 8th ed., Philadelphia: W.B. Saunders Company, 1992.

Puckett, R.P. and Brown, S.M.: Shands Hospital at the University of Florida Guide to Clinical Dietetics, 5th ed., Dubuque: Kendall/Hunt Publishing Co., 1993.

Thomas Jefferson University Hospital Nutrition Manual, Department of Nutrition and Dietetics, Philadelphia, Pennsylvania: 1993.

William S. Rodwell: Nutrition and Diet Therapy, 7th ed., Mosby-Yearbook, Inc.: 1993

▶ LIBERALIZED DIETS FOR OLDER ADULTS ◀ IN LONG-TERM CARE

Long-term care includes a continuum of health services ranging from rehabilitation to supportive care. As defined by the American Health Care Association (1), long-term-care services target persons who have lost the capacity to function on their own as a result of chronic illness or conditions that require intervention for an extended period. The primary users of long-term care are older adults, that is, persons aged 65 years and older.

Care for older adults in long-term care must meet 2 goals: maintenance of health through medical care and maintenance of quality of life. However, these goals often seem to compete, resulting in the need for a unique approach to medical nutrition therapy.

Typically, medical nutrition therapy includes assessment of nutritional status and development of an individualized nutrition intervention plan that frequently features a therapeutic diet appropriate for managing a disease or condition (2). Medical nutrition therapy must always address medical needs and individual desires, yet for older adults in long-term care this balance is especially critical because of the focus on maintaining quality of life. Thus, for older adults, overall health goals may not warrant the use of a therapeutic diet because of its possible negative effect on quality of life. Often, a more liberalized nutrition intervention that allows an older adult to participate in his or her diet-related decisions can provide for the person's nutrient needs and allow alterations contingent on medical conditions while simultaneously increasing desire to eat and enjoyment of food. This ultimately decreases the risks of weight loss and undernutrition.

Position Statement

It is the position of The American Dietetic Association (ADA) that the quality of life and nutritional status of older residents in long-term-care facilities may be enhanced by a liberalized diet. The Association advocates the use of qualified dietetics professionals to assess, monitor, and evaluate the need for medical nutrition therapy according to each person's needs and rights.

Environment and Trends in Long-Term Care

In 1990, 1.5 million persons—5% of all Americans aged 65 years and older—lived in nursing homes (3). When broken down by age group, the percentage increased dramatically by age, ranging from 1% for persons aged 65 to 74 years, 5% for those aged 75 to 84 years, to 25% for persons aged 85 years and older (3). Older adults in 1990 faced a 43% probability of needing at least 1 type of long-term-care facility in their life (4). More than half of those who entered long-term-care facilities remained in the facility for at least 1 year and 21% remained 5 years or longer (4). By 1996, the trend was to decrease the number of nursing home beds for those adults not needing full-time nursing care and to promote assisted living, retirement, or adult family homes. The impetus for this trend was to decrease the Medicare/Medicaid costs and to increase the quality of life in a less restrictive setting.

Older adults in long-term-care facilities are more chronically ill and require more care than most community-dwelling older adults. Of the 1.5 million people who reside in nursing homes, 70% have some organic brain disorder usually accompanied by dementia (3). The single most common symptom is confusion, which afflicts 44% of all residents (5). These residents may also suffer from anorexia and involuntary weight loss, conditions that occur more frequently outside the long-term-care facility (66%) before their admission (5). Diabetes, congestive heart failure, chronic obstructive pulmonary disease, dysphagia, depression, and hypertension are common medical diagnoses for older adults in an institutional setting.

Currently, the trend is toward improving quality of care and residents' quality of life, and increasing each resident's role in making informed care decisions. These factors are outlined in the federal regulations issued by the Health Care Financing Administration as a result of the 1987 Omnibus Budget Reconciliation Act (6).

Current regulations protect a resident's right to refuse services or treatments and to choose alternatives. The law defines resident rights as the right to be free of interference, coercion, discrimination, and reprisal from the facility in exercising his or her rights. According to the Code of Federal Regulations, "The resident has the right to be fully informed in language that he/she can understand of his/her total health status, (includes functional status, medical care, nursing care, nutritional status, rehabilitation and restorative potential, etc) including but not limited to medical condition" (6). A resident has the right to refuse such treatment; however, it is the responsibility of the facility health care team to explain to the resident, family, and/or guardian the risks and benefits of refusing treatment. The risks and benefits of declining medical nutrition therapy need to be documented and signed by the resident (or, if the resident is deemed incompetent, by the legal guardian or other substitute decision maker) in the medical record indicating that he or she understands the consequences of the choice. Facilities must support the resident's decision regarding choice and must serve as an advocate for the resident at all times. As long as the resident is deemed competent, his or her decision stands.

Institutionalized Older Adults and the Risk of Malnutrition

Older adults in long-term-care settings are often among the frail elderly (7). They are more likely to experience a number of problems—physical and social, acute and chronic—that exacerbate poor health and compromise quality of life. Nutrition care is well recognized as an important factor in improving longevity and quality of life, but nutrient requirements of this population are not yet well understood (8). Good nutritional status in older adults benefits both the individual and society: health is improved, dependence is decreased, time required to recuperate from illness is reduced, and use of health care resources is contained (2,9). Conversely, undernutrition adversely affects the quality and length of life and, therefore, has aroused the concern of geriatric health professionals (10). Estimates of malnutrition in institutionalized older adults vary tremendously, from 10% to 85%, making malnutrition one of the most serious problems facing health professionals working in long-term care (11). Dietetics professionals working with institutionalized older adults must overcome many hurdles to obtain good nutritional status. Barriers to adequate nutrition in older adults can generally be divided into 2 broad categories: physical problems and psychosocial concerns.

Common physical problems that affect nutritional status include poor appetite, weight loss, pressure ulcers, chronic disease, eating dependency, sensory loss, and poor oral health. In addition, older adults are often taking several different medications at once, a situation that may affect their nutrient intake. All of these problems can lead to or exacerbate existing malnutrition.

Poor appetite is a widespread complaint in long-term care. In 1 study, more than 33% of residents interviewed complained of poor or variable appetite (12). This phenomenon appears to occur with equal frequency in men and women (5). As appetite diminishes, intake of total energy, protein, vitamins, and minerals is reduced, depleting the body of necessary nutrients. This predisposes older adults to an increased risk of illness and infection. Point-in-time surveys show that 15% to 20% of nursing home residents have active infections of the urinary tract, respiratory tract, skin, or eye (10). At the same time, infections may lead to a higher metabolic rate, increasing the person's total energy and protein needs. A vicious circle ensues. Stringent diet restrictions that limit familiar foods and eliminate or modify seasonings in foods may contribute to poor appetite and decreased food intake and increased risk of illness and infection.

Weight loss in residents is another challenge for dietetics professionals working in long-term care. Weight loss in institutionalized older adults may be the result of a number of circumstances, both physical and emotional. One study found that 70% of the residents in a nursing home had lost more than 10 lb during their stay at the facility (13). Unintentional weight loss has been correlated with increased mortality, compromised ability to resist infections, and increased incidence of pressure ulcers (13). When trying to minimize weight loss, limiting particular foods that appeal to these persons may be counterproductive.

Another consideration is the fact that 50% of the pressure ulcers reported by long-term-care facilities occur in residents over the age of 70 years (14). Among older adults in nursing homes, pressure ulcers are associated with a fourfold increased risk of death (15). Although pressure ulcers have multiple causes, nutritional status is a contributing factor. Bergstrom et al (16) have shown that baseline nutritional status is one of the best predictors in pressure ulcer healing.

Older adults also suffer from a higher incidence of chronic disease, most notably stroke, arthritis, Parkinson's disease, diabetes, and dementia. Some diseases, such as chronic obstructive pulmonary disorder and congestive heart failure, may result in increased metabolic demands and diminished appetite. Dementia syndromes, such as Alzheimer's disease may impair self-feeding, alter appetite, and increase energy needs. Nutrition restrictions may make it more difficult for the resident to eat, resulting in diminished intake and weight loss.

Long-term-care residents ingest an average of 8 medications per day. Of the more frequently used medications, 23 are known to cause reduced food intake and have side effects such as anorexia, nausea, vomiting, food aversions, somnolence, and disinterest in food (16). Accommodating food preferences may be essential to counteract the effects of polypharmacy in long-term-care residents.

Incidence of eating disability in nursing homes is high. One survey documented that 50% of skilled nursing facility residents required eating assistance. A decline in functional ability can be a factor in accessing adequate nutrition. The problem is enhanced by staff shortages and the length of time required to feed a totally dependent resident. In addition, many residents require coaxing and encouragement to eat, increasing the staff time requirement (17).

Sensory loss is common with the aging process. Visual impairment can diminish the appreciation of the color of foods and the ability to recognize them. Similarly, the role of aroma to stimulate appetite is diminished with the loss of olfactory ability. The flavor of foods may be altered for older adults because of loss of both olfactory and taste perception (18).

In addition, as many as 50% of Americans have lost all their teeth by the age of 65 years (13). Lack of teeth or poor oral health reduces chewing ability and limits food selection. Poor dentition or use of dentures affects the ability to perceive food flavor as well (18). Dysphagia also contributes to the decline in oral intake and enjoyment of eating. It is estimated that 40% to 60% of older adults in long-term-care facilities may experience dysphagia symptoms during the eating process. Nutrition restrictions, coupled with sensory losses, may result in limited food enjoyment and compromised food intake.

The link between psychiatric well-being, food intake, and nutritional status is evident in persons of all ages and particularly in older adults (11). Depression among institutionalized older adults is common and can be caused by several factors, including loss of loved ones, loss of independence, loneliness, and failing health. These factors can contribute to a resident's lack of attention to their nutrition needs and food preferences, which results in a decrease in food intake.

The Role of Medical Nutrition Therapy in Long-Term Care

Given the numerous problems faced by dietetics professionals who work with institutionalized older adults, it is necessary to evaluate the role of therapeutic diets in this population. The following questions need attention: Are restricted diets necessary? Do the diets offer health benefits to justify their use? Which residents will benefit from a therapeutic diet? These questions must be answered on an individual basis. A number of studies on the effectiveness of nutrition restrictions on specific conditions common to older adults have been conducted, but controversy continues over their application.

Both ADA and the American Diabetes Association emphasize the importance of individual nutrition assessment in determining the nutrition needs of persons with diabetes (19). The goals of nutrition intervention should include the improvement of overall health through optimal nutrition. Experience has shown that institutionalized older adults eat better when they are given a less restricted diet of "regular" foods rather than an energy-controlled diet (20).

The metabolic impact of prescribed diabetic diets vs regular institutional diets in 18 nursing home residents with type 2 diabetes mellitus showed that good glycemic control could be achieved with a regular diet (21). Benefits of "regular" institutional diets include consistent mealtimes and portion sizes, which are important to diabetes management (20,22). Another benefit is the potential to improve quality of life as well as intake. A key element in the use of "regular" menus in long-term-care facilities is consistency in carbohydrate intake at meals and snacks. Such an approach incorporates sucrose-containing foods as part of the carbohydrate intake (20). This is in keeping with the current nutrition recommendations regarding sucrose intake (19).

Older adults with diabetes on any type of meal plan should have their blood glucose levels monitored to evaluate the effectiveness of the nutrition intervention on glucose control. Those who do not tolerate a less restrictive approach need to be reevaluated by their dietetics professional; recommendations for adjustment of diabetes medication or individualization to a more controlled diet can be made using results of capillary blood glucose monitoring (20).

Available epidemiologic evidence indicates that as age increases above 44 years, the importance of elevated serum cholesterol levels as a risk factor for coronary heart disease decreases and virtually disappears after the age of 65 years (23). Therefore, the appropriateness of low-cholesterol diet prescriptions for older adults in long-term-care facilities is questionable (24–26).

Low-sodium diets are often poorly tolerated in older adults and may lead to loss of appetite, hyponatremia, or confusion (27). A decrease in food intake in reaction to a low-sodium diet has the potential to worsen a person's nutritional status and facilitate the onset of cardiac cachexia, respiratory infections, or pressure ulcers. Diets low in sodium may be perceived as bland and tasteless, diminishing the pleasurable experience of eating and promoting unnecessary weight loss. Congestive heart failure in older adults could be controlled with the use of drug therapy and a mild sodium restriction of 4 to 6 g/day (no added salt) instead of the 2 g sodium diet prescription (27–30).

Dietetics professionals must help residents and health care team members assess the risks vs benefits of therapeutic diets. Optimal nutritional status ultimately depends on adequate intake of food. A diet cannot be effective if it is not eaten. If a resident is noncompliant and does not support the prescribed medical nutrition therapy, the diet may be ineffective and frustrating for both the resident and the health care team. In addition, if a resident's appetite is extremely poor or if substantial weight loss is a problem, treatment of malnutrition may override concern for an elevated serum cholesterol level or a history of hypertension. Also, restricting food in an effort to control blood glucose is not appropriate because of the risk of malnutrition; instead, medication changes are more important.

Food has emotional as well as physical importance. The relationship of food to culture, ethnicity, religion, or personal meaning is a special consideration in any nutrition intervention (11). The pleasurable experience of food and eating can contribute notably to a person's quality of life and nutritional status. Dietetics professionals must help residents and health care team members prioritize any nutrition problems and recommend the nutrition intervention that balances both medical and quality-of-life needs. Thus, it may not be advantageous to initiate a restrictive nutrition prescription for a resident who suffers from poor appetite and substantial, unintentional weight loss.

The Role of Dietetics Professionals in the Management of Medical Nutrition Therapy for Long-Term-Care Residents

Dietetics professionals' primary role in the management of medical nutrition therapy for long-term-care residents is to develop a nutrition care plan consistent with each resident's nutritional status, overall medical condition, and personal preferences and needs. Dietetics professionals can implement medical nutrition therapy in the following steps:

1. *Assess nutritional status.* The dietetics professional should work with the health care team to evaluate all aspects of the resident's nutritional status. The dietetics professional should also determine the resident's goals and desires relating to the medical nutrition therapy.

2. *Determine appropriate nutrition intervention.* After gathering information from the assessment, the dietetics professional recommends the appropriate nutrition intervention. Interventions should address medical, psychosocial, and quality-of-life needs. The dietitian and foodservice manager should work closely to develop menu offerings and dining experiences to increase the enjoyment of eating. Efforts should be made to provide a pleasurable dining experience that preserves resident dignity and accommodates preferences. Together, the dietetics professional and manager should coordinate a dining environment that enables residents to maximize their potential to enjoy meals and the associated social aspects of dining.

3. *Collaborate with the health care team.* During this phase, the dietetics professional should integrate the nutrition care plan with the interdisciplinary plan of care. The purpose of care planning is to identify existing or potential problems and to develop goals and methods to address these problems. The resident and his or her family are encouraged to participate in the care planning conference and assist in the development of goals and approaches. Interdisciplinary care plans are developed from a federally mandated Resident Assessment Instrument known as the Minimum Data Set and the Resident Assessment Protocol, along with additional in-depth assessments by long-term-care professionals. The Minimum Data Set and Resident Assessment Protocol include nutrition assessment and monitoring as part of an interdisciplinary evaluation. The health care team, including the dietetics professional, needs to take into consideration the resident's wishes, assessed needs, and quality of life to develop an acceptable approach. Implementing, monitoring, and evaluating the nutrition intervention also involves an interdisciplinary team approach. It is important that the health care team supports the resident's decision and continues to be an advocate for the resident at all times.

4. *Provide patient education.* The health care team, including the dietetics professional, must educate the resident and/or his or her family/guardian about the nutrition intervention. To help the resident make informed decisions, the dietetics professional should explain the type of medical nutrition therapy indicated and the result of forgoing the recommended therapy.

5. *Monitor and evaluate outcomes.* The dietetics professional, with assistance from other members of the health care team, must monitor the outcomes of the medical nutrition therapy. The dietetics professional needs to provide ongoing assessment of the resident's nutrition needs throughout the year. This includes continued education for the resident about his or her individual nutrition needs, and allowing the resident the opportunity to change his or her mind regarding treatment at any time. As long as the resident is deemed competent, his or her decision stands and must be acknowledged.

Summary

Malnutrition, weight loss, and resident satisfaction are serious issues that need to be addressed by dietetics professionals working in long-term-care facilities. Medical nutrition therapy for older adults in long-term care is multifaceted and critical to reducing the risks of malnutrition and weight loss. To meet the needs of every resident, dietetics professionals must consider each person holistically, including personal goals, overall prognoses, benefits and risks of treatment, and perhaps most important, quality of life. For some long-term-care residents the use of liberalized diets, when appropriate, can enhance both quality of life and nutritional status, thus increasing the resident's satisfaction with the meals provided and reducing the risks of malnutrition and weight loss.

References

1. American Health Care Association. *Compilation of Facts and Trends: The Nursing Facility Source Book.* Washington, DC: American Health Care Association; 1996: 36–37.

2. Position of The American Dietetic Association: cost-effectiveness of medical nutrition therapy. *J Am Diet Assoc.* 1995;95:88–91.

3. *A Profile of Older Americans.* Washington, DC: American Association of Retired Persons, Administration on Aging. 1992:2–4.

4. US Bureau of the Census. Sixty-five plus in the United States, Statistical Brief. <http://www.census.gov/ftp/pub/socdemo/www/agebrief.html> Accessed June 6, 1996:1–7.

5. Bartlett BJ. Characterization of anorexia in nursing home patients. *Educ Gerontol.* 1990;16:591–600.

6. Medicare and Medicaid programs: survey, certification and enforcement of skilled nursing facilities; final rule. 42 CFR § 483. 10.

7. Hogstel MO, Robinson NB. Feeding the fragile elderly. *J Gerontol Nurs.* 1989;15:16–20.

8. Food and Nutrition Board. *Recommended Dietary Allowances.* 10th ed. Washington, DC: National Academy Press; 1989.

9. Gallagher-Allred CR, Voss AC, Finn SC, McCamish MA. Malnutrition and clinical outcomes: the case for medical nutrition therapy. *J Am Diet Assoc.* 1996;96:361–369.

10. Abbasi AA, Rudman D. Observations on the prevalence of protein-calorie undernutrition in VA nursing homes. *J Am Geriatr Soc.* 1993;41:117–121.

11. Kerstetter JE, Holthaussen BA, Fitz PA. Malnutrition in the institutionalized older adult. *J Am Diet Assoc.* 1992;92:1109–1115.

12. Keller H. Malnutrition in institutionalized elderly: how and why? *J Am Geriatr Soc.* 1993;41:1212–1218.

13. Fisher J, Johnson M. Low body weight and weight loss in the aged. *J Am Diet Assoc.* 1990;90:1697–1706.

14. Peterson NC, Bittman S. The epidemiology of pressure sores. *Scand J Plast Reconst Surg Hand Surg.* 1971;5:62–66.

15. Michocki RJ, Lamy PP. The problem of pressure sores in a nursing home population: statistical data. *J Am Geriatr Soc.* 1976;24:323–328.

16. Bergstrom N, Braden BJ, Laguzza A, Holman V. The Braden Scale for predicting pressure sore risk. *Nurs Res.* 1987;36:205–210.

17. Varma RN. Risk for drug-induced malnutrition is unchecked in elderly patients in nursing homes. *J Am Diet Assoc.* 1994;94:192–194.

18. Bartoshuk LM, Duffy VB. Taste and smell in aging. In: Masoro EF, ed. *Handbook of Physiology.* New York, NY: Oxford University Press; 1995:363–375.

19. American Diabetes Association. Nutrition recommendations and principles for people with diabetes mellitus. *J Am Diet Assoc.* 1994;94:504–506.

20. Schafer RG, Bohannon B, Franz M, Freeman J, Holmes A, McLaughlin S, Haas LB, Kruger DF, Lorenz RA, McMahon MM. Translation of the diabetes nutrition recommendations for health care institutions: technical review. *J Am Diet Assoc.* 1997;97:43–51.

21. Coulston AM, Mandelbaum D, Reaven GM. Dietary management of nursing home residents with non-insulin-dependent diabetes mellitus. *Am J Clin Nutr.* 1990;51:67–71.

22. Davis M. Application of the 1994 nutrition recommendations to the elderly population and long term care facilities. *On the Cutting Edge, a newsletter of the Diabetes Care and Education dietetic practice group.* 1995;16:29–30.

23. Allred JB, Allred CG, Bowers DF. Elevated blood cholesterol: a risk factor for heart disease that decreases with advanced age. *J Am Diet Assoc.* 1990;90:574–575.

24. Morley JE, Solomon DH. Major issues in geriatrics over the last five years. *J Am Geriatr Soc.* 1994;42:218–225.

25. Hurley SB, Newman TB. Cholesterol in the elderly. Is it important? *JAMA.* 1994;272:1372–1373.

26. Krumholtz HM, Seeman TE, Merrill SS, deLeon M, Vaccarino V, Silverman D, Tsukchara R, Ostfeld A, Berkman L. Lack of association between cholesterol and coronary heart disease mortality and morbidity and all-cause mortality in persons older than 70 years. *JAMA.* 1994;272:1335–1340.

27. Luchi RJ, Taffet GE, Teasdale TA. Congestive heart failure in the elderly. *J Am Geriatr Soc.* 1992;40:1109–1116.

28. Hajjar R, Morley J. Blood pressure disorders in the nursing home resident. *Nurs Home Med.* 1996;4:111–119.

29. Buckler D, Kelber S, Goodwin J. The use of dietary restrictions in malnourished nursing home patients. *J Am Geriatr Soc.* 1994;42;1100–1102.

30. Dracup K, Dunbar S, Baker D. Heart failure. *Am J Nurs.* 1995;7:22–27.

▶ ADA position adopted by the House of Delegates on October 26, 1997. This position will be in effect until December 31, 2001. ADA authorizes republication of the position statement/support paper, *in its entirety,* provided full and proper credit is given. Requests to use portions of the position must be directed to ADA Headquarters at 800/877–1600, ext. 4896 or hod@eatright.org

▶ Recognition is given to the following for their contributions:
Authors:
Pam Womack, RD; Carolyn Breeding, MS, RD, FADA
Reviewers:
American College of Health Care Administrators; American Diabetes Association (Becky Schafer, MS, RD); American Medical Directors Association (Steven A. Levenson, MD); Consultant Dietitians in Health Care Facilities dietetic practice group (Carol P. Deering, MS, RD; Carlene Russell, MS, RD, FADA); Sharon Emley, MS, RD; Gerontological Nutritionists dietetic practice group (Connie L. Codispoti, MS, RD; Sylvia Escott-Stump, MA, RD)

 ## ▶ HIGH CALORIE HIGH PROTEIN DIET ◀

Description

A High Calorie High Protein diet is a modification of the Regular diet which includes high protein snacks and/or supplements. This is prescribed for individuals who may be in "negative nitrogen balance", where the body is breaking down protein tissue faster than it is being replaced. Certain conditions such as trauma, stress, surgery, malignant diseases, and evidence of cachexia predispose individuals to negative nitrogen balance.

The purpose of this diet is to promote anabolism, wound healing, and/or weight gain. For adults it typically includes a minimum of 2500 kilocalories daily. It should provide a minimum protein level of 1.5 gm/kg of ideal body weight. For adults the range is usually between 100–125 grams of protein daily. At least 60 percent of the protein should be of high biological value which is found in eggs, milk, cheese, meat, poultry, and fish. High protein supplements such as milkshakes, and instant breakfast may be included.

Adequacy

This diet meets the 1989 Recommended Dietary Allowance for all nutrients when a variety of foods are consumed in adequate amounts.

Sample Menu

Breakfast	Lunch	Supper
½ c. Orange Juice 1 c. All Bran 1 Scrambled Egg 1 Slice Toast–1 tsp. Margarine 1 tsp. Jelly 1 c. Milk Coffee–1 tsp. Cream 1 tsp. Sugar	½ c. Cranberry Juice 3 ounces Fried Chicken ½ c. Mashed Potatoes ½ c. Broccoli 1 c. Tossed Salad with 1 Tbsp. Dressing 1 slice Bread-1 tsp. Margarine ½ c. Chocolate Pudding 1 c. Milk	1 c. Cream of Pea Soup with Crackers 3 ounces Tenderloin Steak ⅓ c. Buttered Rice ½ c. Spinach 1 Muffin–1 tsp. Margarine ½ c. Fruit Cocktail 1 c. Milk
10:00 a.m.	**2:00 p.m.**	**8:00 p.m.**
1 c. Commercial high protein drink	½ c. Cottage Cheese ½ c. Pineapple Juice	Ham Sandwich with 2 oz. of Meat 2 Slices of Bread 1 tsp. Mayonnaise

Reference

Puckett, R.P. and Brown, S.M.: Shands Hospital at the University of Florida Guide to Clinical Dietetics. 5th ed., Dubuque: Kendall/Hunt Publishing Co., 1993.

▶ VEGETARIAN DIETS* ◀

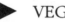

Description

Perceiving plant foods as beneficial because they are high in dietary fiber and, generally, lower in saturated fat than animal foods, many people turn to vegetarian diets.

Vegetarian diets are indicated for persons who restrict food of animal origin.

Vegetarians have been classified to the types of animal foods they restrict in their diets. The extent to which animal foods are avoided varies:

A. Lacto-Ovo-Vegetarian–avoidance of red meat, poultry, and fish.
B. Lacto-Vegetarian–avoidance of red meat, poultry, fish, and eggs.
C. Vegan–avoidance of all animal foods.

It should be noted that animal protein is of high biological value. This is commonly referred to as "complete protein". Plant protein is of lower biological value and is commonly referred to as "incomplete protein". Foods containing incomplete proteins may be served together to form complete proteins. The combinations of incomplete protein which will form complete proteins are called "complimentary proteins". Proper selection of complimentary proteins is a very important aspect of vegetarian diets.

Adequacy

Vegetarian diets can be nutritionally adequate if they provide adequate calories and include unrefined grains, legumes, nuts, seeds, a variety of leafy green vegetables and fruits, and dairy products. Diets excluding dairy products may be inadequate in protein, vitamin D, iron, zinc, and calcium. The vegan diet is also inadequate in vitamin B_{12}, which can result in irreversible nerve deterioration.

*See Position of the American Dietetic Assoc. Vegetarian Diet JADA Vol. 97 No. 11 pp 1317–1321

Replacement of Animal Sources of Nutrients

Vegetarians who eat no animal products need to become aware of what foods to eat to replace nutrients that are reduced. Nutrients most likely be be lacking and some non-animal sources are:

▶ Protein—tofu and other soy-based products, legumes, nuts, seeds, grains and vegetables
▶ Vitamin B_{12}—fortified soy beverages and cereals
▶ Vitamin D—fortified soy beverages and sunshine
▶ Calcium—tofu processed with calcium, broccoli, seeds, nuts, kale, bok choy, greens, legumes (beans and peas), lime-processed tortillas, soy beverages, grain products, and orange juice enriched with calcium
▶ Iron—legumes, tofu, green leafy vegetables, dried fruit, whole grains, and iron fortified breads and cereals, especially whole wheat
▶ Zinc—whole grains (especially the germ and bran), whole wheat bread, legumes, tofu and nuts

Specifics of the Diet

Following are suggested adaptations of the "Basic Food Groups" for vegetarian diets.

Lacto-Ovo-Vegetarian

▶ **Meat Group**—Replace meat, fish and poultry with eggs (4 per week) and generous amounts of legumes, nuts, wheat and/or soy meat analogs, and other formulated plant proteins (1–2 servings per day). Spun soy isolates should be fortified with iron and B vitamins to replace meat on a comparative basis.
▶ **Milk Group**—Fortified milk, yogurt and cheeses are used to provide protein, vitamin B_{12}, and vitamin D. Use amounts recommended in the "Basic Food Groups".
▶ **Bread and Cereal Group**—Increase amounts to 3–6 servings per day. Use cereals and whole grain products for provision of protein, iron and B vitamins.
▶ **Fruit and Vegetable Group**—Provide 2–3 servings of fruit per day and 3 servings of vegetables per day of the variety recommended in the "Basic Food Groups".

Lacto-Vegetarian

Same as in lacto-ovo-vegetarian recommendations with the exception of eggs in the Meat Group.

Vegan

▶ **Meat Group**—Same as in lacto-ovo-vegetarian recommendations with the exception of eggs.
▶ **Milk Group**—Substitute fortified soybean milk (2 cups per day) to supply protein, calcium, riboflavin, and vitamin B_{12}.
▶ **Bread and Cereal Group**—Same as in lacto-ovo-vegetarian recommendations including 3–5 servings of whole grains and one serving of seeds in addition to 3 or more slices of bread.
▶ **Fruit and Vegetable Group**—At least 4 servings of vegetables and 2–4 servings of fruit, including a good source of vitamin C daily. Good sources of calcium and riboflavin are dark green leafy vegetables, legumes, nuts and dried fruits.

Sufficient protein can be achieved in vegetarian diets by consuming a variety of plant protein with complimentary amino acids. The following table can be used for complimentary protein combinations:

► AMINO ACID CONTENT AND COMPLIMENTARY PROTEIN ◄ COMBINATIONS IN VEGETARIAN FOOD GROUPS

Food Group	Limiting Amino Acids	Abundant Amino Acids	Examples of Complimentary Protein Combinations
Legumes	Methionine Tryptophan	Lysine Threonine Isoleucine	Kidney beans and rice; soybeans, rice and wheat; black bean soup and corn tortillas; lima beans and corn; chickpeas and sesame seeds: lentils and cheese
Grains	Lysine Isoleucine Threonine	Methionine Tryptophan	Rice and black-eyed peas; brown bread and baked beans; brown rice and tofu; wheat bread and peanut butter with milk; macaroni and cheese
Vegetables	Methionine Isoleucine	Lysine Tryptophan	Broccoli and sesame seeds; cauliflower and cheese; Brussel sprouts and rice; corn and milk
Nuts and Seeds	Lysine Isoleucine	Methionine Tryptophan	Sesame seeds and black-eyed peas; sunflower seeds and cheese

Source: Massachusetts General Hospital Department of Dietetics, Boston: Diet Reference Manual. Boston: Little, Brown and Company, 1984.

Sample Menu
Lacto-Ovo-Vegetarian
(For Lacto-Vegetarian and Vegan diets, make substitutions listed previously)

Breakfast	Lunch	Supper
Orange Juice	Vegetable Lasagna	Lite Cheese Quiche
Oatmeal	Spinach Salad	Green Beans
Scrambled Egg	Wheat Roll	Fruit Gelatin Salad
Bran Muffin	Angel Food Cake	Lowfat Frozen Yogurt
Margarine	Margarine	Whole Grain Bread
2% Milk	2% Milk	Margarine
Coffee	Iced Tea	Iced Tea
Creamer	Sugar	Sugar
Sugar		

Protein Complements

Dairy products, soy products, fish, poultry, and meat are complete proteins—that is, they contain all the essential amino acids that the body requires to build proteins in our bodies. Nuts and seeds, grains, vegetables, and legumes are incomplete proteins. An incomplete protein has only some of the essential amino acids that the body requires. Therefore, incomplete proteins may combine with each other or a complete protein to become a complete protein.

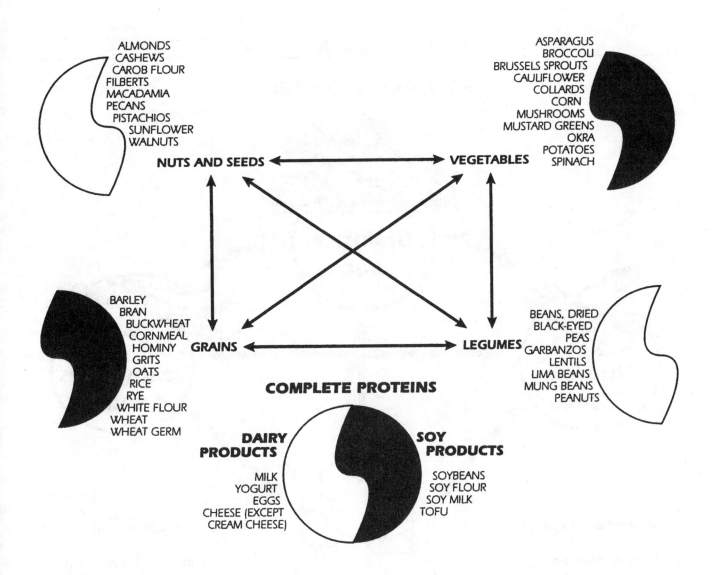

ALMONDS
CASHEWS
CAROB FLOUR
FILBERTS
MACADAMIA
PECANS
PISTACHIOS
SUNFLOWER
WALNUTS

NUTS AND SEEDS

ASPARAGUS
BROCCOLI
BRUSSELS SPROUTS
CAULIFLOWER
COLLARDS
CORN
MUSHROOMS
MUSTARD GREENS
OKRA
POTATOES
SPINACH

VEGETABLES

BARLEY
BRAN
BUCKWHEAT
CORNMEAL
HOMINY
GRITS
OATS
RICE
RYE
WHITE FLOUR
WHEAT
WHEAT GERM

GRAINS

LEGUMES

BEANS, DRIED
BLACK-EYED
PEAS
GARBANZOS
LENTILS
LIMA BEANS
MUNG BEANS
PEANUTS

COMPLETE PROTEINS

DAIRY PRODUCTS

SOY PRODUCTS

MILK
YOGURT
EGGS
CHEESE (EXCEPT
CREAM CHEESE)

SOYBEANS
SOY FLOUR
SOY MILK
TOFU

PROTEIN COMBINING

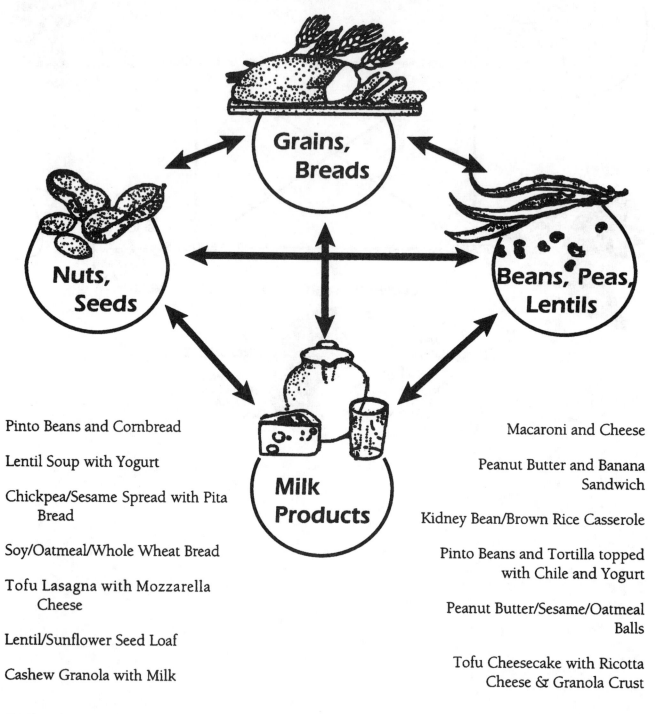

Pinto Beans and Cornbread

Lentil Soup with Yogurt

Chickpea/Sesame Spread with Pita Bread

Soy/Oatmeal/Whole Wheat Bread

Tofu Lasagna with Mozzarella Cheese

Lentil/Sunflower Seed Loaf

Cashew Granola with Milk

Macaroni and Cheese

Peanut Butter and Banana Sandwich

Kidney Bean/Brown Rice Casserole

Pinto Beans and Tortilla topped with Chile and Yogurt

Peanut Butter/Sesame/Oatmeal Balls

Tofu Cheesecake with Ricotta Cheese & Granola Crust

References

American Dietetic Association: Manual of Clinical Dietetics, Chicago: 1988.

Aspen Reference Group: Dietitian's Patient Education Manual. Sara Nell DiLima, ed., Gaithersburg: Aspen Publishers, Inc., 1993.

Circulation, October 1996; AHA Press Release 10/1/96; AHA Scientific Position: "Dietary Guidelines for Healthy American Adults".

Dallas–Fort Worth Hospital Council: Dallas–Fort Worth Hospital Council Diet Manual. Irving: 1992.

Puckett, R.P. and Brown, S.M.: Shands Hospital at the University of Florida Guide to Clinical Dietetics, 5th ed., Dubuque: Kendall/Hunt Publishing co., 1993.

Rodwell, W.S.: Nutrition and Diet Therapy, 7th ed., St. Louis: Mosby-Yearbook, Inc., 1993.

▶ REGULAR PEDIATRIC DIET ◀

Description

This diet is designed to meet the nutritional needs of growing children 4 years and older. All foods and beverages are allowed except coffee, strong tea and those foods highly seasoned. Foods should be prepared in a variety of ways with moderate seasonings.

Adequacy

This diet meets the 1989 Recommended Dietary Allowance for good nutrition as established by the Food and Nutrition Board of the National Research Council when the types of foods and amounts suggested are included daily.

Type of Foods	Foods Allowed	Foods Not Allowed
Milk (3 or more cups)	Milk (all types), yogurt	None
Meat, Fish, Poultry, and Meat Substitutes (4 ounces or more daily)	Lean tender beef, chicken, turkey, pork and veal; fish without small bones, mild cheeses, peanut butter, hot dogs cut into strips	Highly seasoned meats or any with small bones, whole hot dogs
Eggs (Limit to 4 per week)	Eggs prepared any way except raw and soft cooked	Raw
Fruits (2 or more servings–include citrus daily)	All fruit juices; fresh, frozen or canned fruits	Fruits with seeds or tough skin, whole grapes*
Vegetables (2 or more servings—Include a dark green leafy or deep yellow vegetable 3–4 times daily)	Fresh, frozen or canned vegetables or juices	Raw carrot* or celery sticks*
Bread, Cereal, Rice and Pasta (6 or more servings)	Any whole grain or enriched breads or crackers	Excessive use of sweet rolls and doughnuts
	Any whole grain or enriched cereal (cooked or ready-to-eat)	Excessive use of presweetened cereals; any dry coarse cereal containing nuts* or hard, dry fruit*; highly seasoned rice or pasta mixtures
Fats and Oil	Margarine or butter, cream, gravy, oil, lard, vegetable shortening, mayonnaise, salad dressings, olive*	Excessive use of fats
Soups	Any made with allowed foods	Any highly seasoned soups made with foods to be omitted
Desserts (use in moderation)	Cakes, cookies, puddings, custards, gelatin, ice cream, sherbet, and pie	Excessive use of desserts; any with nuts*

Type of Foods	Foods Allowed	Foods Not Allowed
Beverages	Water, fruit juice, fruit drink, and carbonated beverages (limited)	Coffee, tea, and excessive use of carbonated beverages and sweetened fruit flavored drinks
Miscellaneous	Salt, sugar, honey, jelly, syrup, chocolate, cocoa, catsup, mustard, pickles and vinegar; condiments, herbs, mild spices, and cream sauce	Excessive amounts of pepper, spices, salt or sugar

*These foods may be appropriate for older school age children if caution is used to avoid choking and ensure food safety.

Sample Menu

Breakfast	Lunch	Supper
Orange Juice	Sloppy Joe on Bun	Roast Turkey
Oatmeal	Carrot Slices	Buttered Rice
Scrambled Egg	Tossed Salad with	Green Peas
Toast–Margarine	French Dressing	Roll–Margarine
Jelly	Peach	Custard
Milk	Milk	Milk

References

Dallas–Fort Worth Hospital Council: Dallas–Fort Worth Hospital Council Diet Manual. Irving: 1992.

Puckett, R.P. and Brown, S.M.: Shands Hospital at the University of Florida Guide to Clinical Dietetics, 5th ed., Dubuque: Kendall/Hunt Publishing Co., 1993.

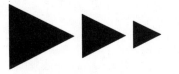

Modification for Consistency/Texture

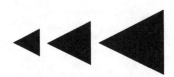

▶ SOFT DIET ◀

Description

This diet is designed for patients who are unable to chew or swallow hard or coarse foods. The soft diet can be used for a postoperative patient who is too ill to tolerate a regular diet. Tender foods are used (not ground or pureed) unless the individual needs additional modifications. Most raw fruits and vegetables and coarse breads and cereals are eliminated. Fried foods and highly seasoned foods are limited based on individual tolerance. Food tolerances vary with individuals; therefore, it is important that food selection be guided by individual tolerances.

Adequacy

This diet meets the 1989 Recommended Dietary Allowances for good nutrition as established by the Food and Nutrition Board of the National Research Council when the types of foods and amounts suggested are included daily.

Type of Foods	Foods Allowed	Foods Not Allowed
Milk (2 or more cups daily)	Milk–any kind, yogurt–with allowed fruits, hot chocolate and milk beverages	None
Meat, Poultry, Fish and Meat Substitutes (6 ounces daily)	Baked, broiled, roasted, or stewed tender and mildly seasoned meat, s hellfish, poultry. Smooth peanut butter. Cottage cheese, creamed and American cheeses if tolerated; soybean, tofu and other meat substitutes. Casseroles and meat salads (no pickles or raw fruit or vegetables)	Fried and tough or fibrous meats, poultry and fish; highly seasoned, cured or smoked meats, fish or poultry such as; corned beef, ham, luncheon meats, frankfurters, and other sausages; sardines anchovies, strongly flavored cheeses and chunky peanut butter
Eggs	Eggs, including fried if tolerated	Fried eggs, unless tolerated
Fruits (2 or more servings daily–include citrus daily)	All fruit juices; cooked, canned or frozen fruits without skins or seeds, such as apples, apricots, cherries, peaches, pears, orange and grapefruit sections without membranes; fresh ripe banana, peeled ripe pears and peaches	All other fresh and dried fruits
Vegetables (3 or more servings daily–1 serving dark green leafy or deep yellow vegetables 3–4 times weekly)	All vegetable juices; cooked or canned vegetables as tolerated; lettuce, tomato (no skin or seeds) in small quantities. Potatoes: (white or sweet) without skin-baked, mashed or boiled. Limit strongly flavored vegetables as tolerated: broccoli, brussel sprouts, cabbage, onions, cauliflower, cucumbers, rutabagas, turnips, green pepper and sauerkraut.	All other raw vegetables; dried peas and beans. Potato chips, fried potatoes, and potato skins

Type of Foods	Foods Allowed	Foods Not Allowed
Bread, Cereal, Rice, and Pasta (6 or more servings daily)	Enriched, refined white, whole wheat or rye breads, rolls, biscuits, plain muffins, saltines, graham crackers, rusk, melba toast, Zwieback® crackers, cornbread, waffles, French toast	Coarse, whole grain breads with seeds, nuts, raisins or dried fruits; other hot breads; all other crackers and popcorn.
	Enriched, refined, cooked or ready-to-eat cereals (corn, oats, rice, wheat), which do not contain coconut, nuts, dried fruits and seeds	Whole grain, bran and granola type cereals
	Enriched rice, spaghetti, noodles, macaroni and other pastas	Wild rice
Fats and Oil	Fortified margarine or butter, oils, mayonnaise, mild salad dressings, cream, crisp bacon, mildly flavored gravies, non-dairy creamers	Strongly flavored salad dressings and gravies, nuts
Soups	Broth, bouillon and consomme; cream and broth based soups made with allowed ingredients	Highly seasoned soups
Desserts	Plain cakes and cookies (thinly iced if desired), plain puddings, custards, ice cream, sherbet, soft brownies made without nuts and plain gelatin or made with allowed foods	Pastries, pies and desserts containing nuts, coconut, dried fruits and seeds
Beverages	Regular and decaffeinated coffee and tea; carbonated beverages and fruit drinks	None
Miscellaneous	Salt, flavorings, mildly flavored sauces pepper, herbs, spices, catsup, mustard vinegar (in moderation), whipped toppings, syrup, honey, jelly, hard candies, plain chocolate candies, molasses and marshmallows	Strongly flavored seasonings and condiments such as garlic barbeque sauce, chili sauce, chili pepper and horseradish; pickles, relishes, olives, nuts, coconut, jams, preserves and marmalades

Sample Menu

Breakfast	Lunch	Supper
Orange Juice	Cream of Mushroom Soup	Sliced Turkey
Cornflakes	Roast Beef	Yellow Rice
Poached Egg	Baked Potato (no skin)	Spinach
Toast–Margarine	Green Beans	Bread–Margarine
Jelly	Dinner Roll–Margarine	Orange Sherbet
Milk	Peach Halves	Iced Tea–Sugar
Coffee–Sugar	Milk	
	Iced Tea–Sugar	

References

American Dietetic Association: Manual of Clinical Dietetics. Chicago; 1988.

Mahan, K. and Arlin, M.: Krause's Food, Nutrition and Diet Therapy. 8th ed., Philadelphia: W.B. Saunders Company, 1993.

Pemberton, C., Moxness, K., German, M., Nelson. J., and Gastineau, C.: Mayo Clinic Diet Manual A Handbook of Dietary Practices. 6th ed. Toronto: B.C. Decker, Inc., 1988.

Puckett, R.P. and Brown, S.M.: Shands Hospital at the University of Florida Guide to Clinical Dietetics. 5th ed. Dubuque: Kendall/Hunt Publishing Co., 1992.

► SURGICAL SOFT DIET ◄

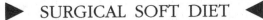

Description

This diet is designed to provide foods that are easy to chew and are moderately low in fiber or connective tissue. The surgical soft diet may be used as a progression from liquids to regular diet following surgery or G.I. disturbance. It consists of foods that require only minimal or moderate amounts of digestive activity. Fried foods, most raw fruits and vegetables, coarse breads and cereals, and very highly seasoned foods are omitted.

Adequacy

This diet meets the 1989 Recommended Dietary Allowance for good nutrition as established by the Food and Nutrition Board of the National Research Council when the types of foods and amounts suggested are included daily. Females, ages 11–50 should include a good source of iron daily.

Type of Foods	Foods Allowed	Foods Not Allowed
Milk (2 or more cups daily)	Milk, buttermilk, milkshakes, eggnogs, yogurt with allowed fruit and milk products	None
Meat, Poultry, Fish and Meat Substitutes (6 ounces daily)	Baked, broiled, roasted, or stewed tender meat, fish, shellfish, poultry. Smooth peanut butter. Cottage cheese, creamed and mildly flavored American cheeses if tolerated; soybean and other meat substitutes	Fried and tough or fiberous meats, poultry and fish; highly seasoned, cured or smoked meats, fish or poultry such as; corned beef, ham, luncheon meats, hot dogs, frankfurters and other sausages; sardines, anchovies, strongly flavored cheeses and chunky peanut butter
Eggs	Egg substitute, or eggs	Fried eggs
Fruits (2 or more servings daily include citrus daily)	All fruit juices; cooked, canned or frozen fruits without skins or seeds, such as apples, apricots, cherries, peaches, pears, fresh ripe banana	All other fresh and dried fruits

Type of Foods	Foods Allowed	Foods Not Allowed
Vegetables (3 or more servings–1 serving dark green leafy or deep yellow vegetable 3–4 times weekly)	All vegetable juices; well cooked asparagus, beets, green or waxed beans, carrots, tender green peas, spinach, and winter squash. Potatoes: baked (without skin), boiled, mashed, or creamed	Raw vegetables, dried peas and beans, corn, gas-forming vegetables such as broccoli, brussel sprouts, cabbage, onions, cauliflower, cucumbers, rutabagas, turnip, and sauerkraut. Potato chips, fried potatoes
Bread, Cereal, Rice, and Pasta (6 or more servings daily)	Enriched, refined white, whole wheat or rye breads, plain muffins, saltines, graham crackers, rusk, melba toast, Zwieback® crackers	Coarse, whole grain breads with seeds, nuts, raisins or dried fruits; hot breads; all other crackers and popcorn
	Enriched, refined, cooked or ready-to-eat cereals (corn, oats, rice, wheat), which do not contain coconut, nuts, dried fruits, seeds, and bran	Whole grain, bran and granola type cereals
	Enriched rice, spaghetti, noodles, and macaroni	Wild rice and other not listed as allowed
Fats and Oil	Fortified margarine or butter, oils, mayonnaise, cream	Strongly flavored salad dressings, nuts, and bacon
Soups	Broth, bouillon, and consomme; cream and broth based soups made with allowed ingredients	Highly seasoned soups and those made with foods omitted
Desserts	Plain cakes and cookies (thinly iced if desired), plain puddings, custards, ice cream, sherbet, and gelatin made with allowed foods	Pastries, pies, and desserts containing nuts, coconut dried fruits, or seeds
Beverages	Coffee, coffee substitute, tea, carbonated beverages, fruit flavored beverages	None
Miscellaneous	Salt, flavorings, mildly flavored gravies, or sauces, pepper, herbs, spices, catsup, mustard, vinegar (in moderation), whipped toppings, syrup, honey, jelly hard candies, plain chocolate candies, molasses and marshmallows	Strongly flavored seasonings and condiments such as garlic, barbeque sauce, chili sauce, chili pepper, and horseradish; pickles, relishes, olives, nuts, coconut, jams, preserves, and marmalades

Sample Menu

Breakfast	Lunch	Supper
Orange Juice	Cream of Tomato Soup	Sliced Turkey
Cornflakes	with Crackers	Yellow Rice
Scrambled Egg	Roast Beef	Carrots
Toast–Margarine	Baked Potato (no skin)	Bread–Margarine
Jelly	Green Beans	Orange Sherbet
Milk	Dinner Roll–Margarine	Iced Tea–Sugar
Coffee–Sugar	Peach Halves	
	Milk	
	Iced Tea–Sugar	

References

Mahan, K. and Arlin, M.: *Krause's Food, Nutrition and Diet Therapy*. 8th ed., Philadelphia: W.B. Saunders Company, 1992.

Pemberton, C., Moxness, K., German, M., Nelson, J., and Gastineau, C.: *Mayo Clinic Diet Manual A Handbook of Dietary Practices*. 6th ed. Toronto: B.C. Decker, Inc., 1988.

▶ MECHANICAL SOFT DIET ◀

Description

The mechanical soft diet is designed for individuals with poor dentition, difficulty swallowing, and stomatitis. The soft diet serves as the basis for planning the diet with certain modifications in consistency. Depending upon patient tolerance, tender whole, chopped, ground, or pureed foods may be required. The patient must be visited by the dietitian to determine the required consistency of foods.

Adequacy

This diet meets the 1989 Recommended Dietary Allowance for good nutrition as established by the Food and Nutrition Board of the National Research Council when the types of foods and amounts suggested are included daily.

Sample Menu

Breakfast	Lunch	Supper
Orange Juice	Cream of Tomato Soup	Meatloaf
Oatmeal	with Crackers	Buttered Rice
Scrambled Egg	Chopped Chicken and Gravy	Asparagus with Cheese Sauce
Toast–Margarine	Mashed Potatoes	Bread–Margarine
Jelly	Buttered Carrots	Chocolate Pudding
Milk	Dinner Roll–Margarine	Milk
Coffee–Sugar	Peach Halves	Iced Tea–Sugar
	Milk	
	Iced Tea–Sugar	

References

American Dietetic Association: *Manual of Clinical Dietetics*. Chicago: 1988.

Pemberton, C., Moxness, K., German, M., Nelson, J., and Gastineau, C.: *Mayo Clinic Diet Manual A Handbook of Dietary Practices*. 6th ed., Toronto: B.C. Decker, Inc., 1988.

Puckett, R.P. and Brown, S.M.: *Shands Hospital at the University of Florida Guide to Clinical Dietetics*. 5th ed., Dubuque: Kendall/Hunt Publishing Co., 1993.

▶ PUREED DIET ◀

Description

This diet is designed to provide foods that require minimal or no chewing and to increase the ease of swallowing food. All foods are blenderized or strained unless already in a comparatively smooth form such as pudding or mashed potatoes.

Adequacy

This diet meets the 1989 Recommended Dietary Allowance for good nutrition as established by the Food and Nutrition Board of the National Research Council when the types of foods and amounts suggested are included daily.

Type of Foods	Foods Allowed	Foods Not Allowed
Milk (2 or more cups daily)	Skim milk, 1% and 2% milk, whole milk, plain yogurt, cocoa, and milk beverages	All others
Meat, Poultry, Fish and Meat Substitutes (6 oz. daily)	Beef, lamb, veal, liver, lean pork, chicken, turkey, fish without bones (all should be pureed or strained and may be served in broth or cream sauce); mild cheddar or processed cheese may be melted and served in a sauce, souffles made with strained meats	Meat, fish, poultry not prepared as indicated; fatty pork, ham or bacon; spiced or smoked meat or fish; sharp or strongly flavored cheese; crunchy peanut butter
Eggs	Eggs	Fried eggs
Fruits (2 or more servings daily)	Fruit juices and nectars; mashed banana; all other fruits that are cooked and pureed	Tart fruit juice which is irritating to mouth or throat; raw fruit except banana; fruit that is not pureed
Vegetables (3 or more servings daily–include a dark green leafy or deep yellow vegetable 3–4 times weekly)	All vegetable juices; cooked and pureed asparagus, beets, green and wax beans, carrots, corn, lima beans, peas, pumpkin, spinach, squash, tomatoes; souffles made with allowed strained vegetables; mashed or well cooked white potatoes and mashed sweet potatoes	All raw vegetables; all others Potatoes with skin, prepared in highly spicy sauces or fried; all others
Breads, Cereals, Rice, and Pasta (6 or more servings daily)	Enriched white bread or toast, saltines, and graham crackers if tolerated Refined cooked cereals such as cornmeal, farina, rice, and oatmeal Hominy, rice, spaghetti, macaroni, or noodles if pureed and thinned with a sauce	All breads unless tolerated Whole grain cereals except oatmeal; other prepared cereals unless tolerated All others
Fats and Oil	Butter, margarine, cream, vegetable shortening and oils, lard, bland salad dressing, and white sauce	Strongly flavored salad dressings and nuts

Type of Foods	Foods Allowed	Foods Not Allowed
Soups	Cream soups made with pureed foods, broth type soups (strained)	Spicy soups or those containing pieces of whole meat or vegetables
Desserts	Plain cornstarch, rice and tapioca puddings; custards, ice cream, sherbert gelatin desserts; fruit whips, fruit ice and popsicles	Pastries, pies; any desserts containing nuts, raisins, coconut, or fruit that is not pureed
Beverages	Coffee, tea, jello, water, cereal beverages, or any liquids tolerated by the patient	All others not tolerated by patient
Miscellaneous	Salt, mild flavorings, cinnamon, chocolate and cocoa in moderation, cream sauce, gravy, sugar, syrup, honey, clear jelly and plain candies	Horseradish, pepper, nuts, coconut, olives, pickles, relish, catsup, mustard, popcorn, vinegar, chili sauce, excessive amounts of spices or herbs; jam, preserves and candies containing nuts, seeds or tough skins

Sample Menu

Breakfast	Lunch	Supper
Strained Orange Juice	Strained Cream of Pea Soup	Strained Cream of Tomato Soup
Cream of Wheat	Pureed Lamb	Alaskan Seafood Souffle
Soft Scrambled Egg	Mashed Potatoes	Mashed Potatoes
Bread–Margarine	Pureed Carrots	Pureed Beets
Milk	Ice Cream	Baby Peaches
Coffee–Sugar	Bread–Margarine	Bread–Margarine
	Milk	Milk
	Iced Tea–Sugar	Iced Tea–Sugar

References

Chicago Dietetic Association and South Suburban Dietetic Association, *Manual of Clinical Dietetics,* American Dietetic Association, Chicago, 1988.

Puckett, R.P. and Brown, S.M.: *Shands Hospital at the University of Florida Guide to Clinical Dietetics,* 5th ed., Dubuque: Kendall/Hunt Publishing Co., 1993.

▶ FULL LIQUID DIET ◀

Description

This diet provides foods that are liquid to semi liquid at room or body temperature. It is used for patients postoperatively, esophageal or stomach disorders, mastication problems, dysphagia, testing of gastric motility, dental surgery, those patients who can not tolerate regular solid foods, and to provide a transitional diet between clear liquids and solid foods. This diet consists of a large percent of milk and milk based products and may not be tolerated by patients who have a lactose intolerance.

Adequacy

This diet may be inadequate in fiber, niacin, folacin and iron according to the National Research Council's Recommended Dietary Allowances. The nutritional adequacy of the diet may be improved with the use of a high protein, high calorie supplement. Because this diet is inadequate in fiber, constipation may result from its prolonged use. A fiber rich liquid supplement may be useful. Lactose free beverages/supplements should be used for patients with lactose intolerance. A nutritional consult with the dietitian is recommended if a full liquid diet is to be used for longer than three days. If the diet is used for an extended period of time, two–three weeks, a vitamin/mineral supplement in a liquid form is recommended.

Type of Foods	Foods Allowed	Foods Not Allowed
Milk (3 or more cups/day)	All milk and milk drinks such as milkshakes and eggnogs made from commercial mix, yogurt–plain or flavored without seeds or fruit pieces	None
Meat, Fish, Poultry and Meat Substitutes	Puree meat may be added to broth or cream soup	All others
Eggs	Eggs in custard	Raw eggs
Fruits (2 or more servings/day, include citrus daily)	All fruit juices	All others
Vegetables (3 or more servings daily)	All vegetable juices (regular or low sodium), puree vegetables, or mashed potatoes added to broth or cream soup	All others
Bread, Cereal, Rice and Pasta (1 or more serving/day)	Strained whole grain cereals, gruels, refined cooked cereals	All others
Fats and Oils (as desired)	Butter or fortified margarine, cream, vegetable oil, non-dairy creamer, whipped topping, gravy	All others
Soups (at least 2 servings/day	Broth, bouillon, strained cream soup	All others
Dessert (at least 3 servings/day	Custard, ice cream, pudding, sherbet, plain flavored gelatin, Junket, popsicles, Bavarian cream, frozen yogurt (without fruit pieces and nuts), clear candies	All others and any made with coconut, nuts, seeds or whole fruit

Type of Foods	Foods Allowed	Foods Not Allowed
Beverages (as desired)	All beverages, coffee, tea (regular and decaffeinated), carbonated beverages (regular or diet), cocoa, fruit drink, cereal drink, High protein–High calorie liquid supplements	None
Miscellaneous (as desired)	Salt, spices in moderation, flavorings, syrups, sugar, honey	Pepper, chili powder, meat sauces and all other seasoning and condiments

Sample Menu

Breakfast	Lunch	Supper
Orange Juice Cream of Wheat Milk Coffee–Sugar	Strained Cream Soup Low Sodium Tomato Juice Flavored Gelatin Milk Tea–Sugar	Strained Cream Soup Ice Cream Milk Apple Juice Coffee–Sugar–Cream

Between meal snack may be appropriate especially if additional protein, vitamins and minerals are required.

References

American Dietetic Association: *Manual of Clinical Dietetics,* Chicago, 1988.

Dallas–Fort Worth Hospital Council: *Dallas–Fort Worth Hospital Council Diet Manual.* Irving: 1992.

Florida Dietetic Association, *Diet Manual, Manual of Clinical Dietetics,* 1990.

Mahan, K. and Arlin, M.: *Krause's Food, Nutrition and Diet Therapy,* 8th. ed., Philadelphia: W.B. Saunders Co., 1992.

Puckett, R.P. and Brown, S.M.: *Shands Hospital at the University of Florida Guide to Clinical Dietetics.* 5th ed., Dubuque: Kendall/Hunt Publishing Co., 1993.

Thomas Jefferson University Hospital Nutrition Manual, Department of Nutrition and Dietetics, Philadelphia, Pennsylvania, 1993.

University of Michigan Hospitals, Food and Nutrition Services, *Guidelines for Nutritional Care,* Ann Arbor, 1995.

William S. Rodwell, *Nutrition and Diet Therapy,* 7th. Edition, Mosby Yearbook, Inc., 1993.

▶ CLEAR LIQUID DIET ◀

Description

This diet provides oral liquid foods that are easily digested and leave a minimal residue in the gastrointestinal tract. Indications for use are preparation for surgery or diagnostic test, post operative patients, nausea, diarrhea, partial intestinal obstruction, relief of thirst and minimized stimulation of the gastrointestinal tract. All foods are liquid at room and/or body temperature. Recent evidence suggests chemically formulated nutritional residue supplements (such as *Ensure, *Ensure Plus, *Sustacal and *Sustacal HC) may be used in certain diagnostic test procedures and preoperatively for bowel surgery in place of or in addition to a clear liquid diet.

Adequacy

This diet is inadequate when compared to the 1989 Recommended Daily Allowances for calories, protein, calcium, phosphorous, thiamine, iron, riboflavin, niacin, and Vitamins A and D. In general, this diet should be used no longer than two days. If a clear liquid diet is to be used longer than three days, it is recommended that a multi-vitamin and mineral supplement in a liquid form be used and a nutrition consult with a dietitian be ordered.

Type of Foods	Foods Allowed	Foods Not Allowed
Milk	None	All
Meat, Fish, Poultry and Meat Substitutes	None	All
Eggs	None	All
Fruits	All strained fruit juices (apple, pineapple, orange, grapefruit, cranberry, grape, blended)	Fruit juice with pulp, nectars and all fruits
Vegetables	None	All
Bread, Cereal, Rice and Pasta	None	All
Fats and Oil	None	All
Soup	Clear broth, consomme, bouillon	All others
Desserts	Plain and flavored gelatin, ices, popsicles, clear candies	All others
Beverages	Tea and coffee (regular or decaffeinated), gingerale, *7-Up, *Gatorade, Kool-Aid, *Citrotein (high protein, high calorie oral supplement), fruit flavored drinks	All others
Miscellaneous	Salt, sugar, lemon juice, sugar substitute	All others

*Registered trademark-Brand name used for clarification and does not constitute endorsement of the product.

Sample Menu

Breakfast	Lunch	Supper
Strained Orange Juice	Strained Pineapple Juice	Strained Apple Juice
Beef Broth	Chicken Broth	Beef Broth
Gelatin	Gelatin	Gelatin
Coffee–Sugar	Iced Tea–Sugar	Iced Tea–Sugar

References

American Dietetic Association: *Manual of Clinical Dietetics,* Chicago, 1988.

Dallas–Fort Worth Hospital Council: *Dallas–Fort Worth Hospital Council Diet Manual.* Irving: 1992.

Florida Dietetic Association, *Diet Manual, Manual of Clinical Dietetics,* 1990.

Mahan, K. and Arlin, M.: *Krause's Food, Nutrition and Diet Therapy,* 8th. ed., Philadelphia: W.B. Saunders Co., 1992.

Puckett, R.P. and Brown, S.M.: *Shands Hospital at the University of Florida Guide to Clinical Dietetics.* 5th ed., Dubuque: Kendall/Hunt Publishing Co., 1993.

Thomas Jefferson University Hospital Nutrition Manual, Department of Nutrition and Dietetics, Philadelphia, Pennsylvania, 1993.

University of Michigan Hospitals, Food and Nutrition Services, *Guidelines for Nutritional Care,* Ann Arbor, 1995.

William S. Rodwell, *Nutrition and Diet Therapy,* 7th. Edition, Mosby Yearbook, Inc., 1993.

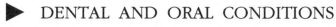

► DENTAL AND ORAL CONDITIONS ◄

Description

Clues to the general health and nutritional status of the patient are often provided by a careful examination of the teeth, gums, and soft tissues of the mouth and jaw. Nutritional deficiency states may manifest from dental caries, gingivitis, periodontal disease, stomatitis, glossitis, cheilosis, xerostomia, glossopyrosis or other conditions. Rarely, can these conditions be found to be directly related to a specific mineral deficiency or an avitaminosis. Usually, the condition involves the deficiency of several nutrients.

Many of the above oral conditions may lead to nutritional deficiency states by preventing the proper mastication of food. People with a diminished ability to chew properly are more prone to nutritional deficiencies, not because the foods eaten are incompletely digested, but because of their inadequate food selection process. For instance, an elderly patient with poorly fitting dentures may be more likely to select a diet based largely on milk products, which are low in iron.

Depending on the dietitian's analysis of the patient's nutritional status and the patient's dental and oral health, prescribed diets may range from full liquid to regular and include the use of nutritional supplements.

Adequacy

A nutrition consultation should be completed so that the registered dietitian can individually evaluate each patient's case. Recommendations for the use of nutritional supplements administered orally or enterally may be necessary to ensure adequate intake.

Common Oral Problems that Diminish Masticatory Ability

Absence of Teeth
▶ Edentulism without dentures
▶ Partial edentulism
▶ Ill-fitting dentures

Recent Trauma and Painful Dental Treatments
▶ Orthodontic manipulations
▶ Oral surgery, including jaw immobilization, mouth-open wounds (post extractions), radical cancer surgery

Hereditary and Developmental Jaw Deformities
▶ Cleft lip and palate
▶ Tooth malformations
▶ Ankyloglossia (tongue-tied)

Periodontal Disease
▶ Mobile teeth
▶ Sore, bleeding gums
▶ Periodontitis

Painful Oral Lesions and Infections
▶ Herpetic ulcers/aphthae
▶ Periodontal abscesses
▶ Vitamin deficiencies–especially B and C
▶ Gum changes in leukemia
▶ Uncontrolled diabetes
▶ Chemical burns, food burns, or abrasions
▶ Neoplasia
▶ Salivary gland infection (mumps)
▶ Stomatitis from chemotherapy
▶ Partially erupted teeth

Masticatory Muscle Pain/Hypofunction
▶ Malocclusion
▶ Arthritis
▶ Limited jaw opening
▶ Muscle atrophy

Neurological Disorders
▶ Glossodynia
▶ Facial paralysis
▶ Glossopyrosis (burning tongue syndrome)
▶ Cerebral palsy
▶ Trigeminal neuralgia

For further information about Dental and Oral Conditions, refer to the recent American Dietetic Association Report entitled:

Position of the American Dietetic Association: Oral Health and Nutrition, February, 1996, Volume 96, Number 2, pg. 184–189, Journal of the American Dietetic Association.

References

Pemberton, C.M., Moxness, K.E., German, M.J., Nelson, J.K., Gastineau, C.F., *Rochester Methodist Hospital and Saint Marys Hospital, Mayo Clinic Diet Manual: A Handbook of Dietary Practices,* (6th ed), B.C. Decker, Inc., Toronto, pp. 53–54, 1988.

Puckett, R.P. and Brown, S.M.: *Shands Hospital at the University of Florida Guide to Clinical Dietetics.* 5th ed., Dubuque: Kendall/Hunt Publishing Co., 1993.

▶ DIETS FOR OTORHINOLARYNGOLOGICAL DISORDERS ◀

This section of the manual contains diets which are frequently used in the care of patients with otorhinolaryngological disorders. The dietary needs of these patients are special because of the nature of these illnesses. Nutritional intake is often inadequate due to:

1. Loss of appetite.
2. Chewing and swallowing difficulties.
3. Interference of sensory mechanisms (diminished taste and smell).
4. Patients' psychological reaction to change in body image or temporary dysfunction of aerodigestive tract.

The chart below is a guide for the various diets ordered in the care of patients with head and neck disorders. The diet is dependant upon the physician's order and the patient's tolerance.

Surgical Procedure	Appropriate Diet Order
Laryngectomy	Tube feedings, High Protein
Hemilaryngectomy	High Calorie Liquid, Soft
Tonsillectomy—Adult,	T&A Liquid, no citrus, no hot food,
Pediatric	T&A Soft
Repairs of:	
Zygomatic Fractures	High Protein High Calorie Dental Liquid
Trimalar Fractures	
Maxillary Fractures	
Mandibular Fractures	
Nasal Fractures	
Reconstructive Procedures:	
Verminellimectomy	High Protein High Calorie Dental Liquid
Mandibulectomy	Tube Feeding, High Protein High Calorie Dental Liquid
Palate Resection	Tube Feeding, High Protein High Calorie Dental Liquid
Rhytidectomy	High Protein High Calorie Liquid, Soft
Septoplasty	High Protein High Calorie Liquid, Soft
Facial Plastic	High Protein High Calorie Dental Liquid
Post Head & Neck Radiation	High Protein High Calorie Dental Liquid
Epitaxis	High Protein High Calorie Dental Liquid, Mechanical Soft, Soft

► HIGH CALORIE HIGH PROTEIN DENTAL LIQUID ◄

Description

This diet is indicated following surgical wiring of the oral cavity and following facial trauma or oral reconstructive surgery. This diet requires a minimal amount of chewing for those patients with intramaxillary facial trauma. Foods must be pureed and thinned. It is high in protein and calories. There is an increased need for dietary protein (1.2–2.0 gm/kg current body weight) and calories (35–45 kcal/kg current body weight) to promote proper wound healing and prevent protein depletion.

Adequacy

This diet meets the 1989 Recommended Dietary Allowance for good nutrition as established by the Food and Nutrition Board of the National Research Council when the types of foods and amounts suggested are included daily.

Type of Foods	Foods Allowed	Foods Not Allowed
Milk (2 or more cups milk daily)	Milk, milk drinks, milkshakes, plain yogurt, hot chocolate (4% milk suggested)	None
Meat, Poultry, Fish and Meat Substitutes (6 ounces daily)	Strained, pureed meats, or cheese thinned with gravy, broth or milk; commercially strained baby meats	All others
Eggs (1 daily)	Cooked, blenderized, and thinned with milk or cream	All others, raw eggs
Fruits (2 or more servings–include citrus daily)	Strained fruit juices; blended and strained fruit; commercially strained baby fruit	All others, juice or fruit containing pulp
Vegetables (3 or more servings–include a dark green leafy or deep yellow vegetable 3-4 times weekly)	Strained vegetables thinned with strained vegetable juice, cream or milk; commercially strained baby vegetables and blended potatoes	All others
Breads, Cereals, Rice, and Pasta	Cream of wheat, farina, grits, cream of rice or strained cooked cereals thinned with water, milk, or cream	All others
Fats and Oil	Cream, butter, margarine, plain gravy, cooking oils, mayonnaise, non-dairy creamer	All others
Soups	Strained or cream soups without solids	All others
Desserts	Plain pudding, custard, junket, ice cream, sherbet, gelatin, frozen yogurt, ice milk	All others
Beverages	Coffee, tea, soft drinks, soft drink mixes	None
Miscellaneous	Sugar, honey, syrup, jelly, salt, pepper herbs, spices, mustard, catsup	All others

Note: Regular foods may be blenderized until liquified in form if desired.

Sample Menu

Breakfast	Lunch	Supper

Apple Juice
Cream of Wheat
  make with Margarine and Milk
Coffee
Sugar
Whole Milk
	Strained Tomato Soup
	  mixed with pureed meat
	Mashed Potatoes thinned
	  with Milk & Margarine
	Pureed Carrots with Margarine
	Ice Cream
	Whole Milk
		Pureed Fruit, thinned
		  with Nectar
		Cream of Chicken Soup
		  mixed with pureed Chicken
		Pureed Green Beans with
		  Margarine
		Pudding, thinned with Milk
		Whole Milk

Mid–Morning/Mid–Afternoon Snack	Evening Snack
Commercial Milkshake Grape Juice	Commercial Milkshake Ice Cream

Reference

Dallas–Fort Worth Hospital Council: *Dallas–Fort Worth Hospital Council Diet Manual.* Irving: 1992.

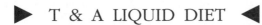

▶ T & A LIQUID DIET ◀

Description

    This diet is for patients who have had a tonsillectomy. The diet is designed to replace fluids, relieve thirst, provide comfort, and help protect against bleeding in the surgical area. A full liquid diet can be served; however, hot beverages and citrus juices must be omitted.

    It should be noted that due to the short convalescent period post-tonsillectomy, the above described diet can be progressed after the first 24 hours. The following are guidelines for feeding post-tonsillectomy:

▶ FOODS BEST TOLERATED POST-OPERATIVELY ◀

First 24 Hours	Greater Than 24 Hours
Cold Milk Milkshakes Eggnog (made with pasteurized eggs) Plain Ice Cream Fruit Ices Sherbet Peach, Pear, or Prune Juice Popsicles	Warm Beverages as tolerated Soft Foods Warm or Hot Foods as tolerated

Adequacy

    This diet may be planned to meet the 1989 Recommended Dietary Allowances for good nutrition as established by the Food and Nutrition Board of the National Research Council if the diet is to be used for an extended period of time.

Sample Menu

Breakfast	Lunch/Supper
Pear Nectar	Gelatin
Gelatin	Ice Cream
Eggnog (made with pasteurized eggs)	Milk
Milk	

Reference

Mahan, K. and Arlin, M.: *Krause's Food, Nutrition and Diet Therapy,* 8th ed., Philadelphia: W.B. Saunders Company, 1992.

► T & A SOFT DIET ◄

Description

This diet is designed for the patient following a tonsillectomy as a progression from the T&A Liquid Diet. The diet is mechanically non-irritating to prevent pharyngeal abrasions and/or unnecessary roughness when swallowing foods. The patient should be instructed to chew foods well. Extra fluids should be provided.

Adequacy

This diet does not meet the 1989 Recommended Dietary Allowance for ascorbic acid as established by the Food and Nutrition Board of the National Research Council.

Type of Foods	Foods Allowed	Foods Not Allowed
Milk (2 or more cups/day)	Milk, milk drinks, yogurt	Hot chocolate
Meat, Poultry, Fish and Meat Substitutes (6 ounces or more daily)	Any ground meat. Very soft ground meat or cheese casseroles, cottage cheese	All others
Eggs (1 daily)	Eggs or Egg Substitute	Fried eggs
Fruits (2 or more servings daily)	Canned peaches, pears or applesauce. Any strained pureed fruit or juice (no citrus)	Citrus and all others not listed
Vegetables (3 or more servings–include a dark green leafy or deep yellow vegetable 3-4 times weekly)	Any pureed vegetable	All others. Tomato or V-8 Juice*
Breads and Cereals	Enriched strained cooked cereals	All others
Fats and Oil	Cream, margarine, butter, plain gravy, cooking oils, mayonnaise, cream cheese, non-dairy creamer	All others
Soups	Any strained or cream soups without solids	All others

Type of Foods	Foods Allowed	Foods Not Allowed
Desserts	Plain jello, pudding, custard, ice cream, and sherbet	All others
Beverages	Carbonated beverages, lukewarm or iced coffee, coffee substitute and tea	All hot beverages, alcohol
Miscellaneous	Salt, seasonings and spices, sugar, honey, syrup, jelly, sauces without solids, plain chocolate and hard candies	All others

Sample Menu

Breakfast	Lunch	Supper
Apple Juice	Strained Cream of Mushroom Soup	Strained Chicken Noodle Soup
Strained Oatmeal	Ground Beef with Gravy	Ground Chicken with Gravy
Scrambled Egg	Mashed Potatoes	Mashed Potatoes
Margarine	Pureed Carrots	Pureed Green Beans
Milk	Margarine	Margarine
	Custard	Applesauce
	Iced Tea–Sugar	Milk
		Iced Tea–Sugar

*Registered trademark. Brand names are used for clarification and do not constitute endorsement of that product.

References

Mahan, K. and Arlin, M.: *Krause's Food, Nutrition and Diet Therapy,* 8th ed., Philadelphia: W.B. Saunders Company, 1992.

Mayo Clinic Diet Manual A Handbook of Dietary Practices, 6th ed., Toronto: B.C. Decker, Inc., 1988.

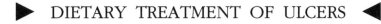

► DIETARY TREATMENT OF ULCERS ◄

Rationale

Research does not support previously held concepts regarding dietary treatment of ulcer disease. Traditionally, milk was advocated for management of patients with peptic–ulcer disease. One study concerning the effect of milk on gastric–acid secretion reported that milk caused a significant increase in acid secretion and its frequent ingestion by ulcer patients should be questioned.

The rationale for the Strict Bland Diet is not supported adequately by scientific data. Therefore, the strict bland diet is no longer included in this manual. The American Dietetic Association Position Paper: Bland Diet in the Treatment of Chronic Duodenal Ulcer Disease (J. Am. Diet. Assoc. 59:244, 1971) discusses controversies related to the treatment of patients with chronic ulcer disease. The diet usually used for ulcers is a regular diet omitting caffeinated and decaffeinated coffees and sodas, alcohol, black pepper, chili powder, and caffeine.

References

American Dietetic Association: *Manual of Clinical Dietetics.* Chicago: 1988.

Dallas–Fort Worth Hospital Council: *Dallas–Fort Worth Hospital Council Diet Manual.* Irving: 1992.

Ippoliti, A.F., et al: *The Effect of Various Forms of Milk on Gastric-Acid Secretion;* Annals of Internal Medicine 84:286; 1976.

Mahan K. and Arlin, M.: *Krause's Food, Nutrition and Diet Therapy.* 8th ed., Philadelphia: W.B. Saunders Company, 1992.

▶ LIBERAL BLAND DIET ◀

Description

This diet limits the few items known to be stimulators of gastric acid secretion. Alcohol, decaffeinated and caffeinated coffees, and caffeinated beverages are known to stimulate gastric secretion. Black pepper, chili powder, garlic and cloves are agents which can irritate gastric mucosa. All other foods, regardless of texture have not been shown to be irritants of gastric mucosa.

Snacks between meals and at bedtime are not recommended as this can cause further acid production, unless relief is gained by small frequent meals. Any food that causes individual distress should not be used. Good nutritional habits will aid greatly in the healing and prevention of ulcers. Avoid foods that may make patient feel worse.

Adequacy

This diet meets the 1989 Recommended Dietary Allowance for good nutrition as established by the Food and Nutrition Board of the National Research Council when the types of foods and amounts suggested are included daily.

Type of Foods	Foods Allowed	Foods Not Allowed
Milk (2 or more cups daily)	Whole, 2%, 1%, skim, and milk drinks	None
Meat, Poultry, Fish and Meat Substitutes (6 ounces daily)	All meats as tolerated	Any that cause individual distress
Eggs	Egg or egg substitute	Any that cause individual distress
Fruits (2 or more servings–include citrus daily)	All fruits and juices	Any that cause individual distress
Vegetables (3 or more servings–include a dark green leafy or deep yellow vegetable 3–4 times weekly)	Any as desired	Any that cause individual distress
Bread, Cereal, Rice and Pasta (6 or more servings daily)	Any bread or cereal product	Any that cause individual distress
Fats and Oils	Any in moderation	Any that cause individual distress
Soups	Any as desired	Any that cause individual distress
Desserts	Any in moderation	Any that cause individual distress
Beverages	Weak tea and all beverages except those omitted	All coffee, soda, alcohol, other beverages containing caffeine
Miscellaneous	Any condiments or spices except those omitted	Black pepper, chili powder, chocolate, garlic, cloves and any spices that cause individual distress

Sample Menu

Breakfast	Lunch	Supper
Grapefruit Juice	Vegetable Soup	Roast Beef
Oatmeal	Tuna Fish on Whole	Parsleyed Noodles
Scrambled Egg	Wheat Bread/Sandwich	Cooked Carrots
Toast–Margarine	Sliced Tomatoes	Tossed Salad
Jelly	Canned Peaches	Bread–Margarine
Milk	Milk	Sherbet
Weak Tea–Sugar	Weak Tea–Sugar	Weak Tea–Sugar

References

Chicago Dietetic Association and South Suburban Dietetic Association, *Manual of Clinical Dietetics,* American Dietetic Association, Chicago, 1988.

Dallas–Fort Worth Hospital Council: *Dallas–Fort Worth Hospital Council Diet Manual.* Irving: 1992.

Mahan, K. and Arlin, M.: *Krause's Food, Nutrition and Diet Therapy,* 8th ed., Philadelphia: W.B. Saunders Company, 1992.

Puckett, R.P. and Brown, S.M.: *Shands Hospital at the University of Florida Guide to Clinical Dietetics,* 5th ed., Dubuque: Kendall/Hunt Publishing Co., 1993.

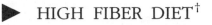 ▶ HIGH FIBER DIET[†] ◀

Description

This diet is indicated primarily for the prevention and treatment of constipation, encopresis, diverticulosis and irritable bowel syndrome. Fiber adds bulk and helps in the functioning of the peristaltic action of the intestine. Eating foods high in fiber may also reduce the risk of cancers of the colon and rectum. Dietary fiber is a valuable therapeutic tool in treatment of diabetes, hyperlipidemia, and obesity. Dietary fiber may also aid in the treatment of hypertension and coronary heart disease. Emphasis is on the following foods:

▶ ***Whole Grain and Bran Cereals***–Shredded Wheat®, All-Bran®, Oatmeal, Fiber-One®, Ralston®, Wheatena® (1–2 servings per day)

▶ ***Whole Grain Breads***–Whole Wheat, Whole Rye, Wheat Germ, Oatmeal, Pumpernickel, Bran, Cracked Wheat (3 or more servings per day)

▶ ***Raw and Dried Fruits with Skin and Seeds*** (2 or more per day)

▶ ***Raw or Slightly Cooked Vegetables***–Carrots, Cauliflower, Tomatoes, Broccoli, Green Beans (2 or more servings per day)

▶ ***Dried Peas, Beans, and Lentils*** (cooked)

▶ ***High Fiber Snacks***–Nuts, Seeds, Popcorn, Fresh and Dried Fruit, Whole Grain Crackers

Unprocessed bran is recommended several times a day before meals or with the first course. It can be taken dry, mixed in beverages, cereals, soups, vegetables, and other foods.

Fluid intake should be increased to at least 8 cups daily. Prune juice may be included to encourage regular elimination. High fiber foods should be added gradually to the diet until a high fiber diet is achieved.

Many foods are now being fortified with psyllium. Psyllium is a supplement that acts like high fiber.

[†]See Position Paper of American Dietetic Assoc." Health Implications of Dietary Fiber, J. Am. Diet. Assoc. 1997:97:1157.

Adequacy

This diet will provide approximately 20–35 grams of fiber per day. The diet meets the 1989 Recommended Dietary Allowance for good nutrition as established by the Food and Nutrition Board of the National Research Council when the types of foods and amounts suggested are included daily.

Sample Menu

Breakfast	Lunch/Supper
Prune Juice	Meat
Bran Cereal	Potato (preferably with skin) or Substitute
Egg	Cooked Vegetable
Whole Wheat Toast	Raw Salad with Dressing
Butter or Margarine	Bran Muffins
Jam	Butter or Margarine
Milk	Raw Fruit
Beverage/Cream/Sugar	Milk if desired
	Beverage/Cream/Sugar

*Registered Trademark—Brand names are used for clarification and do not constitute endorsement of the product.

Gastrointestinal Responses to the Ingestion of Dietary Fiber

▶ Increased fecal bulk
▶ Greater frequency of defacation
▶ Reduced intestinal transit time
▶ Delayed gastric emptying
▶ Increased postprandial satiety

▶ Reduced glucose absorption
▶ Alterations in mineral balances
▶ Changes in intestinal enzyme activity
▶ Increased bile acid excretion
▶ Decreased intraluminal pressure

References

American Dietetic Association: *Manual of Clinical Dietetics,* Chicago: 1988.

Bourquin, L.D., Titgemeyer, E.C., Fahey, C. Jr., Garleb, K.A., Fermentation of dietary fiber by human colonic bacteria: disappearance of short-chain fatty acid production from, and potential water-holding capacity of, various substrates. *Scand J Gastroenterol.* 1993;28:249–255.

Dallas–Fort Worth Hospital Council: *Dallas–Fort Worth Hospital Council Diet Manual.* Irving: 1992.

Larson, D.E. Mayo Clinic Family Health Book 2nd ed., NY William Morrow & Co, Inc. 1996

Mahan, K. and Arlin, M.: *Krause's Food, Nutrition and Diet Therapy.* 8th ed., Philadelphia: W.B. Saunders Company, 1992.

▶ RESIDUE AND FIBER RESTRICTED DIET

Description

This diet is designed to avoid blockage of a stenosed gastrointestinal tract and to reduce fecal output. It is indicated on a short term basis during acute phases of diverticulitis, imflammatory bowel disease (i.e. Ulcerative colitis or Chrohn's disease), infectious enterocolitis; before or after bowel surgery; during radium implantation; and/or radiation enteritis.

Adequacy

This diet will provide approximately 8–10 gm fiber per day. It meets the 1989 Recommended Dietary Allowance for good nutrition as established by the Food and Nutrition Board of the National Research Council when the types of foods and amounts suggested are included daily. Females age 11–50 years need to include a good source of iron daily.

Type of Foods	Foods Allowed	Foods Not Allowed
Milk (limit to 2 cups daily)	Whole, 2%, 1%, skim, yogurt–plain or with allowed fruits only	Yogurt containing omitted fruits
Meat, Fish, Poultry and Meat Substitutes (6 ounces daily)	Tender beef, veal, lamb, liver, lean pork, poultry, fish (baked, broiled, stewed, roasted, grilled or steamed), cottage cheese cream cheese, American and mild cheeses: 1 oz. may be substituted for 1 cup milk; smooth peanut butter	Cured meats, luncheon meats, frankfurters, shellfish; all fried foods; hard or sharp cheese or any with herbs or seeds; crunchy peanut butter; dried beans, peas, lentils, and legumes
Eggs	Hard boiled, scrambled, creamed, omelet, or souffle	Fried eggs
Fruits (2 servings–include citrus daily)	Fruit juice, applesauce, canned peaches, pears, apricots (without skin), Royal Anne cherries, orange and grapefruit sections (without membrane), any pureed fruits, ripe bananas	Raw fruits except bananas; all fruits with skins or seeds; dried fruits, raisins, dates, figs, prunes, prune juice, canned berries, plums, fruit cocktail, pineapple or strawberries
Vegetables (2 servings–include a dark green leafy or deep yellow vegetable 3–4 times weekly)	Well cooked asparagus tips, beets and carrots, green beans, wax beans, and spinach; pureed: peas squash and pumpkin; vegetable juices (no limit), white potato (no skin) and pureed/mashed sweet potato	Raw vegetables; all vegetables not listed; all fried vegetables; potato chips
Bread, Cereal, Rice and Pasta (6 or more servings daily)	Enriched white or refined bread, saltines, melba toast, rusk, soda crackers, Zwieback® and vanilla wafers	Bread or crackers containing whole grain flour, bran, nuts or seeds, hot breads, pancakes, waffles, muffins, cornbread, quick breads, popcorn
	Rice, macaroni, noodles, or spaghetti	Whole grain rice
	Cooked refined corn, wheat and rice cereals, strained oatmeal, hominy grits and farina; commercially prepared cereals from corn and rice such as cornflakes, Rice Krispies* and puffed rice	Bran and whole grain cereals, any cold cereal not listed
Fats and Oil (in moderation)	Butter, margarine, vegetable oils, and lard; cream or half and half, sour cream (no more than ½ c. daily); crisp bacon, mild salad dressing, white sauce in moderate amounts; non dairy creamers	Spicy dressing, nuts, olives, and spicy gravies

Type of Foods	Foods Allowed	Foods Not Allowed
Soups	Clear broth, bouillon, consomme, strained cream soup made from allowed vegetables and milk allowance	Highly seasoned soups, soups made with whole vegetables
Desserts	Custard, pudding, ice cream, sherbet, gelatin, plain cookies, plain cake (all without nuts, spices or coconut)	Rich pastries, pies and tarts that contain nuts, raisins and coconut
Beverages	Coffee, tea, cocoa, carbonated beverages	Alcohol, unless ordered by physician
Miscellaneous	Hard candies, sugar, jelly, syrup, molasses, honey, salt, vinegar, lemon	Spices, pepper, gravies, rich sauces, rich honey, candies, preserves, jams, marmalades

*Registered Trademark: Brand names are used for clarification and do not constitute endorsement of the product.

Sample Menu

Breakfast	Lunch	Supper
Orange Juice	Cream of Tomato Soup	Strained Cream of Corn Soup
Cream of Wheat	Roast Beef	Lamb Chop
Scrambled Egg	Mashed Potato	Buttered Noodles
White Toast–Margarine	Green Beans	Pureed Peas
Jelly	Saltine Crackers	Saltine Crackers
½ cup Cream	White Toast–Margarine	White Toast–Margarine
Coffee–Sugar	Canned Peach Halves	Sugar Cookies
	Iced Tea–Sugar	Iced Tea–Sugar

Note: Milk is not found in sample menu because it is incorporated in the food.

References

American Dietetic Association: *Manual of Clinical Dietetics*. Chicago: 1988.

Dallas–Fort Worth Hospital Council: *Dallas–Fort Worth Hospital Council Diet Manual*. Irving: 1992.

Mahan, K. and Arlin, M.: *Krause's Food, Nutrition and Diet Therapy*, 8th ed., Philadelphia: W.B. Saunders Company, 1992.

▶ GASTROESOPHAGEAL REFLUX ◀

Description

This diet is indicated for individuals with persistent and severe symptoms of gastroesophageal reflux (GER) caused by a dysfunction of the lower esophageal sphincter (LES) mechanism. GER and its major symptoms of heartburn and acid regurgitation are prevalent in our population. Other symptoms that may occur include esophagitis, hoarseness, and dysphagia. Patients with a hiatal hernia commonly have GER.

GER is usually a mild condition that can be managed medically. However, if chronic reflux leads to esophagitis, hemorrhage or stricture formation, surgical intervention may be indicated.

Non-dietary factors which may reduce GER include elevation of the head of the bed, cessation of smoking and not wearing tight fitting clothes. Changing of an infant's diaper should be completed prior to feeding to eliminate or reduce GER.

The following guidelines are used for patients experiencing symptoms of GER:

▶ Consume a high protein diet to increase LES pressure. (A source of protein should be consumed at each meal).

▶ Fat intake should be limited to 45–50 gram/day.

▶ Avoid foods that decrease LES pressure such as peppermints, chocolate, alcohol and coffee.

▶ Avoid acidic or spicy foods or any other foods that regularly cause heartburn.

▶ Eat five to six small meals each day and remain in an upright posture during and after eating.

▶ Achieve and maintain ideal body weight.

▶ Provide foods that are easily masticated and moist.

▶ Drinking liquids between meals instead of at mealtime helps many patients decrease their symptoms.

▶ Stop smoking.

▶ Eat three meals a day and cut down on portion size. Do not eat anything 2–3 hours before going to bed.

▶ Take medications with plenty of water.

▶ ESOPHAGEAL REFLUX DIET ◀

Food Group	Include	Avoid
Beverages	All except those avoided	Coffee (regular and decaffeinated) alcohol, carbonated beverages, chocolate drinks
Dairy products	Skim milk, low-fat dairy products	Whole milk
Meats, Meat Substitutes	Baked, boiled and grilled meats	Processed meats, cold cuts
Breads, cereals, starches	All except those avoided	Pancakes, waffles
Vegetables	All except those avoided	Tomato, onion, red pepper
Fruits	All except those avoided	Citrus fruits and juices
Desserts, sweets	Low-fat desserts	Chocolate, ice cream, rich pastries, frosted cakes
Fats	Limit to 45 to 50 g/day	None
Miscellaneous	All except those avoided	Chocolate, mint, chewing gum

Adequacy

This diet meets the 1989 Recommended Dietary Allowance for good nutrition when a variety of foods are consumed in adequate amounts. Due to some good sources of vitamin C being restricted, vitamin C intake may be inadequate and should be supplemented if needed. Iron status should be monitored if prolonged antacid use has occurred which decreases iron absorption.

References

Castrell, D., Holtz, A., Gastroesophageal reflux: Don't forget to ask about heartburn, *Post-graduate Medicine*, 86(5), pp. 141–144, 1989.

Larson, D.E. Mayo Clinic Family Health Book 2nd ed. NY William Morrow Co. Inc. 1996

Puckett, R.P. and Brown, S.M.: *Shands Hospital at the University of Florida Guide to Clinical Dietetics*, 5th ed., Dubuque: Kendall/Hunt Publishing Co., 1993.

University of Michigan Hospitals, Food and Nutrition Services, *Guidelines for Nutritional Care*, Ann Arbor, Michigan, 1995.

▶ POSTGASTRECTOMY DIET (ANTI-DUMPING DIET) ◀

Description

The post-gastrectomy diet is designed for those individuals who have had surgical procedures that decrease the normal emptying time of the stomach: vagotomy, pyloroplasty, hemigastrectomy, total gastrectomy, Whipple's procedure or gastroenterostomy. The dumping syndrome is a phenomenon that can occur after the previously mentioned surgical procedures and is characterized by weakness, sweating, abdominal distress, dizziness, abdominal discomfort, vomiting and diarrhea after meals. Symptoms usually appear about 10–15 minutes after ingestion of a meal and are caused by the rapid flow of food from the stomach into the jejunum (small intestine) which is unable to accommodate it.

The occurrence and severity of post gastrectomy symptoms will vary depending on the location and extent of the gastric resection. The diet must take into consideration individual patient tolerances.

Carbohydrate containing foods are restricted because they are more rapidly hydrolyzed to osmotically active substances than are proteins and fats. Simple carbohydrates are eliminated. Liberalization of the diet should occur as adaptive changes take place and the patient's tolerance is improved.

Adequacy

When sufficient calories are consumed this diet meets the 1989 Recommended Dietary Allowances for all nutrients with the exception of iron in women of childbearing age.

Specifics of the Diet

Recommendations for reducing the occurrence and severity of dumping syndrome:

1. Avoid concentrated forms of carbohydrates. (limit sweets)
2. Initiate small frequent meals. (6–8 meals per day)
3. Do not drink fluids with meals or within thirty minutes before or after each meal.
4. Relax at mealtimes and eat slowly.
5. Chew foods well.
6. Drink hot or cold fluids slowly.
7. Include a protein source with each meal.
8. Limit milk and milk products. Fermented milk products such as cheese or yogurt are usually tolerated.
9. Vitamin and mineral supplement as needed.

Type of Foods	Foods Allowed	Foods Not Allowed
Milk* (if tolerated)	Whole, lowfat, and skim milk (tolerance to milk and milk products should be tested); buttermilk	Milk in all forms if not tolerated; chocolate milk, hot chocolate
Meat, Fish, Poultry and Meat Substitutes (6 ounces or more daily)	All	None
Eggs	All	None

Type of Foods	Foods Allowed	Foods Not Allowed
Fruits (2 or more servings daily–including citrus daily)	All unsweetened fruits and fruit juices* except those omitted	Persimmons, apple skins, berries, figs, grapes, citrus fruit; dried fruit, fruits cooked, canned or frozen with sugar
Vegetables (3 or more servings daily–include dark green leafy or deep yellow vegetable 3–4 times weekly)	All except those omitted	Potato skins, broccoli, brussel sprouts, dry beans, celery stalks, lettuce, spinach, or any to which sugar has been added
Bread, Cereal, Rice and Pasta (6 or more servings daily)	Enriched white, wheat, rolls, or crackers; melba toast, graham crackers; all cooked and ready-to-eat cereals except those not allowed; macaroni, noodles, rice, spaghetti grits	Sweetened breads; cereals containing dried fruit, coconut, cereals coated or flavored with sugar or honey; popcorn
Fats and Oil	Butter, cream, margarine, oils, fats, mayonnaise, salad dressing, crisp bacon, olives, nuts, gravy	Poppy seeds, sweetened whipped toppings, coconut
Soups*	Soups made with allowed ingredients	Soups made from ingredients not allowed
Desserts	Unsweetened yogurt, pudding or baked custard made without sugar; artificially sweetened or plain gelatin	Ice cream and all other desserts
Beverages*	Coffee, tea, decaffeinated beverages, dietetic carbonated or powdered beverages	Sweetened beverages; alcoholic beverages
Miscellaneous	Salt, saccharin, aspartame, condiments, seasonings, spices, horseradish, unsweetened pickles and relish, sugar-free jam, jelly, syrup, sauce	Candies, sweetened pickles and relishes, honey, jam, jellies, marmalade, syrup

*Consider as Fluid

Sample Menu

Breakfast	Lunch	Supper
2 Diet Peach Halves, Drained 1 Slice Whole Wheat Bread 1 Scrambled Egg 1 tsp. Margarine 1 Strip Bacon	3 oz. Roast Beef ½ c. Mashed Potatoes ½ c. Green Beans, Drained 1 Slice Bread 2 Pineapple Slices, Drained 1 tsp. Margarine	3 oz. Baked Chicken ½ c. Yellow Rice ½ c. Carrots, Drained ½ c. Unsweetened Applesauce 2 tsp. Margarine
Mid-Morning Snack	**Mid-Afternoon Snack**	**Evening Snack**
1 Slice American Cheese 6 Saltines	¼ c. Cottage Cheese 1 Half Unsweetened Peach 6 Saltines	1 oz. Roast Beef 1 Slice Bread 1 Tbsp. Mayonnaise

Note: Additional calories and nutrients will be contributed by milk, fruit juice, etc. which are not allowed at meal time.

References

American Dietetic Association: *Manual of Clinical Dietetics.* Chicago: 1988.

Dallas–Fort Worth Hospital Council: *Dallas–Fort Worth Hospital Council Diet Manual,* Irving: 1992.

Mahan, K. and Arlin, M.: *Krause's Food, Nutrition and Diet Therapy,* 8th ed., Philadelphia: W.B. Saunders Company, 1992.

Puckett, R.P. and Brown, S.M.: *Shands Hospital at the University of Florida Guide to Clinical Dietetics,* 5th ed. Dubuque: Kendall/Hunt Publishing Co., 1993.

▶ DIET RESTRICTIONS FOR OSTOMY PATIENTS ◀

Description

This diet is ordered when a n ileostomy or colostomy is performed on a patient for the treatment of colon cancer, Crohn's Disease or ulcerative colitis. If the patient is not on a restricted diet for another condition, all foods can safely be consumed as tolerated.

The dietary restrictions are based solely on the individual's tolerance to different food items. A trial and error period is necessary to identify troublesome foods that should be avoided.

Eat foods at a regular time each day. Eating 4 to 6 smaller meals may help to promote a regular bowel pattern. Try eating the main meal at noon and a smaller meal in the evening. This helps reduce the stool output at night.

The ostomy patient's primary concerns include gas, odor and diarrhea. Greater comfort to the patient is usually obtained by simply avoiding foods that are gas and odor producing, as well as foods that produce excessive, loose stools.

It is rare that a patient with a well functioning ostomy becomes nutritionally depleted, but there is a concern to be closely monitored. The ileostomy frequently causes excessive loss of fluids and electrolytes requiring the use of extra salt on foods and including at least 2 servings of high potassium foods in their daily diet (See chapter on high potassium foods).

Drinking plenty of water, 2 to 3 quarts per day, and other fluids should be stressed. A common concern of the patient is that excessive fluid intake will make diarrhea worse. The patient must be reassured that excessive fluid intake above and beyond output will be absorbed by the kidney and will not make diarrhea worse.

Very fibrous vegetables should be avoided due to the concern that a food bolus may partially obstruct the ileum at the point where it narrows as it enters the abdominal wall. Also, it should be stressed that foods must be chewed thoroughly.

The following chart lists foods that tend to be gas producing or irritating and also foods that are helpful in controlling diarrhea and constipation.

Gas-Producing Foods

Dried beans and peas	Rutabaga	Turnips	Melons
Broccoli	Asparagus	Cucumbers	Sugar, sweets
Brussels sprouts	Sweet potatoes	Fish	Beer or
Cabbage	Parsnips	Roquefort cheese	carbonated
Cauliflower	Onions	Bleu cheese	beverages
Radishes	Eggs	Milk	Nuts
	Sauerkraut	Kohlrabi	Apple juice

High Fiber Foods That May Cause Irritation or Food Blockage

Seeds	Strawberries	Carrots	Chinese vegetables	Cucumbers
Corn	Coleslaw	Popcorn	Tomatoes	Green peppers
Skins	Salad greens	Nuts	Mushrooms	Olives
Membrane on oranges	Celery	Coconut	Relishes	Pickles
Pineapple	Raisins or dried fruit	Highly seasoned foods	Peas	

Foods That May Contribute to Diarrhea

Spinach, greens	Raw fruits	Excessive coffee	Red Wine
Broccoli	Highly seasoned foods	Hot beverages or soups	Chocolate
Dried beans, baked beans	Prunes	Licorice	Beer

Foods That May Control Diarrhea

Bananas	Rice	Pretzels	Tapioca	Bread
Applesauce	Marshmallows	Creamy peanut butter	Pasta	Cheeses

Measures to Help Control Mild Constipation

Increase fluids	Increase fruit juice	Increase cooked fruits and vegetables

Odor-Producing Foods

Asparagus	Fish	Onions
Eggs	Garlic	

Adequacy

This diet meets the 1989 RDA's for all nutrients when a variety of foods are consumed in adequate amounts. If specific foods groups are eliminated due to intolerances, a vitamin and mineral supplement may be beneficial. Fluid and electrolyte replacement may also be necessary if excessive losses occur.

References

Cataldo, C.B., Nyenhuis, J.R., Whitney, E.N., *Nutrition and Diet Therapy,* 2nd ed, West Publishing Company, New York, pp. 341–370, 1989.

Jackson Gastroenterology, http://www.gicare.com, 1998, Camp Hill, PA.

Krause, M.V., Mahan, L.K., *Food, Nutrition and Diet Therapy,* 6th ed, W.B. Sanders, Philadelphia, pp. 687–688, 1979.

Pemberton, C.M., Moxness, K.E., German, M.J., Nelson, J.K., Gastineau, C.F., *Rochester Methodist Hospital and Saint Marys Hospital, Mayo Clinic Diet Manual: A Handbook of Dietary Practices,* 6th ed., B.C. Decker, Inc., Toronto, pp. 177–183, 1988.

Puckett, R.P., and Brown, S.M.: *Shands Hospital at the University of Florida Guide to Clinical Dietetics,* 5th ed., Dubuque: Kendall/Hunt Publishing Co., 1993.

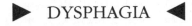

▶ DYSPHAGIA ◀

Description

The dysphagia diet is indicated for patients who have difficulty in swallowing liquid or solid foods because of decreased oral or pharyngeal function. Dysphasia most often occurs in patients following cerebrovascular accidents or in such conditions as multiple sclerosis, poliomyelitis, muscular dystrophy, Parkinson's disease, cerebral palsy, Wilson's disease, head injury, brain tumors, spinal cord injury, Alzheimer's disease or head and neck cancer/surgery.

There are four phases of swallowing that the patient needs to be evaluated for to obtain the phase and nutrition therapy applicable for oral intake for that individual. The four phases of swallowing include;

▶ **Preparatory Phase**—Mastication and manipulation of the food to form a bolus.

▶ **Oral Phase**—Chewing mixes the food with saliva and forms a bolus which the tongue moves to the back of the mouth. Pharyngeal swallowing is then triggered. Potential problems in this phase include drooling and retention of food in mouth due to improper lip closure or cheek tension.

▶ **Pharyngeal Phase**—The pharyngeal swallow response is initiated and carries the food into the esophagus. Sensory receptors in the tongue and pharynx close off the trachea. This phase has the potential for the patient to loss control of the bolus and trigger coughing, choking, gurgling voice quality, or aspiration.

▶ **Esophageal Phase**—Peristaltic waves carry the bolus through the esophagus into the stomach. Problems may arise from food becoming lodged in the esophagus due to obstruction or decreased esophageal peristalsis. Reflux of food is also a concern.

Patients entering the hospital with dysphagia being the primary complaint usually exhibit marked malnutrition which is the most serious consequence of the condition. Due to this high incidence of malnutrition, many patients require enteral or parenteral nutrition support. The consistency of the diet will require adjustment as swallowing function improves. Coordination between the registered dietitian and the swallowing clinicians (speech-language pathologists or occupational therapists) is necessary to maximize intake and minimize the risk of aspiration.

A National Dysphagia Diet is being coordinated by a group of dietitians, food scientist, and speech language pathologist. The diet includes a science based measurement for food and liquid textures (rheological properties) along with prescriptive component for swallowing therapists that will allow therapist to make a diet prescription based upon a patients diagnosis, swallowing and cognitive abilities. Standard terminology for diet texture will also help continuity of care as patients transfer across the continuum of care. Currently the rheological properties are still being identified. Check out this web site **www.dysphagia-diet.com**

The diet categorizes foods by consistency and type of oral and pharyngeal actions needed for safe mastication and swallow. The food groups are as follows with examples of each group:

Liquids

▶ **Thin liquids:** Thin liquids do not require mastication. Tongue control is required to form a bolus and move the liquids through the oral cavity. Since thin liquids descend by gravity once the swallow reflex is completed, they require minimal pharyngeal or esophageal peristalsis. Examples of these include water, milk, broth, fruit juices, coffee, soft drinks, sherbet, melted ice cream and eggnog.

▶ **Thick liquids:** Thick liquids do not require mastication. Tongue control to form and propel the bolus through the oral cavity is needed. To prevent the formation of a mass that gets stuck in the throat, some pharyngeal and esophageal peristalsis is required. Examples of these include fruit nectars, vegetable juices, thick milkshakes, and strained cream soups.

Solids

▶ **Mashed solids:** These foods do not require mastication. The mashed solids contain more bulk than liquids, but they are easily controlled by the tongue. More pharyngeal and esophageal action is required. Examples of these include plain or flavored yogurt without solids, pureed meats, pureed fruit, applesauce, thinned mashed potatoes, cream or wheat or rice, margarine, gravy, custard or pudding.

▶ **Semi-solids:** These foods require some mastication. The semi-solid foods form a very soft mass that can be held and controlled by the tongue. Good pharyngeal movement is necessary to complete the swallow. Examples of these include plain or flavored yogurt without solids, cottage cheese, minced meat, soft scrambled egg, soft mashed fruit, soft mashed vegetables, cooked cereals, margarine, gravy, sour cream, custard and pudding

▶ **Soft chunks:** These foods require mastication, but do not lead to early fatigue. These foods usually stick together creating a cohesive bolus which may cause the pharyngeal swallow response. Soft chunk foods will not adhere to the palate or teeth and are easy for the tongue to control. Good pharyngeal action is required to complete the swallow. Examples of these include all yogurts except those with skins, seeds, nuts or coconut; soft and semi-soft cheese, minced meat, scrambled, poached or hard boiled eggs; canned fruit without skin or seeds, mashable vegetables; bread, toast, pasta, rice, noodles, smooth peanut butter, and plain soft cookies.

The patient must be monitored continuously for hydration and nutritional status. Due to liquids being avoided frequently, inadequate fluid intake can become a problem, consequently fluid intake and output must be closely monitored. Calorie counts should be implemented to determine the adequacy of the individual's oral intake.

The registered dietitian may want to provide consultation to the patient and patient's family as to the proper food preparations and techniques to be used at home. Include instructions on methods to increase energy and protein intake and the progression of consistency as the patient tolerance increases. Some of the important guidelines for patient instruction should include;

▶ The patient should be allowed sufficient time to eat in a relaxed environment.

▶ Positioning the patient to eat is very important. Sitting in an upright position with feet flat on the floor and the head slightly forward decreased the risk of aspiration. If the patient is bedridden, elevate the head of the bed or use pillows to achieve the correct position.

▶ Fluids should be introduced cautiously because they tend to be difficult for the patient to tolerate. Commercial thickeners are available to stabilize the consistency of liquids and these include Diafoods® and Thick-It®.

▶ Foods should be mildly spiced and if needed only moderately sweet.

▶ To stimulate chewing and swallowing, foods should be slightly colder or warmer than body temperature.

▶ Crumbly foods or small pieces of food tend to form pockets in the cheeks and increase the risk of choking.

▶ Moisten foods with gravy, milk, margarine or broth to avoid crumbling and possible aspiration.

▶ Do not eat sticky foods that adhere to the roof of the mouth.

▶ Dairy products, except yogurt, cause increased mucous production in the mouth and throat so consequently should be limited.

▶ For patients with poor appetites and/or consume their meals very slowly, six small meals instead of three regular meals is recommended. If the appetite is poor, oral nutritional supplements may be required.

Adequacy

This diet may be inadequate depending on the patient fatigue during meal time and the ability to consume the appropriate balanced dietary intake when only easily swallowed foods are consumed. A multiple vitamin and mineral supplement is often recommended. If the patient is unable to tolerate dairy products, the diet may be inadequate in calcium and phosphorus. Constipation may result from the change in food consistencies leading to less dietary fiber intake.

References

Hynak-Hankinson, M.T., Agin, M., Gardner, C., Jones, P.L., Lichtenstein, S., Peiffer, S., Rao, P., Dysphagia evaluation and treatment: The team approach, part II, *Nutrition Support Services,* 4(6), pp. 30–33, 1984.

Logemann, J.A., Evaluation and Treatment of Swallowing Disorders. San Diego, CA: College-Hill Press Inc.; 1983.

Morrell, R.M., *Neurologic disorders of swallowing., Dysphagia Diagnosis and Management.,* Boston, MA: Butterworth Publishing Co; 1984:37–54.

Podell, S.K., Intermittent tube feedings and gastroesophageal reflux control in head-injured patients, *Journal of the American Dietetics Association,* 89(1), pp. 102–103, 1989.

Puckett, R.P., and Brown, S.M.: *Shands Hospital at the University of Florida Guide to Clinical Dietetics.* 5th ed. Dubuque: Kendall/Hunt Publishing Co., 1993.

University of Michigan Hospitals, Food and Nutrition Services, Guidelines for Nutritional Care, Ann Arbor, Michigan, 1995.

Welnetz, K., Maintaining adequate nutrition and hydration in the dysphagic ALS patient. *Canadian Nurse.* 1983;79:30–34.

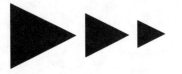

Module 2

Modification for Seasoning

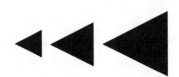

▶ SODIUM RESTRICTED DIETS ◀

Salt intake is usually the result of taste and custom and is often in excess of physiologic need. When the function of homeostatic mechanisms is impaired so that urinary excretion of sodium is limited, restriction of dietary sodium may help control edema. The usual daily intake for an adult in the U.S. has been approximately at 130–300 mEq (3–7 grams) of sodium.

Description

The purpose of sodium restricted diets is to reduce the sodium content of the tissues and to promote loss of body water. A sodium restriction may be useful in the treatment of cardiovascular diseases such as congestive heart failure and hypertension; diseases associated with fluid retention or electrolyte imbalance such as renal disease or cirrhosis; toxemia of pregnancy, and diseases requiring treatment with sodium retaining hormones or drugs such as corticosteroid therapy.

Salt substitute is composed of potassium chloride and may be contraindicated for some patients.

The level of sodium should be specified (mg or mEq) when ordering sodium restricted diets. The level of sodium restriction will determine the nutritional adequacy of the diet.

▶ **4 gram Sodium** (174 mEq)—Minimal Sodium Restriction

Foods high in sodium are avoided. Up to one-half teaspoon of table salt is allowed for cooking. Salt should not be added to food after cooking.

▶ **3 gram Sodium** (130 mEq)—Mild Sodium Restriction

Foods high in sodium are avoided. Up to one-fourth teaspoon of table salt is allowed for food preparation. Salt should not be added to food after cooking.

▶ **2 gram Sodium** (87 mEq)—Mild Sodium Restriction

Foods high in sodium are omitted. Salt should not be used in the preparation of food or at the table. Canned or processed foods with salt or sodium are omitted.

▶ **1 gram Sodium** (43 mEq)—Moderate Sodium Restriction

Foods high in sodium are omitted. Salt should not be used in the preparation of food or at the table. Canned or processed foods with salt or sodium are omitted. This diet may be difficult for most patients to follow at home.

▶ **500 mg Sodium** (22 mEq)—Strict Sodium Restriction

Foods high in sodium are omitted. Salt should not be used in the preparation of foods or at the table. Canned or processed foods with salt or sodium are omitted. Foods naturally high in sodium are omitted. This diet is unpalatable and should only be used for short periods of time.

▶ **250 mg Sodium** (11 mEq)—Severe Sodium Restriction

THIS DIET IS NOT RECOMMENDED, BUT COULD BE USED FOR SHORT TERM OR TESTS ONLY. Foods high in sodium are omitted. Salt should not be used in the preparation of foods or at the table. Canned or processed foods with salt or sodium are omitted. Foods naturally high in sodium are omitted. Protein containing foods are limited. Low sodium milk replaces regular milk.

Conversion of Sodium

1. To convert from milligrams (mg) to milliequivalents (mEq) use the following:

$$\frac{mg \times valance}{atomic\ weight} = mEq \qquad\qquad Example: \frac{1000\ mg\ Na+}{23} = 43.5\ mEq\ Na+$$

$$\frac{mEq \times atomic\ weight}{valence} = mg \qquad\qquad Example: 43.5\ mEq \times 23 = 1000\ mg.\ Na+$$

2. To convert specific weight of Na+ to NaCl, multiply by 2.54
    Example: 1000 mg. Na+ × 2.54 = 2540 mg NaCl
3. To convert specific weight of NaCl to Na+, multiply by .393
    Example: 2.5 mg NaCl × 0.393 = 1000 mg Na+

Sources

Food

Although a number of compounds may be used in food preparation and processing, NaCl (table salt) is usually the major source of dietary sodium.

For example:

1 tsp. of table salt contains 2000 mg sodium (87 mEq)

1 tsp. of baking soda (sodium bicarbonate) contains 1000 mg sodium (43 mEq)

As a rule, processed foods contain more sodium than do fresh foods. Good protein sources (milk, eggs and meat) are higher in sodium. Fats, oils, sugar, and fruits are lowest in natural sodium content.

Additives that Contain Sodium

Baking Powder	Sodium Cyclamate
Baking Soda	Sodium Benzoate
Brine (Salt & Water)	Sodium Hydroxide
Disodium Phosphate	Sodium Propionate
Monosodium Glutamate	Sodium Saccharin
Sodium Alginate	Sodium Sulfite

Medicine

Some medicines contain large amounts of sodium. Some of these are: alkalizers, laxatives, cough medicines, sedatives, antacids.

Water

Water may contribute significant amounts of sodium to the diet. The water supply should be investigated if a strict sodium restriction must be followed. If a municipal source is used, the Department of Public Health can usually provide information as to sodium content. If the content exceeds 40 parts per million (2 mEq or 40 mg of sodium per liter), distilled water should be used.

Other

▶ Eliminate or limit alcohol intake to < 1 drink per day
▶ Encourage activity—such as walking
▶ Eliminate smoking
▶ Follow diet and medication regimens.

▶ **ALLOWED SERVINGS FROM FOOD GROUPS PER SODIUM RESTRICTION** ◀

Food Group	Serving Size	Sodium Content	Servings Allowed Per Day				
			250 mg	500 mg	1,000 mg	2,000 mg	3,000 mg
Milk, Milk Products	1 c. varies	120 mg	0	2	2	2	2
Low Sodium	1 cup	7 mg	2	0	0	0	0
Meat, Fish, Poultry	1 oz.	25 mg	3	4	4	6	6
Salted	1 oz.	100 mg	0	0	0	0	0
Egg	1	70 mg	1	1	1	1	1
High Sodium Meats	1 oz.	300 mg	0	0	0	0	0
Fruits & Fruit Juices	1/2 cup	2 mg	3	3	3	3	3
Vegetables, Unsalted	1/2 cup	15 mg	2	3	3	3	As desired
Salted	1/2 cup	250 mg	0	0	0	0	3
Breads/Starches							
Salt-Free	1/2 cup or 1 slice	10 mg	4	4	6	4	As desired
Regular, Salted	1/2 cup or 1 slice	150 mg	0	0	3	6	6
Fats							
Salt-Free	1 tsp.	5 mg	3	3	6		
Salted	1 tsp.	50 mg	0	0	0	6	6
Desserts							
Salt-Free	Varies	15 mg	1	1	2	As desired	As desired
Regular	Varies	250 mg	0	0	0	1	2
Sugars, Sweets	Unlimited	trace	As desired	As desired	As desired	As desired	As desired
Total mg sodium per day			265	531	1031	2001	2916

▶ **TABLE SALT EQUIVALENTS** ◀

Amount	mEq Na+	mg Na+
1/8 tsp.	11	250
1/4 tsp.	22	500
1/2 tsp.	43	1000
3/4 tsp.	65	1500
1 tsp.	87	2000

4 Gram Sodium Diet (170 Milliequivalents)

Description

Mild sodium restriction. The "No Added Salt" diet is indicated for patients with mild sodium and fluid retention associated with cardiovascular, hepatic, or renal diseases, and/or treatment with sodium-retaining hormones such as corticosteroids.

Adequacy

This diet meets the 1989 Recommended Dietary Allowances for good nutrition as established by the Food and Nutrition Board of the National Research Council when the types of foods and amounts suggested are included daily.

Principles

1. Salt may be used moderately in cooking.
   Do not exceed 1/2 teaspoon salt total in a day for cooking.
2. Add no salt at the table.

▶ FOODS TO AVOID ◀

Meats	Other Foods	Seasonings
Salted, smoked, canned and cured Meats	Bouillon	Seasoned Salts:
Salted, smoked or cured Fish	Consomme	Garlic Salt
Bacon and Bacon Fat	Canned salted Soups	Onion Salt
Ham	Dried Soup Mixes	Celery Salt
Salt Pork	Breads and Rolls with salted tops	Sea Salt
Sausage	Salted Crackers	Rock Salt
All Luncheon Meats	Snack Foods:	Kosher Salt
Chipped and Corned Beef	Pretzels	Meat Tenderizer
Frankfurters	Potato Chips	Monosodium Glutamate
Meat Extracts	Salted Popcorn	Catsup
Kosher Meat	Salted Nuts	Soy Sauce
Anchovies	Olives, Pickles and Relishes	Worcestershire Sauce
Caviar and Roe	Sauerkraut and other vegetables prepared in brine	Prepared Mustard
Dried Cod		Chili Sauce
Herring		BBQ Sauce and other Meat Sauces
Sardines	Commercial Rice, Pasta, Stuffing, and Casserole Mixes	
Pickled Meat		
Pickled Eggs		

Sample Menu

Breakfast	Lunch	Supper
Orange Juice	S.F. Vegetable Soup	Baked Chicken
Grits	Roast Beef	Baked Potato
Scrambled Egg	Rice	Green Beans
Toast–Margarine	Tomato & Lettuce with French Dressing	Bread–Margarine
Jelly	Roll–Margarine	Angel Food Cake with Peaches
Milk	Apple	Iced Tea–Sugar
Coffee–Sugar	Milk	Pepper
Pepper	Iced Tea–Sugar	
	Pepper	

S.F. = Salt-Free

3 Gram Sodium Diet (130 Milliequivalents)

Description

The 3 gram sodium diet is indicated for the patient with fluid and sodium retention associated with cardiovascular, renal, and hepatic disease, and/or treatment with sodium retaining hormones such as corticosteroids. It is a mild sodium restriction. Foods may be lightly seasoned with salt in cooking. (Do not exceed 1/4 teaspoon salt total in a day on cooking.) Do not use salt at the table. Foods high in sodium are to be avoided.

Adequacy

This diet meets the 1989 Recommended Dietary Allowance for good nutrition as established by the Food and Nutrition Board of the National Research Council when the types of foods and amounts suggested are included daily. Females, ages 11–50, need to include a good source of iron daily.

Type of Food	Foods Allowed	Foods Not Allowed
Milk (limit to 2 cups daily)	Any milk, chocolate milk, malted milk, ⅓ cup condensed milk, instant cocoa mix	Buttermilk
Meat, Poultry, Fish and Meat Substitutes (limit to 6 ounces daily)	All fresh or fresh frozen meats, poultry, fish: beef, lamb, veal, fresh pork, chicken, turkey, liver, heart, brains, duck, quail, rabbit, cod, flounder, halibut, trout, bass, bluefish, catfish, clams, crabs, lobster, oysters, low sodium salmon and tuna, shrimp and sole. Cheese: swiss, cheddar, mozarella, ricotta and cream; peanut butter (2 Tbsp. = 1 oz.)	Cured, canned or smoked meats, poultry and fish; chipped or corned beef, ham luncheon meats, bacon, frankfurters, sausages, sardines, anchovies, Koshered meats, salt pork, smoked tongue, kidneys, caviar, salted and dried cod, herring, processed cheese, cheese spreads, Roquefort, Camembert or Gorgonzola cheese; meat substitutes (soy)
Eggs (limit to 1 serving)	Eggs; egg substitute	None
Fruits (2 or more servings daily—include citrus daily)	All fruit juices; fresh, frozen, canned or sun dried fruit	Any fruit which has salt or sodium added (read label)
Vegetables (3 servings daily—include a dark green leafy or deep yellow vegetable 3–4 times weekly)	Fresh, frozen or canned vegetables; regular tomato juice or vegetable juice (Limit to ½ cup per day) Fresh potatoes, sweet potatoes, and yams; salt free potato chips	Sauerkraut or pickled vegetables prepared in brine Potato chips and other salted snack foods

Type of Food	Foods Allowed	Foods Not Allowed
Bread, Cereal, Rice and Pasta (limit to 6 servings daily)	Whole grain or enriched breads, rolls, muffins, biscuits, hamburger buns and crackers made without salt toppings; rice, noodles, spaghetti and other enriched pastas, (limit use of instant or commercial rice, noodle, and stuffing to one serving a day), graham crackers, vanilla wafers, rusk, cornbread, pancakes, waffles, hot breads and quick breads.	Salted or soda crackers, pretzels, and bread products made with salt toppings; salted popcorn
	All whole grain or enriched cooked and dry cereals except those omitted As desired:	Instant hot cereals or quick cooking cereals that have a sodium compound added (read label)
	Low sodium bread, crackers, matzo, melba toast, hot water cornbread, biscuits, pancakes and waffles made with low sodium baking powder; salt free popcorn	
Fats and Oil (limit to 6 servings daily— (1 tsp. = 1 serving)	Regular butter or fortified margarine, cream, cream substitutes, vegetable oils, mayonnaise, and unsalted nuts	Other salad dressings, bacon fat and salted nuts
	1 Tbsp. French, Blue Cheese or Roquefort dressings may be used in place of 3 fat servings. 1 Tbsp. 1000 Island dressing may be used in place of 2 fat servings.	
	Limit French, Blue Cheese, Roquefort and 1000 Island salad dressings to 1 Tbsp. per day. S.F. salad dressing may be used as desired.	
Soups	Salt free cream soup (made from allowed milk); special low sodium soups and low sodium broth	Commercially canned soups, bouillon cubes, consomme and broth
Desserts	All sweets and desserts made with allowed foods (For milk based desserts, an equal amount of milk should be omitted from the daily milk allowance.)	Desserts made with foods omitted
Beverages	Coffee, coffee substitutes, tea, and carbonated beverages	None
Miscellaneous	Pepper, spices, flavorings, vinegar, lemon juice, vanilla and peppermint extract, sugar, honey, dry mustard, pure horseradish, maple syrup, low sodium catsup, low sodium chili sauce, low sodium mustard, low sodium pickles, tabasco sauce, hard candy	Regular catsup, chili sauce, mustard, pickles, relishes, olives; celery salt, onion salt, garlic salt, sea salt, rock salt, Kosher salt, monosodium glutamate (Accent*), Kitchen Bouquet*, barbecue sauce, soy sauce, teriyaki sauce, steak and worcestershire sauce; sodium based antacids

Sample Menu

Breakfast	Lunch	Supper
½ c. Orange Juice	3 oz. Broiled Chicken	3 oz. S.F. Hamburger
½ c. Oatmeal	½ c. Mashed Potatoes	⅓ c. Rice
1 Scrambled Egg	Tomato and Lettuce	½ c. Carrots
1 Slice Toast	Salad with Mayonnaise	1 Slice Bread
2 tsp. Margarine	1 Slice Bread	2 tsp. Margarine
Jelly	1 tsp. Margarine	½ c. Canned Peaches
1 cup Milk	Yellow Cake with Icing	1 cup Milk
Coffee–Sugar	Tea–Sugar	Tea–Sugar
Pepper	Pepper	Pepper

*Registered Trademark: Brand names are used for clarification and do not constitute endorsement of that product.

2 Gram Sodium Diet (87 Milliequivalents)

Description

The 2 gram sodium diet is a mild sodium restriction indicated for the patient with fluid and sodium retention associated with cardiovascular, renal, or hepatic disease and/or treatment with sodium retaining hormones such as corticosteroids. Certain foods containing high levels of salt or sodium are eliminated and/or restricted. Foods canned or processed with large amounts of sodium or salt are omitted. It is necessary to read labels. Salt should not be used in preparation of food or at the table.

Adequacy

This diet meets the 1989 Recommended Dietary Allowance for good nutrition as established by the Food and Nutrition Board of the National Research Council when the types of foods and amounts suggested are included daily. Females, ages 11–50, need to include a good source of iron daily. The diet may be deficient in iodine due to the elimination of iodized salt, especially in areas with iodine deficient soil.

Type of Food	Foods Allowed	Foods Not Allowed
Milk (limit to 2 cups daily)	Any milk, chocolate milk, instant cocoa mix, yogurt, and eggnog Substitute 8 oz. of milk for one of the following: 4 oz. evaporated milk 4 oz. condensed milk 1/3 c. dry milk powder	Malted milk, buttermilk, and milkshakes
Meat, Poultry, Fish and Meat Substitutes (limit to 6 ounces daily)	All fresh or fresh frozen meats, poultry, fish prepared without salt, beef, lamb, veal, fresh pork, chicken, turkey, liver, heart, brains, duck, quail, rabbit, cod, flounder, halibut, trout, bass, bluefish, catfish, clams, crabs, lobster, oysters, low sodium salmon and tuna, shrimp and sole. Cheese: swiss, cheddar, mozarella, ricotta, and cream; low sodium cheese as desired; peanut butter (2 Tbsp. = 1 oz.)	Any meat, fish, or poultry that is cured, salted, canned or smoked: chipped beef, corned beef, ham, cold cuts, bacon, hot dogs, and other sausages, sardines, anchovies, marinated herring, pickled meats, regular peanut butter, regular hard and processed cheeses, cheese spreads, regular canned tuna and salmon, frozen dinner entrees and meat substitutes (soy)

Type of Food	Foods Allowed	Foods Not Allowed
Eggs (limit to 1 daily)	egg substitute (omit 1 oz. meat) or eggs	Pickled Eggs
Fruits (2 or more servings daily—include citrus daily)	All fruit juices; fresh, frozen, canned fruits, and sun-dried fruits	Any fruit which has salt or sodium added (read label)
Vegetables (3 servings daily—include a dark green leafy or deep yellow vegetable)	Fresh or frozen vegetables prepared without salt; salt free canned vegetables and salt free tomato juice; white potatoes, sweet potatoes, and yams (all prepared without salt) Salt free potato chips	Frozen lima beans, mixed vegetables and green peas (if prepared with sodium preservative); regular canned vegetables and vegetable juice; sauerkraut, pickled vegetables or others prepared in brine; tomato or V-8 juice*; potato chips and other snack chips, instant potatoes and potato substitute products, canned, frozen, or commercial potato products
Bread, Cereal, Rice and Pasta (limit regular products to 6 servings daily—limit salt-free products to 4 servings daily)	Whole grain or enriched breads, rolls, muffins, biscuits, hamburger buns and crackers made without salt toppings; rice, noodles, spaghetti and other enriched pastas, graham crackers, vanilla wafers, rusk, cornbread, pancakes, waffles, hot breads and quick breads. Cooked cereals without salt, low sodium dry cereals Low sodium bread, crackers, matzo, melba toast, hot water cornbread, biscuits, pancakes and waffles made with low sodium baking powder; salt free popcorn	Salted or soda crackers, "Low Salt" snack crackers, pretzels and bread products made with salt toppings; salted popcorn; frozen or commercial rice and pasta products. Instant hot cereals or quick cooking cereals that have a sodium compound added (read label); dry cereals with added sodium
Fats and Oil (limit to 6 servings daily—1 tsp. = 1 serving)	Regular butter or fortified margarine, cream, cream substitute, vegetable oils, mayonnaise, and unsalted nuts. 1 Tbsp. 1000 Island dressing may be used as 2 fat servings. 1 Tbsp. French, Blue Cheese or Roquefort dressings may be used as 3 fat servings. Limit French, Blue Cheese, Roquefort and 1000 Island salad dressings to 1 Tbsp. per day. S.F. salad dressing may be used as desired	Other salad dressings, bacon fat, salt pork, and salted nuts
Soups	Low sodium bouillon, broth, and consomme, low sodium commercial and dehydrated soups; homemade soups made with allowed vegetables and/or milk All sweets and desserts made with	Regular commercially canned and dried soups, bouillon cubes, consomme, and broth

Type of Food	Foods Allowed	Foods Not Allowed
Desserts	allowed foods. For milk based desserts, an equal an equal amount of milk should be omitted from the daily milk allowance.)	Desserts made with foods omitted
Beverages	Coffee, coffee substitutes and tea; carbonated beverages	Commercially softened water
Miscellaneous	Pepper, spices, flavorings, vinegar, lemon juice, vanilla and peppermint extract, sugar, honey, pure horseradish, dry mustard, maple syrup, low sodium catsup, low sodium chili sauce, low sodium mustard, low sodium pickles, tabasco sauce, hard candy, leavening agents such as ad yeasts, cream of tartar, potassium biocarbonate and sodium free baking powder	Regular catsup, chili sauce, mustard, pickles, relishes, garlic salt, sea salt, rock salt Kosher salt, monosodium glutamate (Accent*), Kitchen Bouquet*, barbecue sauce, soy sauce, teriyaki sauce, steak and worcestershire sauce; sodium based antacids; all commercially prepared or convenience food

Sample Menu

Breakfast	Lunch	Supper
½ c. Orange Juice	1 c. S.F. Vegetable Soup	3 oz. S.F. Hamburger
½ c.S.F. Oatmeal	3 oz S.F. Broiled Chicken	⅓ c. S.F. Rice
1 Scrambled Egg	½ c. S.F. Mashed Potatoes	½ c. Carrots
1 Slice Toast	½ c. c. Green Beans	1 Slice Bread
1 tsp. Margarine	1 Slice Bread	1 tsp. Margarine
Jelly	1 tsp. Margarine	½ c. Canned Peaches
1 cup Milk	Yellow Cake with Icing	1 cup Milk
Coffee–Sugar	Tea–Sugar	Tea–Sugar
pepper	pepper	pepper

Salt substitute may be used on the advice of the physician.   S.F = Salt Free

*Registered Trademark: Brand names are used for clarification and do not constitute endorsement of that product.

1 Gram Sodium Diet (43 Milliequivalents)

Description

The 1 gram sodium diet is indicated for the patient with severe sodium and fluid retention associated with cardiovascular, renal, or hepatic diseases and/or treatment with sodium retaining hormones such as corticosteroids. No salt is used in the preparation of food or at the table. Certain foods containing high levels of salt or sodium are omitted. It is necessary to read labels.

Adequacy

This diet meets the 1989 Recommended Dietary Allowance for good nutrition as established by the Food and Nutrition Board of the National Research Council when the types of foods and amounts suggested are included daily. Females ages 11–50 need to include a good source of iron daily.

Type of Food	Foods Allowed	Foods Not Allowed
Milk (limit to 2 cups daily)	Any milk	Chocolate milk, buttermilk, malted milk, milk mixes, condensed milk
Meat, Poultry, Fish and Meat Substitutes (limit to 4 ounces daily)	All fresh or fresh frozen meats, poultry, fish and shellfish; low-sodium cheese, cream cheese, ricotta cheese, low-sodium peanut butter—(2 Tbsp. = 1 oz. meat), low-sodium tuna and salmon	Any meat, fish, or poultry that is cured, salted, canned or smoked: chipped beef, corned beef, ham, cold cuts, bacon, hot dogs, and other sausages, sardines, anchovies, marinated herring, pickled meats, regular peanut butter, regular hard, processed cheeses, cheese spreads, regular canned tuna and salmon, frozen entrees
Eggs (limit 1 daily)	Eggs	Egg substitutes, pickled eggs
Fruits (2 or more servings daily—include citrus daily)	All fruit juices; fresh, frozen, or canned fruits and sun dried fruits	Crystallized or glazed fruit, maraschino cherries, dried fruits containing a sodium compound (read label)
Vegetables (3 servings daily—include a dark green leafy or deep yellow vegetable 3–4 times weekly)	All fresh, unsalted frozen and unsalted canned vegetables except those listed under Foods Not Allowed; salt-free tomato juice and other low sodium vegetable juices, dried beans, lentils, and peas; fresh potatoes, sweet potatoes, yams, salt free potato chips	Frozen lima beans, mixed vegetables and green peas (if prepared with sodium preservative); all fresh, frozen, canned, or pickled: artichokes, beets, beet greens, celery, swiss chard, dandelion greens, kale, mustard greens, collard greens, sauerkraut, spinach, white turnips and carrots; regular canned tomato or V-8 Juice*; potato chips and other snack chips, instant potatoes, potato substitute products; frozen, canned, or commercial potato products
Bread, Cereal, Rice and Pasta (limit regular products to 3 servings daily—limit salt-free products to 6 servings daily)	Whole grain or enriched breads, rolls, muffins, biscuits, hamburger buns and crackers made without salt toppings; rice noodles, spaghetti and other enriched pastas (all prepared without salt); graham crackers, vanilla wafers, rusk, cornbread, pancakes, waffles, hot breads and quick breads; cooked cereals prepared without salt, puffed rice, puffed wheat, shredded wheat	Salted or soda crackers, "Low Salt" snack crackers, pretzels and bread products made with salt toppings; salted popcorn; frozen or commercial rice and pasta products; instant hot cereals or quick cooking cereals that have a sodium compound added (read label), all other dry cereals
Fats and Oil (limit to 6 servings daily)	Salt-free butter or margarine, cream, cream substitutes, unsalted salad dressing, unsalted salad oil, unsalted shortening unsalted mayonnaise, and unsalted nuts	Salted butter or margarine; regular salad dressings, regular mayonnaise, bacon fat, and salted nuts

Type of Food	Foods Allowed	Foods Not Allowed
Soups	Low sodium bouillon, broth, and consomme, low sodium commercial and dehydrated soups	Regular bouillon, broth, or consomme, regular canned or dehydrated soups
Desserts (limit to 2 servings daily)	Salt-free custard or pudding (made from allowed milk), unsalted fruit pies, unsalted gelatin desserts, unsalted bakery goods made with allowed leavening agents	Commercial ice cream and sherbet; all desserts prepared with salt, baking powder or soda, egg whites or self-rising flour; regular gelatin desserts, instant custard or pudding
Beverages	Coffee, coffee substitutes and tea; carbonated beverage (not to exceed 16 ounces daily)	Commercially softened water; beverages made with commercially softened water
Miscellaneous	Salt substitute with physician's approval; sugar, syrup, honey, jelly, marmalade, jam, hard candies and other sugar candies, molasses, marshmallows; pepper, tobasco sauce, s pices, flavorings, vinegar, and lemon sauce; low sodium catsup, low sodium chili sauce, low sodium mustard, low sodium pickles, and fresh ground horseradish; leavening agents: yeast, cream of tartar, potassium bicarbonate, and sodium free baking powder	Salt, Lite Salt*, regular catsup, chili sauce, mustard, pickles, relishes, olives, and horseradish, celery salt, onion salt, garlic salt, seasoned salt, sea salt, rock salt, kosher salt, and monosodium glutamate; Kitchen Bouquet*, barbecue sauce, soy sauce, teriyaki sauce, steak sauce, and Worcestershire sauce; all commercially prepared or convenience foods

Sample Menu

Breakfast	Lunch	Supper
½ c. Orange Juice	1 c. S.F. Vegetable Soup	3 oz. S.F. Beef Patty
½ c. S.F. Oatmeal	3 oz. S.F. Roast Lamb	⅓ c. S.F. Rice
1 S.F. Scrambled Egg	½ c. S.F. Mashed Potato	Tomato Slices
1 Slice Toast	½ c. S.F. Green Beans	1 tsp. S.F. Margarine
1 tsp. S.F. Margarine	1 Slice Bread	Fresh Fruit
Jelly	1 tsp. S.F. Margarine	1 cup Milk
½ c. Milk	1 S.F. Cupcake	Iced Tea–Sugar
Coffee–Sugar	Iced Tea–Sugar	Pepper
Pepper	½ c Milk	
	Pepper	

S.F. = Salt Free

*Registered Trademark: Brand names are used for clarification and do not constitute endorsement of that product.

500 Milligrams Sodium Diet (21.7 Milliequivalents)

Description

The 500 milligram sodium diet is indicated for the patient requiring very strict limitation of sodium, due to cardiovascular, renal, or hepatic diseases and/or treatment with sodium-retaining hormones such as corticosteroids. It is a strict sodium restriction. No salt is used in the preparation of food or at the table. Certain foods containing high levels of salt or sodium are eliminated. Foods canned or processed with sodium or salt are omitted. It is necessary to read labels.

Adequacy

This diet meets the 1989 Recommended Dietary Allowance for good nutrition as established by the Food and Nutrition Board of the National Research Council when the types of food and amounts suggested are included daily. Females ages 11–50 need to include a good source of iron daily. The diet may be deficient in iodine due to the elimination of iodized salt, especially in areas with iodine deficient soil.

Type of Food	Foods Allowed	Foods Not Allowed
Milk (limit to 2 cups daily)	Milk	Chocolate milk, buttermilk, malted milk, milk mixes, condensed milk
Meat, Poultry, Fish and Meat Substitutes (limit to 4 ounces daily)	All fresh or fresh frozen meats, poultry, fish: beef, lamb, veal, fresh pork, chicken, turkey, liver, cod, flounder, halibut, trout, low sodium salmon and tuna, salt-free cottage cheese, low sodium cheeses, low sodium peanut butter (2 Tbsp = 1 oz.)	Cured, salted, canned, or smoked meats, poultry and fish; chipped and corned beef, ham, luncheon meats, bacon, frankfurters, sausages, sardines, anchovies, Kosher meats, salt pork, smoked tongue, kidneys, brains, caviar, frozen fish fillets, clams, crabs, oysters, scallops or shrimp, all other cheeses, regular peanut butter, meat substitutes (soy)
Eggs (limit 1 daily)	Eggs	Egg substitutes, pickled eggs
Fruits (2 or more servings daily—include citrus daily)	All fruit juices; fresh, frozen, or canned fruits and sun dried fruits	Crystallized or glazed fruit, maraschino cherries, dried fruits containing a sodium compound (read label)
Vegetables (3 servings daily—include a dark green leafy or deep yellow vegetable 3–4 times weekly)	Any fresh, frozen & unsalted canned vegetables (prepared without salt) except those listed under Foods Not Allowed; salt-free tomato juice; dried beans, lentils, peas, fresh potatoes, sweet potatoes, yams, salt-free potato chips	Frozen lima beans, green peas, and mixed vegetables (if prepared with sodium preservative); all fresh, frozen, canned, or pickled: artichokes, beets, beet greens, kale, mustard greens, collard greens, sauerkraut, spinach, white turnips, carrots, celery, swiss chard, dandelion greens; regular canned tomato or V-8 juice; potato chips and other snack chips, instant potatoes, potato substitute products, frozen or commercial potato and rice products, and canned potatoes

Type of Food	Foods Allowed	Foods Not Allowed
Bread, Cereal, Rice and Pasta (limit to 4 servings daily)	Salt-free bread, macaroni, rice, noodles, spaghetti and other enriched pastas (all prepared without salt); low sodium crackers, and pretzels, unsalted popcorn Cooked cereals prepared without salt: grits, oatmeal, cream of wheat, farina, wheatena; puffed rice, puffed wheat, shredded wheat, low sodium corn flakes	Regular bread, salted or soda crackers, "Low Salt" snack crackers, pretzels and bread made with baking powder or soda, egg whites, or self-rising flour; salted popcorn Instant hot cereals or quick cooking cereals that have a sodium compound added (read label); all other dry cereals not listed
Fats and Oil (limit to 3 servings - 1 tsp. = 1 serving)	Salt-free butter or margarine, cream, cream substitutes, unsalted salad dressing, unsalted salad oil, unsalted mayonnaise, and unsalted nuts shortening,	Salted butter or margarine; regular salad dressings, regular mayonnaise, bacon fat, and salted nuts
Soups (limit to 1 serving daily)	Salt-free cream soup (made from allowed milk), special low sodium soups and low sodium broth	Commercially canned or dried soups, bouillon cubes, consomme and broth
Desserts (limit to 1 daily)	Salt-free custard or pudding (made from allowed milk), unsalted fruit pies, unsalted gelatin desserts, unsalted bakery goods made with allowed leavening agent	Commercial ice cream and sherbet; all desserts prepared with salt, baking powder or soda, egg whites or self-rising bakery flour; regular gelatin desserts, instant custard or pudding
Beverages	Coffee, coffee substitutes and tea	Flavored instant coffee, soft water, all carbonated beverages
Miscellaneous	Pepper, spices, flavorings, vinegar, lemon juice, vanilla and peppermint xtract, sugar, honey, pure horseradish, dry mustard, maple syrup, low sodium catsup, low sodium chili sauce, low sodium mustard, low sodium pickles, tabasco sauce, hard candy, leavening agents such as yeast, cream of tartar, potassium bicarbonate, and sodium free baking powder	Salt, lite salt, catsup, chili sauce, prepared mustard, pickles, relishes, olives, celery salt, onion salt, garlic salt, sea salt, rock salt, Kosher salt, monosodium glutamate (accent), Kitchen Bouquet®, barbecue sauce, soy sauce, teriyaki sauce, steak and worcestershire sauce, all commercially prepared or convenience foods; sodium based antacids

Sample Menu

Breakfast	Lunch	Supper
½ c. Orange Juice	2 oz. S.F. Chicken	2 oz. S.F. Roast Beef
1 Scrambled Egg	⅓ c. S.F. Rice	½ c. S.F. Carrots
½ c. S.F. Grits	½ c. S.F. Broccoli	1 Slice S.F. Bread
1 Slice S.F. Bread	1 Apple	½ c. Fresh Fruit Salad
1 tsp. S.F. Margarine	1 tsp. S.F. Margarine	1 tsp. S.F. Margarine
1 cup Milk	Iced Tea–Sugar–Lemon	1 cup Milk
Coffee–Sugar		

S.F. = Salt-Free

250 Milligrams Sodium Diet (10.8 Milliequivalents)

Description

The 250 milligrams sodium diet is indicated for the patient requiring very strict limitation of sodium due to cardiovascular, renal, or hepatic diseases and/or treatment with sodium-retaining hormones such as corticosteroids. It is a severe dietary restriction, not practical outside the hospital. No salt is used in the preparation of food or at the table. Certain foods containing high levels of salt or sodium are eliminated. Foods canned or processed with sodium or salt are omitted. It is necessary to read labels.

Adequacy

This diet does not meet the 1989 Recommended Dietary Allowance for calcium, riboflavin, niacin, and vitamin D as established by the Food and Nutrition Board of the National Research Council. The diet may be deficient in iodine due to the elimination of iodized salt, especially in areas with iodine deficient soil.

Type of Food	Foods Allowed	Foods Not Allowed
Milk (limit to 2 cups daily)	Low sodium milk	Regular milk, buttermilk, chocolate milk, malted milk
Meat, Poultry, Fish and Meat Substitutes (limit to 4 ounces daily)	All fresh or fresh frozen meats, poultry, fish: beef, lamb, veal, fresh pork, chicken, turkey, liver, cod, flounder, halibut, trout, low sodium salmon and tuna, salt-free cottage cheese, low sodium cheeses, low sodium peanut butter (2 Tbsp = 1 oz.)	Cured, salted, canned, or smoked meats, poultry and fish; chipped and corned beef, ham, luncheon meats, bacon, frankfurters, sausages, sardines, anchovies, Kosher meats, salt pork, smoked tongue, kidneys, brains, caviar, frozen fish fillets, clams, crabs, oysters, scallops or shrimp, all other cheeses, regular peanut butter, meat substitutes (soy)
Eggs (limit 1 daily)	Egg	Egg substitutes, pickled eggs
Fruits (2 or more servings daily— include citrus daily)	All fruit juices, any fresh, frozen, canned, or dried fruits	Crystallized or glazed fruit, maraschino cherries, dried fruits containing a sodium compound (read label)

Type of Food	Foods Allowed	Foods Not Allowed
Vegetables (2 servings daily—include a dark green leafy or deep yellow vegetable 2–4 times weekly)	Any fresh, frozen and unsalted canned vegetables except those listed under Foods Not Allowed; salt-free tomato juice; dried beans, lentils, peas, potatoes, sweet potatoes, yams, salt-free potato chips	Frozen lima beans, green peas, and mixed vegetables (if prepared with sodium preservative); all fresh, frozen, canned, or pickled: artichokes, beets, beet greens, kale, mustard greens, collard greens, sauerkraut spinach, white turnips, and carrots; regular canned tomato or V-8 juice; potato chips and other snack chips, instant potatoes, potato substitute products, frozen or commercial potato products, and canned potatoes
Bread, Cereal, Rice and Pasta (limit to 4 servings daily)	Salt-free bread, macaroni, rice, noodles, spaghetti and other enriched pastas (all prepared without salt); low sodium crackers, and pretzels, unsalted popcorn	Regular bread, frozen or commercial macaroni, rice, noodles or spaghetti products. Salted or soda crackers, "Low Salt" snack crackers, pretzels and bread made with baking powder or soda, egg whites or self-rising flour; salted popcorn
	Cooked cereals prepared without salt; grits, oatmeal, cream of wheat, farina, wheatena, and puffed rice, puffed wheat, shredded wheat, low sodium corn flakes	Instant hot cereals or quick cooking cereals that have a sodium compound added (read label), all other dry cereals not listed
Fats and Oil	Salt-free butter or margarine, 1/3 cup cream, cream substitutes, unsalted salad dressing, unsalted salad oil, unsalted shortening, unsalted mayonnaise, and unsalted nuts	Salted butter or margarine; regular salad dressings, regular mayonnaise, bacon fat, and salted nuts
Soups (limit to 1 serving)	Salt-free cream soup (made from allowed milk), special low sodium soups and low sodium broth	Commercially canned or dried soups, bouillon cubes, consomme and broth
Desserts (limit to 1 serving)	Salt-free custard or pudding (made from allowed milk), unsalted fruit pies, unsalted gelatin desserts, unsalted bakery goods made with allowed leavening agents	Commercial ice cream and sherbet; all desserts prepared with salt, baking powder or soda, egg whites or self-rising flour; regular gelatin desserts, instant custard or pudding
Beverages	Coffee, coffee substitutes and tea	Flavored instant coffee, soft water, all carbonated beverages

Type of Food	Foods Allowed	Foods Not Allowed
Miscellaneous	Pepper, spices, flavorings, vinegar, lemon juice, vanilla and peppermint extract, sugar, honey, pure horseradish, dry mustard, maple syrup, low sodium catsup, low sodium chili sauce, low sodium mustard, low sodium pickles, tabasco sauce, hard candy, leavening agents such as yeast, cream of tartar, potassium bicarbonate and sodium free baking powder	Salt, lite salt, catsup, chili sauce, prepared mustard, pickles, relishes, olives, celery salt, onion salt, garlic salt, sea salt, rock salt, Kosher salt, monosodium glutamate (accent), Kitchen Bouquet®, barbecue sauce, soy sauce, teriyaki sauce, steak and worcestershire sauce, all commercially prepared or convenience foods; sodium based antacids

Sample Menu

Breakfast	Lunch	Supper
½ c. Orange Juice	2 oz. S.F. Chicken	2 oz. S.F. Roast Beef
1 Scrambled Egg	½ c. S.F. Mashed Potatoes	⅓ c. S.F. Rice
½ c. S.F. Grits	1 Slice S.F. Bread	½ c. S.F. Broccoli
1 tsp. S.F. Margarine	1 Apple	½ c. Peaches
1 cup S.F. Milk	1 tsp. S.F. Margarine	1 tsp. S.F. Margarine
Coffee–Sugar	Coffee or Tea–Sugar	1 cup S.F. Milk
		Coffee or Tea–Sugar

S.F. = Salt-Free

References

Aspen Reference Group: *Dietitian's Patient Education Manual*. Sara Nell DiLima, ed., Gaithersburg: Aspen Publishers, Inc., 1993.

Mahan, K. and Arlin, M.: *Krause's Food, Nutrition and Diet Therapy*. 8th ed., Philadelphia: W.B. Saunders Company, 1992.

Puckett, R.P. and Brown S.M.: *Shands Hospital at the University of Florida Guide to Clinical Dietetics*. 5th ed., Dubuque: Kendall/Hunt Publishing Co., 1993.

▶ THE SODIUM ALTERNATIVE—SPICE AND HERB CHART ◀

Spices and Herbs	Main Dish	Salad	Sauces	Vegetables
Spices:				
Allspice	Beef pot roast, duck, turkey or chicken, fish	Fruit salad	Tomato	Beets
Cayenne	Beef, stews, chicken, seafood	All varieties except fruit	Meat, vegetable	All Vegetables
Chili powder	Beef, hamburgers, meat loaf, chili con carne	Bean salad	Mexican type	Corn
Cloves	Pork, ham, boiled beef, pot roast		Tomato	
Curry	Meat, fish, poultry, lamb, veal, fish or shrimp chowders	Chicken salad	Vegetable	Rice, creamed onions

Spices and Herbs	Main Dish	Salad	Sauces	Vegetables
Ginger	Pork, chicken	Fruit salad	Dessert	Squash
Mace	Poultry stuffing, veal	Fruit Salad	Fish, poultry, veal	Potatoes
Dry Mustard	Beef, hamburgers, chicken, tuna, egg	Chicken, egg, tuna, macaroni, potato	Fish, Vegetable	Cabbage
Nutmeg	Chicken stew, beef stew, creamed dishes	Fruit Salad	Dessert and fruit sauces, pudding	All vegetables except cabbage family
Paprika	Meat, fish, poultry, veal, creamed dishes	All except fruit salad	All gravies and sauce	All vegetables
Pepper	Meat, fish, poultry, veal	All except fruit salad	All gravies and sauces	All vegetables
Herbs: Basil	Tomato, egg, fish, chicken cacciatore, beef stew	Vegetable salads with marinades	Tomato	Cucumbers, green beans, zucchini, yellow squash
Chives	Creamed dishes, fish, eggs	Potato salad, green salad	Creamed type	Potatoes
Dill	Fish	Potato, vegetable	Creamed type	Green beans, cucumbers, cabbage, carrots
Marjoram	Italian type, tomato, beef, lamb, fish, veal, poultry, eggs	Salad dressings	Tomato, Brown	Broccoli, green beans, peas, eggplant
Oregano	Italian type, tomato, meat loaf, pork, veal, pot roast	Vegetable salads with marinades, bean salad	Tomato, Fish	Tomato, broccoli, zucchini, eggplant
Parsley	All	All except fruit salad	All except fruit	All
Rosemary	Beef, pork, fish, lamb		Vegetable, meat and fish gravies	Cauliflower, potatoes, turnips
Sage	Pork, poultry, goulash, beef stews	Vegetable salads with marinades	Meat, chicken, pork gravies	Mushroom, broccoli, cabbage, onions, cauliflower
Thyme	Beef, pork, chicken, fish, beef stews, fish chowders, fish soups	Vegetable salads with marinades, salad dressings	Brown	Creamed onions
Tarragon	Eggs, poultry, fish	Salad dressings	Creamed type	Potatoes

Reference

Campbell Soup Company, Consumer Nutrition Center, *Your Sodium Intake: Some Basic Steps in the Right Direction,* Camden New Jersey.

Module 3

Modification
for Calories

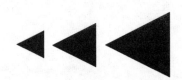

▶ DIABETIC DIETS ◀

Description

The dietary management of Diabetes Mellitus has been recognized as an important part of the total care plan of the patient. A realistic and attractive individualized eating plan is most effective to influence dietary compliance and will contribute to the control of diabetes mellitus. The goals of the diabetic diet are to:

▶ Improve blood glucose and lipid levels
▶ Reduce the potential for acute and/or chronic complications
▶ Achieve and/or maintain desirable body weight
▶ Encourage healthy eating habits
▶ Provide a nutritionally adequate and acceptable diet
▶ Include other nutrient modifications made necessary by coexisting medical conditions
▶ Stop smoking
▶ Exercise as appropriate
▶ Eliminate or limit alcohol intake to less than 1 oz per/day
▶ Increase dietary fiber
▶ Reduce dietary saturated fat and cholesterol

Approximately 16 million people in the United States suffer from the disease, which means that one out of every 20 people has diabetes. An estimated 385,000 people in the U.S. die from the disease every year, making it the nation's sixth leading cause of death by disease.

Clinical classification of diabetes mellitus includes three classes of glucose intolerance: diabetes mellitus (Type I, Type II, and diabetes associated with certain conditions and syndromes), gestational diabetes mellitus and impaired glucose tolerance.

Type I or insulin-dependent diabetes mellitus (IDDM) is a chronic disease in which insulin production is limited or absent. This type occurs frequently in the pediatric population, but may occur at any age. Establishing a consistent food intake pattern is crucial in the care plan for the individual with IDDM. Besides following an established nutrition regimen, exercise and medication (insulin) are primary objectives and achieving a balance among all three.

Type II or non-insulin-dependent diabetes mellitus (NIDDM) is characterized by impaired insulin secretion and diminished tissue sensitivity to insulin (insulin resistance). NIDDM is the most frequently diagnosed type of diabetes, occurring in 85–90% of cases. NIDDM can occur at any age, but the most often diagnosed population is after the age of 40 years. The majority of diagnosed cases occur in the overweight individual, but the diagnosis in non-obese individuals is increasing. The primary treatment is from an established nutrition regimen. Oral hypoglycemic agents or insulin therapy may also be needed to reach blood glucose goals. Parental history and obesity are associated with higher rates of NIDDM.

Gestational diabetes mellitus (GDM) is a glucose intolerance of variable severity with the onset being recognized for the first time during pregnancy. GDM being diagnosed in approximately 2% of pregnancies, can occur at any time during pregnancy, but is diagnosed most often during the second and third trimesters. Early detection, aggressive diet management, insulin if indicated, and appropriate obstetric care can help prevent associated maternal and perinatal risks. After parturition, glucose levels generally return to normal, but with GDM there is an increased risk of developing diabetes later in life. The maintenance of desirable body weight and exercise after delivery helps reduce the risk of the onset of diabetes later in life. Refer to the section on Gestational Diabetic Diet for establishing an appropriate diet regimen.

Impaired glucose tolerance (IGT) is indicated when the plasma glucose levels are above normal, but less than those of diagnosed diabetes. Approximately 25% of individuals with IGT will develop diabetes later in life.

Lifestyle changes for an individual with IDDM should include:

▶ An achieved balance of exercise and insulin action with food absorption and metabolism
▶ Caloric intake appropriate for age, sex and physical activity
▶ Meal composition
▶ Assessment of needs for growth, pregnancy or lactation

Lifestyle changes for an individual with NIDDM should include:

▶ Weight reduction/maintenance
▶ Nutritional balance in diet regimen
▶ Proper meal spacing to reduce demand on the pancreas and balance the action of endogenous insulin
▶ Appropriate physical activity regimen to promote weight management and control of glucose and lipid levels
▶ Coordination of insulin and exercise with meal timing if exogenous insulin is needed

▶ NUTRITION GOALS FOR TREATMENT OF NIDDM AND IDDM ◀

	NIDDM	IDDM
Energy intake:		
Calories	Decrease to achieve weight loss if needed. Adequate to maintain reasonable weight.	Adequate for energy requirements and/or sufficient for growth and development.
Diet composition:		
Protein	Customary American intake is double amount needed. Usual recommendation for people with diabetes is 12% to 20% of total calories.	Same
	RDA for adults is 0.8 g/kg body weight or at least 60 g/day to reduce body protein loss during restriction.	Modify intake for children, pregnancy, lactation, and special medical conditions.
Carbohydrate	Up to 50% to 60% of total calories. Liberalized-with emphasis on complex carbohydrates with fiber and low intake of simple sugars. Sucrose-could be included in individualized diet plan, contingent on good metabolic control.	Same
Fiber	Up to 40 g/day; 25 g/1,000 Kcal for calorie-restricted diets. Emphasize water-soluble fiber.	Same
Fat	Ideally <30% of total calories, although may be difficult and needs to be individualized. Fat breakdown: • Saturated fats: <10% • Polyunsaturated fats: up to 10% • Monounsaturated fats: Remaining percent (10% to 15%)	Same
Cholesterol	<300 mg/day	Same

NUTRITION GOALS FOR TREATMENT OF NIDDM AND IDDM—Continued

	NIDDM	IDDM
Alternative sweeteners	Use is acceptable.	Same
Sodium	Do not exceed 3,000 mg/day. Modify for coexisting medical conditions.	Same
Vitamins/minerals	No evidence of increased need.	Same

The Diet Prescription

The process of developing the diet prescription includes an assessment of desirable weight, calculation of energy requirement, evaluation of patients current food intake (See Food and Nutrition Service Diet History Form), formulation of an initial meal plan and the very important follow-up.

Weight and height should be evaluated in relation to height and frame size. Refer to the appendix for Weight and Height Ranges.

A simple method to determine desirable body weight is the Hamwi formula:

▶ Women: Allow 100 pounds for the first 5 feet, plus 5 pounds for each additional inch over 5 feet

▶ Men: Allow 106 pounds for the first 5 feet, plus 6 pounds for each additional inch over 5 feet

▶ Small frame: Subtract 10%

▶ Large frame: Add 10%

Determine normal daily energy requirements from information charted in the patient diet history form if the patient is maintaining a reasonable weight. If not, use the following method;

▶ Caloric requirement = basal Kcal + activity Kcal

- Basal Kcal:
    IBW (lb) × 10
- Activity Kcal:
    IBW (lb) × 3 for sedentary activity
    IBW (lb) × 5 for moderate activity
    IBM (lb) × 10 for strenuous activity

▶ Add calories for indicated weight gain:
    (+ 500 Kcal/day for anticipated gain of 1 lb/week)

▶ Subtract calories for indicated weight loss:
    (−500 Kcl/day for anticipated loss of 1 lb/week)

A weight loss of 1 to 2½ pounds per week is the maximum recommended.

The "Exchange Lists for Meal Planning", developed by the American Diabetes Association and The American Dietetic Association categorizes foods that are similar in calorie, carbohydrate, protein and fat content into 6 groups. Foods in each group or list can be exchanged for other foods within that group, but never exchanged for foods in other groups. The exchange system is an excellent tool in evaluating the individual's usual intake and in calculating a new meal plan that is a nutritionally adequate and acceptable to the individual.

To obtain more information for customizing the Exchange List for Meal Planning to meet individual needs, call the American Dietetic Association at 1-800-877-1600, Fax–(312) 899-1979 or log on to www.eatright.org.

For the composition of the six groups in the Exchange List, refer to the following.

▶ COMPOSITION OF FOOD GROUPS ◀

Food	Measure	Carbohydrates (g)	Protein (g)	Fat (g)	Calories (Kcal)
Milk (skim)	8 oz.	12	8	0	90
Milk (2%)	8 oz.	12	8	5	120
Milk (whole)	8 oz.	12	8	8	150
Vegetable	½ cup	5	2	0	25
Fruit	1 serving	15	0	0	60
Starch/Bread	1 serving or 1 slice	15	3	0	80
Meat (lean)	1 oz.	0	7	3	55
Meat (medium fat)	1 oz.	0	7	5	75
Meat (high fat)	1 oz.	0	7	8	100
Fat	1 tsp.	0	0	5	45

Adequacy

Diets of 1200 Kcal/day or more for women and 1500 Kcal/day for men, should supply the Recommended Dietary Allowances for all nutrients if a variety of foods are chosen.

Refer to the Diabetic Sample Meal Patterns for appropriate meal planning to meet the individual's needs.

Sample Menu For Diabetic Diet (1200 Calories)

Breakfast	Lunch	Supper	Bedtime Snack
½ c. Orange Juice 1 Slice Toast 1 Scrambled Egg 1 tsp. Margarine 1 c. Skim Milk Coffee or Tea	1 oz. Broiled Chicken ⅓ c. Rice ½ c. Green Beans Tossed Salad with Lemon ½ tsp. Margarine 1 Slice Bread 1 Small Pear Coffee or Iced Tea	2 oz. Roast Beef Small Baked Potato ½ c. Spinach Sliced Tomatoes ½ tsp. Margarine 1¼ c. Strawberries, Whole Coffee or Iced Tea	½ c. Skim Milk 3 Graham Cracker Squares

Sample Menu For Diabetic Diet (1800 Calories)

Breakfast	Lunch	Supper	Bedtime Snack
½ c. Orange Juice 2 Slices of Toast 1 Scrambled Egg 1 tsp. Margarine 1 c. Skim Milk Coffee or Tea	2 oz. Broiled Chicken ⅓ c. Rice ½ c. Green Peas 1 c. Carrot & Celery Sticks 1 tsp. Margarine 1 Slice Bread 1 Small Pear Coffee or Iced Tea	2 oz. Roast Beef Small Baked Potato ½ c. Whole Kernel Corn Sliced Tomatoes 2 tsp. Margarine 1 Slice Bread 1¼ c. Strawberries, Whole 3 Graham Crackers, 2½" Sq. ½ C. Skim Milk	½ c. Skim Milk 6 Saltine Crackers 1 oz. American Cheese 1 Small Apple

Diabetic Replacement Procedures

Unless a large amount of food must be replaced, orange juice will be used. More than 8 ounces of orange juice replacement is not practical. The dietitian should be notified and another replacement will be calculated.

Standard replacements are listed below:

Food to be Replaced	Grams CHO	Orange Juice
1 Slice Bread	15	4 ounces
6 Saltine Squares	15	4 ounces
1 Small Potato	15	4 ounces
1 pkg. Dry Cereal	15	4 ounces
½ cup Cooked Cereal	15	4 ounces
⅓ cup Rice or Substitutes	15	4 ounces
1 cup Milk (Whole, Buttermilk, Skim)	12	4 ounces
1 serving Fruit (Fresh or Diet Pack)	15	4 ounces
2 ounces Meat, Cheese or Egg	none	none
1 pat Butter	none	none

Note: For Renal patients do not use orange juice.
May substitute: ½ cup Apple Juice
or
⅓ cup Cranberry Juice

Diabetic Sample Meal Patterns

Calories	1000	1200	1400	1500	1600	1800	2000	2500
Breakfast								
Starch/Bread	1	1	2	2	2	2	2	3
Meat	1	1	1	1	1	1	1	1
Fruit	1	1	1	1	1	1	1	1
Nonfat Milk	.5	1	1	1	1	1	1	1
Fat	-	1	1	1	1	1	1	1
Lunch								
Starch/Bread	1	2	2	2	2	3	4	4
Meat	1	1	2	2	2	2	2	2
Vegetable	1	1	1	1	1	1	1	2
Fruit	1	1	1	1	1	1	1	1
Nonfat Milk	-	-	-	-	-	-	-	-
Fat	.5	.5	.5	.5	1	1	1	1
Midafternoon Snack								
Starch/Bread	-	-	-	-	-	-	1	2
Meat	-	-	-	-	-	-	1	1
Dinner								
Starch/Bread	1	1	2	3	3	4	4	4
Meat	2	2	2	2	2	2	2	3
Vegetable	2	2	2	2	1	1	1	3
Fruit	1	1	1	1	1	1	1	2
Nonfat Milk	-	-	-	-	.5	.5	-	-
Fat	.5	.5	.5	.5	1	2	1	1

Calories	1000	1200	1400	1500	1600	1800	2000	2500
Bedtime Snack								
Starch/Bread	1	1	1	1	1	1	1	2
Meat	-	-	-	-	1	1	1	1
Fruit	-	-	-	-	1	1	1	1
Nonfat Milk	.5	1	1	1	.5	.5	1	1
Totals								
Starch/Bread	4	5	7	8	8	10	12	15
Meat	4	4	5	5	6	6	6	8
Vegetable	3	3	3	3	3	2	2	5
Fruit	3	3	3	3	4	4	4	5
Nonfat Milk	1	2	2	2	2	2	2	2
Fat	1	2	2	2	3	4	3	3
Carbohydrate	132	159	189	204	214	244	274	349
Protein	54	65	71	81	86	92	105	127
Fat	28.6	39.5	41.3	37.2	45	50	55	68.5
Calories	1002	1207	1440	1500	1605	1794	2011	2521

Adapted from Hart, B.E., Clinical Diet Manual, Food & Nutrition Management Services, Inc., 1993.

Individual Meal Plan

The meal plan is adjusted to individual needs while still maintaining dietary modifications.

Clear Liquid Diabetic Diet

Description

A clear liquid diet should only be used for short periods of time post-operatively, in acute inflammatory conditions of the gastro-intestinal tract, or acute stages of many illnesses. When a clear liquid diabetic diet is ordered, only the total carbohydrate level within the prescribed diet will be achieved.

Full Liquid Diabetic Diet

Description

A full liquid diet should only be used for short periods of time after surgery or as a progression from liquids to a soft diet. When a full liquid diabetic diet is ordered, it will meet the requirements for protein, fat, and carbohydrate for the prescribed level.

Gestational Diabetic Diet

Description

The distribution of carbohydrate, protein, and fat is similar to that for the non-pregnant diabetic. The percentage of calories from protein is higher due to the additional protein needs of pregnancy. Calories are determined on an individual basis.

Typical diet may include:

1. 30–35 kcal/kg ideal (pre-pregnancy) body weight
   50–60% carbohydrate
   20–25% fat
   20–25% protein
2. Four–six feedings per day to prevent hypoglycemia.
3. Pre-natal vitamin/mineral supplement as prescribed by physician.

Unmeasured Diabetic Diet

Description

The Unmeasured Diabetic diet may be ordered if no specific calorie level is desired and for patients who are unable to comprehend the use of the exchange list. Diet will include three meals and a bedtime snack.

Adequacy

This diet will supply the Recommended Dietary Allowances if a variety of food is chosen.

Guidelines

1. Eat a variety of foods at each meal. Choose fresh fruits, vegetables, whole grain breads and cereals, lean meats, and lowfat milk and dairy products.
2. Three balanced meals should be eaten at approximately the same time every day. Do not skip meals.
3. A bedtime snack is recommended. Snack food suggestions are skim milk, cheese, crackers, or cereals.

Avoid
1. Sugar, honey, regular jams or jelly, syrup and molasses
2. Sweet desserts, i.e. cakes, cookies, candy, pies, pastries, donuts
3. Regular canned fruits
4. Sugar-coated cereals
5. Regular soft drinks or pre-sweetened beverages
6. Fried foods

The Following Can Be Used:
1. Sugar substitutes, artificially sweetened jams, jelly or syrup
2. Graham crackers (3 squares) and vanilla wafers (6) can be used as desserts
3. Fresh fruit or fruits canned without sugar or in natural fruit juices
4. Unsugared cereals, i.e. Cornflakes, Bran Flakes, etc.
5. Diet soft drinks or mixes pre-sweetened with a sugar substitute

References

American Diabetes Association—ADA Vital Statistics, 1996.

Mahan, K. and Arlin, M.: *Krause's Food, Nutrition and Diet Therapy*. 8th ed., Philadelphia: W.B. Saunders Company, 1992.

Puckett, R.P. and Brown, S.M.: *Shands Hospital at the University of Florida Guide to Clinical Dietetics*. 5th ed. Dubuque: Kendall/Hunt Publishing Co., 1993.

Dallas–Fort Worth Hospital Council: *Dallas–Fort Worth Hospital Council Diet Manual*. Irving: 1992.

Nutrition Guide for Professionals, Diabetes Education and Meal Planning, Edited by Margaret Towers M.S., R.D., C.D.E..

American Diabetes Association and The American Dietetic Association, 1988.

University of Michigan Hospitals, Food and Nutrition Services, *Guidelines for Nutritional Care,* Ann Arbor, Michigan, 1995.

Powers, M.A. (Ed), *Nutrition Guide for Professionals Diabetes Education and Meal Planning,* American Diabetes Association, Inc. and The American Dietetic Association, 1988.

Beebe, C.A., Pastors, J.G., Powers, M.A., Wylie-Rosett, J., Nutrition management for individuals with non-insulin-dependent diabetes mellitus in the 1990's: A review by the Diabetes Care and Education Dietetic Practice Group, *Journal of the American Dietetic Association,* 91 (2), pp. 196-207, 1991.

Paige, D.M., *Clinical Nutrition,* (2nd ed.), C.V. Mosby Company, St. Louis, Missouri, pp. 628-634, 1988.

Hart, B.E., RD, CD, *Clinical Diet Manual* (9th ed.), Food and Nutrition Management Services, Inc., 1993.

Hamwi, G., Therapy and changing dietary concepts. Danowski, T.S. (Ed), *Diabetes Mellitus: Diagnosis and Treatment,* (Vol. 1), New York, American Diabetes Association, pg. 74, 1964.

▶ HYPOGLYCEMIC DIET ◀

Description

This diet is designed to help prevent fluctuations of blood sugar levels for individuals who have functional or reactive hypoglycemia.

1. Energy content of diet is based on patient's normal requirements.
2. Carbohydrate is restricted to 40–55% of your total calories.
3. Protein—a moderate protein diet 70–130 grams per day is common.
4. Fat—the remaining calories are obtained from fat.
5. The diet for hypoglycemia is calculated using the exchange lists in a procedure similar to the diabetic diet.
6. A diet divided into five or six meals a day containing protein and fiber in each meal will provide a less readily absorbed source of glucose. This helps to maintain blood glucose at a more normal level.

Adequacy

This diet will supply the 1989 Recommended Dietary Allowances for all nutrients if a variety of food is chosen. Here are some simple rules to follow:

1. Concentrated sweets such as table sugar, honey, syrups, jelly, jams and candies are avoided.
2. Foods high in carbohydrates are limited (i.e. breads, fruits and milk).
3. "Free Vegetable" items may be eaten as desired.
4. Select fruits and juices without sugar added.

5. Avoid sweetened carbonated drinks or fruit drinks with added sugar.
6. Beverages containing alcohol or caffeine should be avoided since they may affect blood glucose levels.

Total daily amounts (1750 calories):

2 cups Milk
3 Fruit Choices
6 Bread Choices
2 Vegetable Choices
8 Meat Choices
3 Fat Choices

Sample Menu

Breakfast	Lunch	Supper
½ c. Orange Juice	2 oz. Roast Beef	2 oz. Broiled Chicken
¾ c. Cornflakes	½ c. Mashed Potatoes	Small Baked Potato
1 Scrambled Egg	½ c. Cooked Carrots	½ c. Green Beans
1 Slice Bacon	Tossed Salad (free Veg.)	Tossed Salad (free Veg.)
1 c. Milk	with 1 Tbsp. French Dressing	with Zero Dressing
Decaffeinated Coffee	Small Apple	1 tsp. Margarine
	½ c. Milk	2 Diet Peach Halves
	Decaffeinated Iced Tea	(canned)
	(weak)	½ c. Milk
		Decaffeinated Iced Tea
		(weak)

10:00 a.m. Snack	2:00 p.m. Snack	Bedtime Snack
1 oz. Cheddar Cheese	¼ c. Cottage Cheese	½ Turkey Sandwich:
1 Slice Toast	6 Saltine Crackers	1 oz. Turkey on
		1 Slice Bread

References

Cryer, P.E. and Childs, B.P. American Diabetes Assoc. Complete Guide to Diabetes Bantam Books NY 1996

Mahan, K. and Arlin, M.: Krause's Food, Nutrition & Diet Therapy, 8th ed. Philadelphia: W.B. Saunders Company, 1992.

Florida Dietetic Association Diet Manual, 1988.

▶ DISACCHARIDE RESTRICTED DIET ◀

Description

This diet is designed for individuals who are unable to utilize disaccharides or polysaccharides. In the severe stages of this syndrome, only glucose (dextrose) and fructose are tolerated. As tolerance increases, starches may be added gradually back to the diet. Foods containing sucrose are added next with milk (lactose) containing foods last.

If one of the carbohydrate "breakdown products" is not tolerated, the carbohydrate forming that product must be omitted.

For example:

Starch ————— dextrin ————— maltose ————— glucose & glucose
Sucrose ————— frucose & glucose
Maltose ————— glucose & glucose
Lactose ————— galactose & glucose

Adequacy

The nutritional adequacy of this diet is variable, depending upon the number of foods tolerated.

Type of Foods	Low Disaccharide	Starches Tolerated	Sucrose Tolerated	Milk Solids Tolerated
Meat, Fish, 2 Poultry, Cheese	Fresh beef, chicken, lamb, liver, pork, turkey; fish, and seafood that do not contain fillers, breading, lactose or sucrose	Any that do not contain sucrose or milk solids	Any that do not contain milk solids	Any
Eggs	Eggs with no milk added			Any
Fruits	Unsweetened juice from allowed fruits; unsweetened fresh, frozen or canned fruits; fruits sweetened with dextrose: apples, boysenberries, cranberries, currants, cherries, figs, concord grapes, lemons, loganberries, loquates, papayas, pears, damson grapes, pomegranates, raspberries and strawberries	Other fruits as tolerated		Any
Vegetables	Asparagus, green and waxed beans, cabbage family, carrots, celery, cucumbers, pumpkin, lettuce, rutabaga, squash, tomato; juices from allowed vegetables	Corn, lima beans, boiled or baked	Sweet potato	Any
Breads	None	Breads made with dextrose but without sugar or milk, crackers that do not contain added sugar or milk	Breads and crackers that do not contain milk	Any

Type of Foods	Low Disaccharide	Starches Tolerated	Sucrose Tolerated	Milk Solids Tolerated
Cereals	None	Farina, infant oat and rice cereals, oatmeal, puffed rice, shredded wheat	Any that do not contain milk	Any
Rice and Pasta	None	Hominy, macaroni noodles, spaghetti, rice		Others
Fats	Butter, vegetable oils, margarine without milk solids	Butter, vegetable oils, margarine without milk solids	Butter, vegetable oils, margarine without milk solids	Any
Soups	Any made from allowed vegetables	Any made from allowed foods		Any
Desserts	Gelatin flavored with Kool-Aid* and dextrose	Dextrose-sweetened lemon pudding	Any that do not contain milk or milk products	Any
Beverages	Kool-Aid* or tea sweetened with dextrose, special formula containing monosaccharides (Pregestimil*, CHO-free* with dextrose)	Soft drinks containing corn syrup solids (i.e. 7-Up*)	Beverage containing sucrose if it has been found to be tolerated	Milk
Miscellaneous	Dextrose, fructose, herbs (read labels for other foods not listed above)		Sucrose	Any

* Registered Trademark—
  Brand names are used for clarification and do not constitute endorsement of that product

Sample Menu

Breakfast	**Lunch**	**Supper**
½ c. Unsweetened Apple Juice Scrambled Egg 1 cup Pregestimil	Roast Beef Broccoli Spears Margarine Unsweetened Applesauce 1 cup Pregestimil	Baked Chicken Carrots Lettuce & Tomato Salad with Vinegar and Oil Margarine Unsweetened Pear Halves 1 cup Pregestimil
Mid-Morning Nourishment	**Mid-Afternoon Nourishment**	**Evening Nourishment**
¼ c. Kool-Aid* sweetened with 2 Tbsp. Dextrose	½ c. Kool-Aid* sweetened with Dextrose	1 cup Pregestimil

Reference

Recent Advances in Therapeutic Diets, 3rd ed. Iowa: Iowa State University Press: 1979.

▶ CALORIE CONTROLLED DIET ◀

Description

A calorie controlled diet is utilized when weight loss, weight gain, or weight maintenance is desired. If not already determined, a calorie level should be calculated for the individual to achieve the desired weight goal. The Diabetic Exchange Lists for meal planning will be used as the basis for these diets. The diet should be nutritionally adequate, adapted to individual life style, provide a variety of choices of regular food, consistent with modified eating habits and appropriate for weight maintenance

Adequacy

Diets containing less than 1200 calories per day may not meet the 1989 Recommended Dietary Allowances for all vitamins and minerals. If calorie levels less than 1200 are used, a vitamin and mineral supplement may be required. Females age 11–50 should include a good source of iron daily.

Recommendations

1. An ideal body weight or a realistic weight goal will be determined with the help of the patient.
2. Provide a calorie level to achieve a 1–2 pound weight loss per week. Use the Harris-Bennedict equation with the appropriate activity level and subtract 500–1000 kcal per day.
3. Very low calorie diets (800 or less per day) require that individual be monitored under medical supervision.
4. Adapt the meal plan to the individual's lifestyle, preferences, socioeconomic status, ethnic, or religious influences.
5. Inclusion of extra fiber is recommended to reduce calorie density and promote satiety by prolonging stomach emptying time.
6. Use the Exchange lists to instruct the patient on meal planning. To obtain a copy of the American Dietetic Association Exchange List for Meal Planning call 1-800-877-1600, Fax–(312) 899-1979 or log on to www.eatright.org.

7. No specific distribution is recommended, but a breakdown of 20% protein, 30% fat, and 50% carbohydrate can be used as a guide.
8. Identify the patient's eating habits and discuss techniques for appropriate behavior modification.
9. Exercise is an important part of a weight management program. Increase physical activity to the level recommended by physician.
10. Regain health.

Suggested Menu Patterns For Calorie Controlled Diets
For Use With Food Exchange Lists

Exchanges	800 cal.	1000 cal.	1200 cal.	1500 cal.	1800 cal.
Milk (Skim)	1	1	2	2	2
Vegetable	2	2	2	2	2
Fruit	2	3	3	5	6
Starch/Bread	3	3	4	6	7
Meat	4	5	5	5	7
Fat	1	3	3	4	5
Total Calories	809	1032	1184	1493	1799
Protein, gram	49	56	67	73	92
Fat, gram	25	40	40	45	55
Carbohydrate, gram	97	112	139	199	234

Sample Menu For 1200 Calorie Controlled Diet

Breakfast	Lunch	Supper
½ c. Orange Juice	2 oz. Broiled Chicken	2 oz. Beef Patty
1 Scrambled Egg	Small Baked Potato	⅓ c. Rice
1 Slice Toast	1 tsp. Margarine	1 Slice Bread
1 tsp. Margarine	½ c. Spinach	1 tsp. Margarine
1 c. Skim Milk	Tossed Salad with Lemon	½ c. Carrots
Coffee	1 Small Apple	Tossed Salad with lemon
	Iced Tea	2 Halves Unsweetened Canned Pears
		1 c. Skim Milk
		Iced Tea

References

Dallas–Fort Worth Hospital Council: *Dallas–Fort Worth Hospital Council Diet Manual,* Irving: 1992.

Mahan, K. and Arlin, M.: *Krause's Food, Nutrition, and Diet Therapy,* 8th ed. Philadelphia: W.B. Saunders Company, 1992.

Manual of Clinical Dietetics, *The Florida Dietetic Association Diet Manual,* 1988.

Puckett, R.P. and Brown, S.M.: *Shands Hospital at the University of Florida Guide to Clinical Dietetics,* 5th ed. Dubuque: Kendall/Hunt Publishing Co., 1993.

► WEIGHT MANAGEMENT CONCEPTS ◄

Americans spend more than $33 billion per year on weight control products and services. At any given time, approximately 25% of men and 45% of women are attempting to lose weight. According to the National Health and Nutrition Examination Survey (NHANES), approximately 33% of adults living in the United States are obese. Along with this comes the increased risk of coronary heart disease, dyslipidemias, hypertension, gallstones, diabetes, sleep apnea, osteoarthritis and cancers of the reproductive organs. Medical conditions, that are obesity related, are the second leading cause of death in America resulting in 300,000 lives lost each year.

The treatment for obesity should be refocused from only losing weight to a life-style change of weight management, achieving the best weight possible for the good of overall health. This could be defined as achieving healthful and sustainable eating and exercise behaviors to reduce disease risk and improve feelings of energy and well-being. The achievable lifestyle change should have the goals to: 1) change to a healthful eating style with increased consumption of whole grains, fruits and vegetables; 2) reach a nonrestrictive goal of eating a caloric level that is achieved comfortably and not calculated; and 3) a gradual increase to at least 30 minutes of physical activity almost everyday. Weight management includes a lifelong commitment to a healthful life-style.

Periodically over the years, a lot of attention has been given to the no or low carbohydrate, high protein diet. This diet goes by a variety of names, and often is known by the latest author selling a book about some variation of it. Basically, this type of diet involves eating unlimited amounts of protein foods, such as meats, poultry, fish, cheese, eggs and bacon. With eating only protein foods, a person is eating a diet very high in fat, especially saturated fat. The diet has no or low amounts of carbohydrates that include fruits, vegetables, sweets, rice, pasta, potatoes, breads and milk. The vitamins, minerals and fiber that is beneficial in consuming these types of carbohydrates are almost eliminated causing deficiencies over a period of time.

The theory of why most people on a no or low carbohydrate, high protein diet lose weight initially is primarily due to excessive water loss. A decreased carbohydrate diet causes liver and muscle glycogen depletion, which causes a large loss of water. Three parts of water are stored with one part glycogen magnifying the water loss. Also, restricting carbohydrate intake reduces the kidney's ability to concentrate urine, leading to more excretion of sodium. Taking these factors into consideration cause a powerful, but temporary diuretic. This rapid initial weight loss is assumed to be fat loss, but actually their body fat stores are not effected.

Another explanation for the apparent ease of losing weight on a low-carbohydrate diet is the loss of appetite. The reason eating protein causes the reduction in appetite is because of adjustments your liver is making to handle the large amounts of protein being consumed. There is a considerable amount of evidence from animal studies that feeding a high protein diet inhibits appetite. Feeding a high-protein diet results in a physiological appetite suppression, possibly mediated through branched-chain amino acids. Consequently, the weight loss is the result of a reduced caloric level.

The diet is so limited in food choices that it is very boring and monotonous, so the dieters eat fewer calories than are needed to maintain their weight. One characteristic of human eating behavior is that we crave different foods. If the number of different foods is limited, the amount of the monotonous food consumed is usually decreased. The basis of ketogenic diets is a severe restriction of carbohydrate calories, which causes a net reduction in total calories. Since carbohydrate calories are limited, intake of fat usually increases. This diet high in fat causes ketosis which increases blood ketones from fat breakdown which suppresses hunger and thus contributes to reduced caloric intake.

A ketogenic diet may or may not have side effects, depending on the health of the individual. Complications associated with low carbohydrate, high protein diets include ketosis, electrolyte loss, dehydration, calcium depletion, weakness, nausea and possibly kidney problems. Vitamin and mineral deficiencies are other problems in such unbalanced diet regimens. Another potential side effect is gout since the uric acid in the blood increases as the uric acid competes with ketones for excretion.

Dieters are usually very pleased with the initial weight loss. As soon as dieters begin to increase the amount of carbohydrate in their diets and, consequently, decrease the amount of protein, appetite returns. The caloric intake then increases, glycogen stores get replenished, and the body weight quickly returns to its pre-diet levels.

Dieters on a ketogenic diet are on a more dangerous weight regimen due to its high fat content. A periodic visit to the physician should be done to check for electrolyte depletion and increased blood lipids. They should have periodic blood tests to measure total cholesterol, LDL cholesterol, HDL cholesterol and triglycerides.

Despite the allure of the low carbohydrate diet for weight control, there are no long term follow up studies as to the effectiveness of the diet as a long-term weight management technique. There are so many possible negative side effects for a person to remain on this diet for any length of time. The best advice for long term food consumption is to eat only when hungry, eat lower fat foods, and exercise as much as possible for optimum health.

References

Golay A.: Allis A.F., Morel Y., de Tonic N., Tankova S., Reaven G.: Similar weight loss with low or high carbohydrate diets. Am J Clin Nutr, 1996;63 (2):174-8.

Hannah J.S., Dubey A.K.. Hansen B.C.; Postingestional effects of a high protein diet on the regulation of food intake in monkey; Am J Clin Nutr, 1990;52 (2):320-5.

Kuzmarski R.J., Flegal K.M., Campbell S.M., Johnson C.C.; Increasing Prevalence of Overweight among U.S. Adults: The National Health & Nutrition Examinations Surveys, 1960-1991; JAMA; 1994; 272:205-211.

Levitsky, D.A., Low-Carbohydrate Diets:Heresy or Hype; Cornell Cooperative Extension; http://www.cce.cornell.edu/food/index.html.

Larson Duyff, Roberta, MS, RD, CFCS; The American Dietetic Association's Complete Food & Nutrition Guide, 1998.

Meck Higgins, M.L., Ph.D., RD, LD; No/Low Carbohydrate, High Protein Diets: Kansas State University, Dept. of Human Nutrition; http//www.oznet.ksu.edu/ext_F&N/_Timely/nolov/Carb.htm.

Position of the American Dietetic Association: Weight Management; J Am Diet Assoc.; 1997; 97:71.

▶ WEIGHT REDUCTION DIET FOR CHILDREN ◀

Description

A weight reduction diet may be indicated for children who are above the 75th percentile of weight for length or stature. This diet is designed to provide a decrease in caloric intake and promote weight maintenance or weight loss. The American Dietetic Exchange list is used for meal planning.

The two factors to be modified to bring about reduction of body fat are physical activity and dietary habits. The following guidelines should be followed:

1. Physical activity should be increased to levels similar to non-obese children.
2. Diets should include moderate calorie restrictions that are individualized.
   a. Calorie level should provide adequate amounts of nutrients.
   b. A reduction of 250 calories per day from usual intake should promote a 0.5 pound weight reduction per week.
   c. Rarely should the calorie level be reduced by more than 500 calories per day.
3. Behavior modification is a key to weight maintenance.
4. Weight loss diet should be designed for patient following interview with dietitian.
5. Weight reduction diets are not recommended during peak growth spurts. During this time, weight maintenance is the goal. Maintenance of present weight should lead to a normal weight for height.

Adequacy

For children and adolescents, diets below 1200–1400 calories can not meet the 1989 Recommended Dietary Allowances (RDA's) for nutrient needs and therefore, are not recommended. If diets are below 1400 calories, a multi-vitamin supplement may be indicated. Calorie levels above 1400 calories per day will meet the RDA's if a variety of food is selected in the adequate amounts.

References

Dallas–Fort Worth Hospital Council: *Dallas–Fort Worth Hospital Council Diet Manual*. Irving: 1992.

Mahan, K. and Arlin, M.: *Krause's Food, Nutrition and Diet Therapy*. 8th ed., Philadelphia: W.B. Saunders Company, 1992.

Puckett, R.P. and Brown, S.M.: *Shands Hospital at the University of Florida Guide to Clinical Dietetics*, 5th ed., Dubuque: Kendall/Hunt Publishing Co., 1993.

▶ INSULIN DEPENDENT DIABETIC DIET FOR CHILDREN ◀

Description

To provide adequate calories and nutrients for growth and development of the child with insulin dependent diabetes mellitus.

Composition

Protein	—	20%
Fat	—	30%

(Emphasis on increased intake of mono and polyunsatured fats)

Carbohydrate	—	50%
Cholesterol	—	≤300 mg/day

Calorie level will be calculated by the following formula.

Calculated for ideal weight, age, height, and activity:

Birth–6 months: 108 calories/kg of body weight;

6–12 months: 98 calories/kg of body weight;

1 year and up: 1000 calories/day plus 100 calories for each year up to 11 years;

11 years–15 years: 1000 calories/day: add 100 calories per year for girls and 200 calories for boys.

The food distribution pattern would consist of three meals and three snacks (or two snacks for older children).

The total amount of calories and carbohydrates are divided into tenths.

2/10 Breakfast
1/10 Morning Snack
2/10 Lunch
1/10 Afternoon Snack
3/10 Supper
1/10 Bedtime Snack

Adequacy

This diet meets the 1989 Recommended Dietary Allowances for all nutrients.

Guidelines

1. The American Dietetic Association Exchange List for Meal Planning is used.
2. The dietitian will take a diet history before the meal pattern is planned to take into account the ethnic and cultural dietary habits of the family.

3. The patient and/or family will be instructed on the home diet after orders from the physician are received.
4. Consistency in the eating pattern is important. Meals and snacks should be eaten at approximately the same time each day. Include protein, carbohydrate, and fat in each meal and, preferably, in each snack.
5. Foods or beverages beyond the prescribed meals and snacks are limited to "free" items.
6. Flexibility within exchange lists is encouraged; however, foods cannot be exchanged between food lists.
7. Sucrose containing foods are generally eliminated from the diet. On special occasions (i.e. birthdays or holidays), small servings of these are permissible when calculated into the meal pattern. Sucrose containing foods may be needed for hypoglycemia or strenuous activity.
8. For strenuous exercise additional food may be necessary.
9. Children should always have a source of concentrated carbohydrate with them in the event of an insulin reaction (hypoglycemia). For a mild insulin reaction, 10–15 grams of easily absorbed carbohydrate should be given. This could be four ounces of orange juice or three hard candies. Allow 10–15 minutes for absorption. If there is not adequate improvement, additional carbohydrate can be given. After stabilization a protein containing food should be given to help stabilize the blood glucose.
10. Periods of non-compliance may occasionally occur. However, it is important not to over emphasize mistakes and impose guilt feelings upon the child. It is far better to encourage and support good compliance thereby enhancing the child's self-esteem.

References

Dallas–Fort Worth Hospital Council: *Dallas–Fort Worth Hospital Council Diet Manual.* Irving: 1992.

Puckett, R.P. and Brown, S.M.: *Shands Hospital at the University of Florida Guide to Clinical Dietetics,* 5th ed., Dubuque: Kendall/Hunt Publishing Co., 1993.

▶ PEDIATRIC UNMEASURED DIABETIC DIET ◀ (NO CONCENTRATED SWEETS DIET)

Description

To prevent rapid upswings and downswings of blood sugar levels while providing adequate nutrition for normal growth and development.

Adequacy

This diet meets the 1989 Recommended Dietary Allowance for all nutrients if a variety of foods from all the food groups are consumed in adequate amounts.

Guidelines

1. Meals should be nutritionally adequate to meet the child's energy and growth requirements. The dietitian will obtain a nutrition history to determine if nutrition counseling is required for the parents and/or child.
2. Breakfast, lunch, and dinner are eaten at least four hours apart. Approximately the same amount of food is eaten at the same time each day. However, the child does not have to wait for something to eat when he/she expresses hunger.
3. Children should decide the amount of food they can consume at meals. Second helpings are given freely. Allow approximately 10–15 minutes to pass before a third serving is provided.
4. An afternoon and bedtime snack is necessary. When regular insulin is taken in the morning, a morning snack is also necessary.

5. A snack may be desirable before and/or after a vigorous activity such as gym or athletic competition to prevent hypoglycemic episodes. It is recommended that 10–15 grams of carbohydrates be provided for every 30 minutes of vigorous exercise (i.e. 10–15 grams carbohydrates would be 1/2 cup of orange juice or 1 slice of bread).

6. Snack food suggestions include skim milk, cheese, crackers, nuts, cereals, and sandwiches.

7. Foods containing concentrated sugar, such as regular carbonated beverages, candy bars, chewing gum, sugar, and honey ordinarily should be avoided.

8. Dessert foods (cake, pie, cookies, pudding, ice cream) should be eaten only on special occasions, <u>after</u> a meal with NO second servings, and blood glucose level monitored. Some physicians may prefer that sweets and dessert foods be eliminated.

9. When away from home, children should <u>ALWAYS</u> carry a source of concentrated carbohydrate with them (i.e. sugar, hard candy) in the event of an insulin reaction.

10. For a mild insulin reaction, the recommended amount of carbohydrate to give is 10–15 grams. After 10–15 minutes, it may be necessary to repeat this amount. If there is doubt as to whether the child is having an insulin reaction, it is recommended that he/she immediately be given 10–15 grams of carbohydrate. After stabilization, a protein containing food should be encouraged to assist in maintaining the blood glucose level.

Reference

Puckett, R.P. and Brown, S.M.: *Shands Hospital at the University of Florida Guide to Clinical Dietetics,* 5th ed., Dubuque: Kendall/Hunt Publishing Co., 1993.

▶ ORAL DIABETES MEDICATIONS ◀

Generic Name	Brand Name	Usually Taken	Action Usually Lasts
Metformin	Glucophage	2 or 3 times/day	4 to 8 hours
Repaglinide	Prandin	3 times/day before meals	2 to 6 hours
Acarbose	Precose	3 times/day with meals	4 hours
Troglitazone	Rezulin	Once a day with meal	Up to 24 hours
Glyburide	Diabeta,	1 or 2 times/day	16 to 24 hours
	Micronase	Varies	12 to 24 hours
Glipizide	Glucotrol	1 or 2 times/day	12 to 24 hours
	Glucotrol XL	Varies	Up to 24 hours
Glimepiride	Amaryl	Once a day	Up to 24 hours

Adapted from the American Diabetes Association Complete Guide to Diabetes.

Types of Insulin

Intermediate Acting, NPH (N) or Lente (L) Insulin—Starts working in 1 to 3 hours. Lowers blood sugar most in 6 to 12 hours. Finishes working in 16 to 24 hours.

NPH and Regular Insulin Mixture—Two types of insulins mixed together in one bottle. Starts working in 30 minutes. Lowers blood sugar most in 7 to 12 hours. Finishes working in 16 to 24 hours.

Quick Acting, Insulin Lispro (Humalog)—Prescription Needed—Starts working in 5 to 15 minutes. Lowers blood sugar most in 5 to 90 minutes. Finishes working in 3 to 4 hours.

Short Acting, Regular (R) Insulin—Starts working in 30 minutes. Lowers blood sugar most in 2 to 5 hours. Finishes working in 5 to 8 hours.

Long Acting, Ultralente (U) Insulin—Starts working in 4 to 6 hours. Lowers blood sugar most in 8 to 20 hours. Finishes working in 24 to 28 hours.

Adapted from information from the National Institutes of Health (NIH).

Diabetes Internet Sites Worth Browsing

American Diabetes Association
www.diabetes.org
1-800-DIABETES

Diabetes Digest
www.diabetesdigest.com

Diabetic Lifestyle On-Line
www.diabetic-lifestyle.com

Children with Diabetes
www.childrenwithdiabetes.com

Centers for Disease Control
www.cdc.gov/diabetes

NIDDK
www.niddk.gov

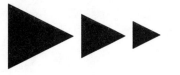

Module 4

Modification for Nutrients

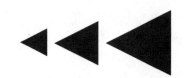

▶ HYPERLIPIDEMIA ◀

Description

Hyperlipidemia (HLP) is a term for higher than normal levels of lipids in the blood. A more general term is dyslipidemia which includes hypertriglyceridemia, low levels of high-density lipoprotein (HDL) cholesterol and/or apoproteins of abnormal composition or amount. Lipids that are measured include cholesterol, triglycerides (TG), and HDL cholesterol. Lipoproteins transport lipids (LDL) cholesterol is a calculated value.

$$\text{LDL Cholesterol} = (\text{Total Cholesterol} - \text{HDL Cholesterol}) - (\text{TG}/5)$$

Dietary management is the primary goal to reduce serum lipid levels. Usually plasma cholesterol and LDL will be lowered by reducing saturated fat and dietary cholesterol. If the patient is overweight, losing weight will also help lower blood cholesterol levels, especially the LDL fraction. To meet the goal of lowering plasma cholesterol, the recommended dietary change is presented in two stages, the Step One and Step Two Diets. (See Dietary Therapy of High Blood Cholesterol later in this chapter)

Premature atherosclerotic vascular disease, a condition characterized by the localized accumulation of lipids in the walls of the arteries, is a leading cause of coronary heart disease (CHD). The major risk factors that have been identified for CHD include:

▶ Male Sex*
▶ Hyperlipidemia
▶ Hypertension
▶ Family history of premature CHD (definite myocardial infarction or sudden death before age 55 in a parent or sibling)
▶ Cigarette Smoking
▶ Alcoholism
▶ Low HDL-cholesterol concentration (below 35mg/dl confirmed by repeat measurement)
▶ Diabetes Mellitus
▶ History of definite cerebrovascular or occlusive peripheral vascular disease
▶ Severe obesity (≥ 30% overweight)
▶ Sedentary lifestyle (physical inactivity)

*Male sex is considered a risk factor because the rates of CHD are 3 to 4 times higher in men than in women in the middle decades of life and roughly 2 times higher in the elderly. Hence, a man with one other CHD risk factor is considered to have a high-risk status. A woman is not unless she has two other CHD risk factors.

The modifiable risk factors are smoking, alcohol use, hypertension, hyperlipidemia, diabetes, obesity and sedentary lifestyle.

In the prevention and treatment of high cholesterol, diet modification is considered to be the cornerstone of therapy. Dietary guidelines set forth by the American Heart Association to reduce the risk of heart disease and lower total serum cholesterol can be summarized by the following guidelines.

▶ A strong emphasis on weight maintenance and physical activity. Eat a diet lower in calories and reduce fat and cholesterol intake.
▶ Limit total daily fat intake to no more than 30% of total calories.
▶ 10 to 15 percent of fat calories should be in the form of monounsaturated fats which include such oils as olive and canola oil.
▶ Cholesterol intake should be less than 300 milligrams daily.
▶ Carbohydrate intake should total 55% to 60% of total daily calories.
▶ Choose a diet moderate in sugar (Changed from avoid foods high in sugar).
▶ Fiber intake from foods, not supplements, should total 25 to 30 grams daily (25-30 grams is about 0.9–1.1 ounces).

▶ Eat five or more servings of fruit and vegetables daily.

▶ Limit salt intake to six grams a day or a little more than one teaspoon. Most salt consumed should be from high-salt cured and processed foods rather than from a salt shaker.

▶ Add the antioxidants, vitamin C, beta-caratene and vitamin E, in the recommended amounts, to your diet to help lower homocysteine levels and reverse the effects of oxidized LDL on your system.

▶ Eat a variety of foods each day, avoiding the consumption of the same foods every day. With the variation of foods allows for a greater intake of the vitamins and minerals the body needs.

If after six months optimal diet therapy is unsuccessful in the treatment of elevated blood cholesterol, it is then recommended that drug therapy, ie cholesterol lowering agent, should be considered based on LDL cholesterol levels and other risk factors.

The recommended goals for LDL cholesterol based on risk are:

▶ <160 mg/dl (<4.15 mmol/l) with < 2 risk factors

▶ <130 mg/dl (<3.35 mmol/l) with ≥ 2 risk factors

The following chart demonstrates the appropriate classification of patients per recommendations of the National Cholesterol Education Program (NCEP)-Adult Treatment Panel. Clinical decisions regarding diet and drug treatment must also take into account the full profile of cardiovascular risk.

Classification Based on Total Cholesterol	Classification Based on LDL Cholesterol
<200 mg/dl (<5.20 mmol/l) desirable blood cholesterol	<130 mg/dl (<3.35 mmol/l) desirable LDL cholesterol
200 to 239 mg/dl (5.20 to 6.15 mmol/l) borderline-high-risk blood cholesterol	130 to 159 mg/dl (3.35 to 4.10 mmol/l) borderline-high-risk LDL cholesterol
≥240 mg/dl (≥6.20 mmol/l) high-risk blood cholesterol	≥160 mg/dl (≥4.15 mmol/l) high-risk LDL cholesterol

When hyperlipidemia is defined in terms of class or classed of elevated plasma lipoproteins, the term hyperlipoproteinemia (HLP) is used. Five hyperlipoproteinemia types have been identified and classified by the National Institutes of Health (NIH) according to the lipid abnormality. The simplest nomenclature for defining the type of lipoprotein(s) present in excess is the phenotyping system of Fredrickson. The Fredrickson classification is not uniformly used and is usually not essential to formulate dietary recommendations.

▶ TYPES OF HYPERLIPOPROTEINEMIA ◀

Fredrickson Type	Lipid Abnormality	Elevated Lipoproteins
I	Hyperchylomicronemia	Chylomicrons
IIa	Hypercholesterolemia	LDL
IIb	Combined hypercholesterolemia and endogenous hypertriglyceridemia	LDL, VLDL
III	Dysbetalipoproteinemia (broad beta pattern)	IDL (intermediate density lipoproteins)
IV	Hypertriglyceridemia	VLDL
V	Hypertriglyceridemia	VLDL, chylomicrons

Adequacy

The American Heart Association's (AHA) Step-One and Step-Two Diets are nutritionally adequate, unless caloric intake levels are less than 1,200 Kcal. A daily multivitamin supplement is recommended to meet the 1989 RDA if less than 1,200 Kcal are consumed daily.

The following Cardiac Diet (300 milligrams or less of cholesterol and 3000 milligrams of sodium) and Low Cholesterol, Low Saturated Fat Diets list the appropriate food items to consume and to avoid for optimal caloric intake.

References

Ernst, N.D., Cleeman, J., Mullis, R., Sooter-Bochenek, J., Van Horn, L., The National Cholesterol Education Program: Implications for dietetic practitioners from the adult treatment panel recommendations, *Journal of the American Dietetic Association,* 88(11),p. 1401, 1988.

Hart, B.E., RD, CD, *Clinical Diet Manual* (9th ed.), Food and Nutrition Management Services, Inc., 1993.

National Cholesterol Education Program. Report of the Expert Panel on Detection, Evaluation, and Treatment of High Blood Cholesterol in Adults. Bethesda, MD: US Dept. of Health and Human Services, Public Health Service, NIH; 1989. NIH Publication 89-2925

National Cholesterol Education Program. Summary of the second report of the National Cholesterol in Adults (Adult Treatment Panel II). Journal American Medical Association. 1993;269:3015-3023.

National Cholesterol Education Program. Report of the Expert Panel on Blood Cholesterol in Children and Adolescents. Bethesda, MD: US Dept. of Health and Human Services, Public Health Service, NIH; 1991. NIH Publication 91-2732.

National Cholesterol Education Program, Report of the expert panel on detection, evaluation, and treatment of high blood cholesterol in adults, Archives of Internal Medicine, 148, p. 36, 1988.

National Heart and Lung Institute, *A Handbook for Physicians and Dietitians: Dietary Management of Hyperlipoproteinemia,* NIH Publication No. 80-110, Bethesda MD, January, 1980.

Puckett, R.P., and Brown, S.M.: *Shands Hospital at the University of Florida Guide to Clinical Dietetics,* 5th ed., Kendall/Hunt Publishing Co., 1993.

▶ DIETARY THERAPY OF HIGH BLOOD CHOLESTEROL ◀

Nutrient	Recommended Intake	
	Step-One Diet	**Step-Two Diet**
Total Fat	Less than 30% of Total Calories	
Saturated Fat	Less than 10% of Total Calories	Less than 7% of Total Calories
Polyunsaturate Fatty Acids	Up to 10% of Total Calories	
Monounsaturated Fatty Acids	10–15% of Total Calories	
Carbohydrates	50–60% of Total Calories	
Protein	10–20% of Total Calories	
Cholesterol	Less than 300 mg/day	Less that 200 mg/day
Total Calories	To achieve and maintain desirable weight	

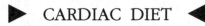

▶ CARDIAC DIET ◀

Description

The purpose of the diet in cardiac disease is to give adequate nourishment with the least possible work effort and muscular strain on the heart, and to prevent or eliminate edema. Loss of weight results in less work for the heart and improved cardiac efficiency. It is recommended that the obese patient lose weight. Those patients of normal weight are permitted calories sufficient to maintain present weight.

The type and amount of fat in the diet influences the serum cholesterol level. It appears that the type of fat in a moderate fat diet (30 percent of total kilocalories) is more important than the amount of fat. By substituting highly unsaturated fats (i.e. safflower, corn, cottonseed and canola oils) for saturated fats (animal or hydrogenated vegetable fats) in human diets, the total amounts of plasma lipids and serum cholesterol are consistently lowered in a high percentage of cases.

Scientific debate over how much trans fatty acids people can healthfully consume continues. Trans fatty acids, also known as trans fats, are found mainly in some margarine, vegetable shortenings, crackers, cookies and snack foods. They are made through the hydrogenation process that solidifies liquid oils. Shelf life and flavor stability is increased in the oils and foods containing them.

Some studies indicate connections between high intakes of trans fatty acids and high cholesterol and heart disease. Other studies have found Americans consume about 5 grams of trans fatty acids per day, amounting to fewer than three percent of their total daily calories and about seven percent of their total fat intake. At this point, there is little scientific evidence to advise the necessity of cutting back on certain foods only because of the trans fatty acid content.

Until more studies show the exact effects of trans fatty acids, it is suggested to consume moderate portions of lean meats, consume low-fat or fat-free dairy products, limit total fat to 30% of total calories, select a wide variety of foods and have a regular physical activity plan.

Edema is the result of impaired cardiac function that causes sodium (and therefore fluids) to accumulate in the tissues. Salt (sodium) and sometimes fluids are restricted and adjusted to the patient's individual needs.

The standard cardiac diet will provide 300 milligrams or less of cholesterol and 3000 milligrams of sodium. Foods high in saturated fat, cholesterol, and sodium are omitted. If the need for a specific calorie level is indicated, it should be ordered by the physician. Up to one-fourth teaspoon of salt daily may be used in cooking.

Adequacy

This diet meets the 1989 Recommended Dietary Allowance for good nutrition as established by the Food and Nutrition Board of the National Research Council when the types of food and amounts suggested are included daily.

Type of Food	Foods Allowed	Foods Not Allowed
Milk (2 or more cups daily)	Skim or 1% lowfat milk, skim milk powder, evaporated skim milk, yogurt made with skim milk, skim milk	Whole milk and whole milk products including: milk, chocolate milk, evaporated condensed milk; buttermilk, 2% milk
Meat, Fish, Poultry and Meat Substitutes (Limit to 6 oz. daily)	Fresh or fresh frozen only. Chicken or turkey (without skin), veal. Clams, crab, scallops, and oysters. Fish: cod, flounder, halibut, trout, bass, mackerel, salmon, water-packed tuna. LIMIT TO 3 oz. 3–4 TIMES PER WEEK: lean beef, lamb, pork (fresh), wild game, shrimp or lobster.	Regular ground beef or hamburger, heavily marbled and fatty meats, spareribs, hot dogs, sausages, luncheon meats and cold cuts, corned beef, goose, duck, poultry skin, shrimp, fish roe (including caviar), sardines, all organ meats (heart, liver, brain, kidney, sweetbreads) commercially fried foods, meats canned or frozen with sauces or gravies, frozen or

Type of Food	Foods Allowed	Foods Not Allowed
Meat, Fish, Poultry and Meat Substitutes—Continued	Old-fashioned peanut butter, (1 T= 1 oz.), skim milk cottage cheese, sapsago cheese, and other lowfat, low cholesterol cheeses (less than 3 gm fat per ounce) or fat free cheese	packaged dinners and prepared products containing fat (unless polyunsaturated fat is indicated), cream cheese, all cheeses made from whole milk, cream, coconut or palm oil
Eggs (Limit to 3 yolks per week)	Egg whites and cholesterol free egg substitute	Egg yolks or whole eggs
Fruits (2 or more servings daily-include citrus daily)	All fruit juices; any fresh, frozen, canned or dried fruits	Dried fruits with sodium preservative
Vegetables (3 or more servings daily-include a dark green leafy or deep yellow vegetable 3-4 times weekly)	Any fresh, frozen, or canned vegetable prepared with allowed foods; salt-free vegetable juice; potatoes, sweet potatoes, yams	Sauerkraut or pickled vegetables prepared in brine. Commercially prepared vegetables with butter, cream or cheese sauce; fried vegetables; pork-and-beans. Regular tomato juice, regular V-8* juice. Instant potatoes, canned potatoes, potato chips, (potato products prepared with whole milk, cream cheese, saturated fats or egg yolk)
Bread, Cereal, Rice and Pasta (6 or more servings daily)	Enriched white, whole wheat, rye, pumpernickel, oatmeal, Italian or French breads; English muffins, matzoth or graham crackers; flour baked goods prepared with allowed foods. Unsalted pretzels, saltines and popcorn.	Egg or cheese bread; commercial #biscuits, #muffins, #sweet rolls, #cornbread, #pancakes, #waffles, #French toast and butter rolls; corn chips, potato chips, cheese or other flavored crackers. Instant hot cereals or quick cooking cereals that have a sodium compound added.
	Any cooked or prepared cereal.	Cereals containing nuts and granola type cereals.
	Enriched rice, macaroni, and noodles prepared with allowed foods. AS DESIRED: Salt-free crackers, salt-free bread, salt-free melba toast	Rice or noodle dishes containing whole milk, cream, egg yolk, etc., egg noodles
Fats and Oil (limit to 5-8 servings daily) Serving Size: 1 tsp. of oil, margarine, and low cholesterol mayonnaise.	Polyunsaturated and monounsaturated oils such as: corn, cottonseed, safflower, soybean, sesame and sunflower, peanut, olive and canola	Other margarines, shortenings and oils; butter & lard, salt pork, suet, meat drippings; commercially prepared gravies, cream and cheese sauces. Powdered cream and

continued

Type of Food	Foods Allowed	Foods Not Allowed
Fats and Oil—Continued 1 tablespoon of salad dressing or reduced calorie margarine. 2 tablespoons reduced calorie salad dressings.	Fortified margarines where the first ingredient listed is liquid polyunsaturated oil. Low cholesterol mayonnaise.	cream substitutes made with saturated fats such as coconut or palm oil; sour cream, mayonnaise and other salad dressings; cashews, macadamia nuts, coconut, bacon
Soups	Salt-free, fat-free bouillon, or fat-free, salt-free vegetable soup. Cream soups made with skim milk (deduct from milk allowance)	Commercial canned soups, dry soup mixes, consomme or regular bouillon
Desserts (Limit to ONE serving daily)	Fruit ices, skim milk sherbet, gelatin, frozen yogurt, pudding popsicles, sorbet, fruit juice bars, ice milk, fudgesicles, Pepperidge Farms* Low Cholesterol Pound Cake, angel food cake, pudding, or junket made from skim milk; baked goods and frostings prepared with allowed ingredients. Deduct from milk allowance for pudding, sherbet, and ice milk.	#Commercial cakes, #pies, #cookies, pastries and mixes; ice cream, and other desserts containing foods omitted
Beverages	Coffee, tea and carbonated beverages	Alcoholic beverages (in excess of 2 oz. ethanol daily)
Miscellaneous	Spices, herbs, cocoa powder, pure sugar candy such as: gum drops, jelly beans, hard candy, marshmallows and mints; jam, jelly, honey, syrup (containing no fat), low low sodium catsup, low sodium mustard, sugar, Molly McButter*, Butter Buds*, carob powder	Chocolate, buttermints, whipped toppings and sweets other than those listed under foods allowed

*Registered Trademark: Brand names are used for clarification and do not constitute endorsement of that product.
#These foods are permitted if prepared with skim milk, margarine, or allowed oils and egg whites or egg substitute.

Sample Menu

Breakfast	Lunch	Supper
Orange Juice	3 oz. Broiled Chicken	3 oz. Baked Fish
Egg Substitute	Baked Potato	Brown Rice
Grits	Broccoli	Steamed Carrots
Toast-Jelly	Fruit Salad	French Bread
2 tsp. Margarine	Hard Roll	1 tsp. Margarine
Skim Milk	1 tsp. Margarine	Fresh Fruit
Coffee-Sugar	Animal Crackers	Sherbet
	Iced Tea–Lemon–Sugar	Skim Milk

References

Journal of the American Dietetic Association, 1999; 99:166–174.

Pemberton, C., Moxness, K., German, M., Nelson, J., and Gastineau, C.: *Mayo Clinic Diet Manual A Handbook of Dietary Practices.* 6th ed., Toronto: B.C. Decker, Inc., 1988.

Puckett, R.P. and Brown, S.M.: *Shands Hospital at the University of Florida Guide to Clinical Dietetics,* 5th ed., Dubuque: Kendall/Hunt Publishing Co., 1993.

▶ LOW CHOLESTEROL LOW SATURATED FAT DIET ◀

Description

This diet provides less than 300 milligrams cholesterol daily. It is designed to reduce the intake of cholesterol, total fat and saturated fats. Foods high in cholesterol (i.e. eggs and organ meats) are omitted. Foods high in saturated fats are limited. Fat intake should be limited to no more than 30% of the total daily calories and saturated fat to less than 10% of total calories. This follows guidelines of the American Heart Association diet.

Adequacy

This diet meets the 1989 Recommended Dietary Allowance for good nutrition as established by the Food and Nutrition Board of the National Research Council when the types of food and amounts suggested are included daily. Females ages 11 to 50 should include a good source of iron daily.

Type of Food	Foods Allowed	Foods Not Allowed
Milk (2 or more cups daily)	Skim milk, 1% lowfat milk, skim milk powder, evaporated skim milk, buttermilk, and yogurt made from skim milk	Whole milk and whole milk products including: chocolate milk, evaporated and condensed milk; buttermilk made from whole milk, 2% milk, milkshakes, and eggnog
Meat, Poultry, Fish and Meat Substitutes (6 ounces daily)	Limit to 3 oz. 3-4 times per week: lean beef, lamb, ham, pork, shrimp, and lobster Fish, clams, crab, scallops, oyster, tuna (packed in water), chicken or turkey (without skin), veal, dried or chipped beef, regular creamed cottage cheese (1/4 c. = 1 oz. meat) 98% fat-free luncheon meats Old-fashioned peanut butter, (1 T- 1 oz.), skim milk cottage cheese, sapsago cheese, and other lowfat, low cholesterol cheeses (Less than 3 gm fat per ounce) or fat free cheese.	Regular ground beef or hamburger, heavily marbled and fatty meats, spareribs, bacon, hot dogs, sausages, luncheon meats and cold cuts, corned beef, goose, duck, poultry skin, fish roe (including caviar), sardines, all organ meats, (heart, liver, brain, kidney, sweetbreads), soy protein meat substitutes, commercially fried foods, meats canned or frozen with sauces or gravies, #frozen or packaged dinners and prepared products containing fat (unless polyunsaturated fat is indicated), cream cheese, all cheeses made from whole milk; coconut, palm oil, or cream

Type of Foods	Foods Allowed	Foods Not Allowed
Eggs	Egg whites and cholesterol free egg substitute as desired	Egg yolks or whole eggs in excess of 3 per week
Fruits (2 or more servings include citrus daily)	All fruit juices, any fresh, frozen, canned or dried fruits	None
Vegetables (3 or more servings daily)	Any fresh, frozen, canned or dried vegetables prepared with allowed foods; vegetable juice, baked beans (no pork), potatoes	Commercially prepared vegetables with butter, cream or cheese sauce; fried vegetables; pork and beans, potato chips
Bread, Cereal, Rice and Pasta (6 or more servings daily)	Enriched white, whole wheat, rye, pumpernickel, raisin, oatmeal, Italian or French breads; English muffins, matzoth, saltines, graham crackers or pretzels, flour; baked goods prepared with allowed foods	Egg or cheese bread; commercial #biscuits, #muffins, sweet rolls, #cornbread, #pancakes, #waffles, #French toast and butter rolls; corn chips, cheese or other flavored crackers
	Any cooked or prepared cereal	Cereals containing nuts and granola type cereal
	Enriched rice, macaroni, spaghetti and noodles prepared with allowed foods	Egg noodles, any prepared with whole milk, cream, cheese, saturated fats, or egg yolk
Fats and Oil (limit to 5-8 servings daily) Serving Size: 1 tsp. of oil, margarine, and low cholesterol mayonnaise. 1 tablespoon of salad dressing or reduced calorie margarine. 2 tablespoons reduced calorie salad dressings.	Polyunsaturated and monounsaturated oils such as: corn, cottonseed, safflower, soybean, sesame and sunflower, peanut, olive and canola	Other margarines, shortenings and oils; butter & lard, salt pork, suet, meat drippings; commercially prepared gravies, cream and cheese sauces.
	Fortified margarines where the first ingredient listed is liquid polyunsaturated oil	Powdered cream and cream substitutes made with saturated fats such as coconut or palm oil; sour cream, mayonnaise and other salad dressings; cashews, macadamia nuts
	Salad dressings, cream substitutes made with allowed oils; low cholesterol mayonnaise and salad dressings made with allowed oils	
	Dry-roasted nuts and olives sparingly	
Soup	Fat-free bouillon or consomme, fat-free vegetable soup, cream soups made with skim milk, packaged dehydrated soups (broth base)	All others
Desserts	Fruit ices, skim milk sherbet, gelatin, fruit whips, meringues, angel food cake, pudding or junket make from skim milk; baked goods and frostings prepared with allowed ingredients; frozen yogurt, pudding popsicles, sorbet, fruit juice bars, low fat ice milk	Commercial #cakes, #pies, #cookies, pastries and mixes; ice cream, and other desserts containing foods omitted

Type of Food	Foods Allowed	Foods Not Allowed
Beverages	Coffee, tea, carbonated beverages	
Miscellaneous	Fat-free or high fat margarine and margarine substitute; fat-free sour cream, cream cheese fat-free mayonnaise and salad dressings; salt, spices, herbs, cocoa powder, pure sugar jelly beans, hard candy, marshmallows marshmellows and mints; jam, jelly, honey, syrup (containing no fat), sugar, catsup, mustard, relishes, pickles, carob powder	Chocolate, buttermints, coconut, whipped toppings and sweets other than those listed under foods allowed candy suckers, gum drops,

#These foods are permitted if prepared with skim milk, egg substitute and allowed fats providing they do not contain more than 30% of their calories from fat.

Sample Menu

Breakfast	Lunch	Supper
½ c. Juice	3 oz. Broiled Chicken Breast	3 oz. Baked Fish
¾ c. Bran Flakes	1 Baked Potato	½ c. Rice
1 Slice Toast, Jelly	½ c. Broccoli	½ c. Steamed Carrots
1 tsp. Margarine	1 Apple	Tossed Salad with
1 c. Skim Milk	1 Hard Roll	Fat-Free Dressing
Coffee—Sugar	1 tsp. Margarine	1 Slice Bread
	Iced Tea—Sugar	1 tsp. Margarine
		1 c. Skim Milk
		1 Peach

References

NIH Publication No. 89-2925, *Detection, Evaluation and Treatment of High Blood Cholesterol in Adults.* 1989.

Puckett, R.P. and Brown, S.M.: *Shands Hospital at the University of Florida Guide to Clinical Dietetics,* 5th ed. Dubuque: Kendall/Hunt Publishing Co., 1993.

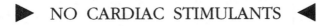 ▶ NO CARDIAC STIMULANTS ◀

Description

This diet may be ordered by the physician for post myocardial infarction patients.

The no cardiac stimulants diet is the American Heart Association's (AHA) Step One Diet (described earlier in this chapter), with the elimination of the following items from the diet.
▶ **Caffeine:** coffee, tea, cola beverages, and other sodas containing caffeine (see Appendix for Caffeine Content of Various Foods)
▶ **Theobromine:** chocolate, cocoa

Adequacy

This diet meets the 1989 RDA for all nutrients when a variety of foods are consumed in adequate amounts.

Reference

Food and Nutrition Services, *Shands Hospital at the University of Florida, Guide to Normal Nutrition and Diet Modification,* (3rd ed), Gainesville, Florida, p. 200, 1983.

 DIET FOR ELEVATED TRIGLYCERIDES ◀

Description

Hypertriglyceridemia may result from dietary factors, as well as from primary or secondary alterations in metabolic pathways. Excessive caloric intake leading to obesity is often associated with hypertriglyceridemia. Liver synthesis of triglycerides may be stimulated by high intakes of both carbohydrates and alcohol.

The primary concern in dietary management of hypertriglyceridemia is to adjust food intake to achieve/maintain desirable body weight. Other factors of concern include limiting total fat to approximately 30% of calories; reducing saturated fat/cholesterol intake; and eliminating simple sugars and alcohol.

Adequacy

This diet meets the Recommended Dietary Allowances for all nutrients with the exception of iron in women of childbearing age.

Type of Food	Foods Allowed	Foods Not Allowed
Milk (2 or more cups daily)	Skim milk, 1% lowfat milk, skim milk powder, evaporated skim milk, buttermilk, and sugar-free yogurt made from skim milk	Whole milk, 2% milk and whole milk products including: chocolate milk, evaporated and condensed milk; buttermilk make from whole milk, milkshakes and eggnogs
Meat, Poultry, Fish and Meat Substitutes (6 ounces daily)	Chicken or turkey (without skin), veal, dried or chipped beef, regular creamed cottage cheese (¼ c. = 1 oz. meat), 98% fat-free luncheon meats Fish, clams, crab, scallops, oyster, tuna (packed in water) Old-fashioned peanut butter, (1 T. = 1 oz.), skim milk, cottage cheese, and other low-fat, low-cholesterol cheese (with less than 3 grams of fat per oz.), fat free cheeses Limit lean red meat to 3 oz. 3-4 times weekly.	Avoid all high fat meats including beef, lamb, ham and pork; regular ground beef or hamburger, heavily marbled and fatty meats, spareribs, bacon, hot dogs, sausages, luncheon meats and cold cuts, corned beef, goose, duck, poultry skin; shrimp, lobster, fish roe (including caviar), and sardines; all organ meats (heart, liver, brain, kidney, sweetbreads), soy protein meat substitutes, commercially fried foods, meats canned or frozen with sauces or gravies, frozen or packaged dinners and prepared products containing fat (unless polyunsaturated fat is indicated), cream cheese, all cheeses made from whole milk; coconut, palm oil or cream

Type of Foods	Foods Allowed	Foods Not Allowed
Eggs	Egg whites and cholesterol free egg substitute as desired	Egg yolks or whole eggs
Fruits (2 or more servings include citrus daily)	All fresh fruit; all unsweetened fruit juice, canned, frozen or dried fruit	Fruit or fruit juices that have added sugar
Vegetables (2 or more servingsdaily)	Any fresh, frozen, canned or dried vegetables prepared with allowed foods; vegetable juice, baked beans (no pork), potatoes	Commercially prepared vegetables with butter, cream or cheese sauce; fried vegetables; pork and beans, potato chips
Bread, Cereal, Rice and Pasta (6 or more servings daily)	Enriched white, whole wheat, rye, pumpernickel, raisin, oatmeal, Italian or French breads; English muffins, matzoth, saltines, graham crackers or pretzels, flour; low sugar baked goods prepared with allowed foods	Egg or cheese bread; commercial biscuits, muffins, sweet rolls, cornbread, pancakes, waffles, French toast and butter rolls; corn chips, cheese or other flavored crackers
	Any low sugar cooked or prepared cereal	Cereals containing nuts, granola, or pre-sweetened cereals
	Enriched rice, macaroni, spaghetti and noodles prepared with allowed foods	Egg noodles, any pasta prepared with whole milk, cream, cheese, saturated fats or egg yolk
Fats and Oil (limit to 5-8 servings daily) Servings Size: 1 tsp. of oil, margarine, and lowcholesterol mayonnaise. 1 tablespoon of salad dressing or reduced calorie margarine. 2 tablespoons reduced calorie salad dressings.	Monounsaturated and polyunsaturated oils such as: corn, cottonseed, safflower, soybean, sesame and sunflower, peanut, olive and canola	Other margarines, shortenings and oils; butter & lard, salt pork, suet, meat drippings; commercially prepared gravies, cream and cheese sauces; powdered cream and cream substitutes made with saturated fats such as coconut or palm oil; sour cream, mayonnaise, and other salad dressings
	Fortified margarines where the first ingredient listed is liquid polyunsaturated oil	
	Cream substitutes made with allowed oils. Low cholesterol mayonnaise and salad dressings made with allowed oils	
	Nuts and olives sparingly	Cashews, macademia nuts
Soup	Fat-free bouillon or consomme, fat-free vegetable soup, cream soups made with skim milk, packaged dehydrated soups (broth base)	All others
Desserts	Sugar-free gelatin, pudding, popsicles, or fruit bars; angel food cake	Commercial cakes, pies, cookies, pastries and mixes; ice cream, ice milk, and other desserts containing foods omitted

continued

Type of Food	Foods Allowed	Foods Not Allowed
Beverages	Coffee, tea, sugar-free carbonated beverages, sugar-free drink mixes	Alcoholic beverages, regular carbonated beverages, drink mixes containing sugar
Miscellaneous	Fat-free or low fat margarine and margarine. substitute; fat-free sour cream, fat-free cream cheese, fat-free mayonnaise and salad dressings; salt, spices, herbs, cocoa powder; artificial sweeteners, sugar-free hard candies; sugar-free syrups, jams, jellies, fruit spreads; catsup, mustard and sugar-free pickles	Chocolate, buttermints, coconut, whipped toppings and sweets other than those listed under foods allowed; sugar, honey, syrup, jam, jelly; candies containing sugar

Sample Menu

Breakfast	Lunch	Supper
Orange Juice	3 oz. Roast Pork	3 oz. Broiled Chicken (no skin)
Oatmeal	Mashed Potato	Rice
Scrambled Egg Substitute	Green Beans	Carrots
Bran Muffin	Tossed Salad with	Fruit Salad
Corn Oil Margarine	Italian Dressing	Bread
Jelly-Diet	Angel Food Cake	Corn Oil Margarine
Skim Milk	Bread	Iced Tea
Coffee	Corn Oil Margarine	Sugar Substitute
Sugar Substitute	Skim Milk	
	Iced Tea	
	Sugar Substitute	

References

Dallas-Fort Worth Hospital Council: *Dallas-Fort Worth Hospital Council Diet Manual.* Irving: 1992.

Pemberton, C., Moxness, K., German, M., Nelson, J., and Gastineau, C.: *Mayo Clinic Diet Manual A Handbook of Dietary Practices,* 6th ed. Toronto: B.C. Decker, Inc., 1988.

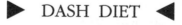

▶ DASH DIET ◀

Description

Elevated blood pressure is a common condition among the population of the United States. About 25% of U.S. adults have hypertension (blood pressure equal to or greater than 140 mm Hg systolic or equal to or greater than 90 mm Hg diastolic or taking antihypertensive medication). A modification in lifestyle, especially dietary modification, is the first approach to reducing higher than optimal blood pressure before medication is prescribed.

In 1992, the National Heart, Lung, and Blood Institute issued a Request for Applications (RFA) inviting researchers to purpose a study to research dietary patterns and high blood pressure. Unlike most previous studies on diet and blood pressure that focused on single nutrients or a few combinations of nutrients, the RFA requested that dietary patterns were to be the focus of the intervention. The study was conducted on an outpatient feeding basis on a large sample size to be able to detect small reductions in blood pressure. From this the "Dietary Approaches to Stop Hypertension"

(DASH) clinical study evolved. The National Heart, Lung, and Blood Institute was both a partner in the research and provided funding for the study.

DASH's final results appeared in the April 17, 1997 issue of The New England Journal of Medicine. The results show that the DASH combination diet lowered blood pressure, so consequently, may help prevent and control high blood pressure.

The combination diet emphasizes fruits, vegetables and low fat dairy foods. The diet is low in saturated and total fat and cholesterol. Nutrients shown to be related to decreased blood pressure include dietary fiber, potassium, calcium, magnesium and moderately high intake of protein. Those related to higher blood pressure include sodium, ratios of cations (such as sodium-to-potassium), fat (usually saturated fat), and alcohol.

The breakdown of % calorie Target levels for a 2000 kcal Combination Diet is as follows.

Nutrient	Target Level
Fat	27%
Saturated Fat	6%
Monounsaturated Fat	13%
Polyunsaturated Fat	8%
Carbohydrates	55%
Protein	18%

The breakdown of the nutrient levels for a 2000 kcal Combination Diet is as follows.

Nutrient	Target Level
Cholesterol	150 mg/day
Potassium	4566 mg/day
Magnesium	484 mg/day
Calcium	1200 mg/day
Sodium	3000 mg/day
Fiber	30 g/day

The diet pattern shown below is the DASH eating plan based on 2,000 calories per day. Depending on caloric levels, the number of daily servings in a food group may vary.

Food Group	Daily Servings	Serving Sizes	Examples and Notes	Significance of each Food Group to the DASH Diet Pattern
Grains and grain products	7–8	• 1 slice bread • ½ C dry cereal • ½ C cooked rice, pasta or cereal	whole wheat bread, English muffin, pita bread, bagel, cereals, grits, oatmeal	major sources of energy and fiber
Vegetables	4–5	• 1 C raw leafy vegetable • ½ C cooked vegetable • 6 oz vegetable juice	tomatoes, potatoes, carrots, peas, squash, broccoli, turnip greens, collards, kale, spinach, artichokes, sweet potatoes, beans	rich sources of potassium magnesium, and fiber

Food Group	Daily Servings	Serving Sizes	Examples and Notes	Significance of each Food Group to the DASH Diet Pattern
Fruits	4–5	• 6 oz fruit juice • 1 medium fruit • ¼ C dried fruit • ½ C fresh, frozen, or canned fruit	apricots, bananas, dates, oranges, orange juice, grapefruit, grapefruit juice, mangoes, melons, peaches, pineapples, prunes, raisins, strawberries, tangerines	important sources of potassium, magnesium, and fiber
Low fat or nonfat dairy foods	2–3	• 8 oz milk • 1 C yogurt • 1.5 oz cheese	skim or 1% milk, skim or low fat buttermilk, nonfat or lowfat yogurt, part skim mozzarella cheese, nonfat cheese	major sources of calcium and protein
Meats, poultry, and fish	2 or less	• 3 oz cooked meats, poultry, or fish	select only lean; trim away visible fats; broil, roast, or boil, instead of frying; remove sin from poultry	rich sources of protein and magnesium
Nuts, seeds, and legumes	4–5 per week	• 1.5 oz or ⅓ C nuts • ½ oz or 2 Tbsp seeds • ½ C cooked legumes	almonds, filberts, mixed nuts, peanuts, walnuts, sunflower seeds, kidney beans, lentils	rich sources of energy, magnesium, potassium, protein, and fiber

Adapted from material from the Harvard University Website, http://pharminfo.com/disease/cardio/Dash_Diet.html

Important eating tips to follow when eating the DASH way includes;
▶ Start small. Make gradual changes in eating habits.
▶ Center the meal around carbohydrates, such as potatoes, pasta, rice, beans or vegetables.
▶ Think of meat as a part of the whole meal and not as the focus.
▶ Use fruits or low fat, low calorie foods such as sugar free gelatin for desserts and snacks.

Adequacy

This diet is adequate for all nutrients according to the 1989 National Research Council's Recommended Dietary Allowances.

Sample Menu for 2,000 Calories

Breakfast	Lunch	Supper
6 oz. Orange Juice	¾ c. Chicken Salad	3 oz. Herbed Baked Cod
1 c. 1% Low Fat Milk	½ large Pita Bread	1 c. White Rice
1 c. Cornflakes with 1 tsp. Sugar	Raw Vegetable Medley:	½ c. Steamed Broccoli
1 medium Banana	3–4 each, Carrot & Celery Sticks	½ c. Stewed Tomatoes
1 slice WW Toast	2 Radishes	Spinach Salad:
1 Tbsp. Jelly	2 leaves iceburg lettuce	½ c. Raw Spinach
1 tsp. Margarine	1.5 oz. Mozzarella Cheese	2 Cherry Tomatoes
Coffee	1 c. 1% Low Fat Milk	2 slices Cucumber
	½ c. Fruit Cocktail/Lite Syrup	1 Tbsp. Lite Italian Dressing
Snack		1 small WW Roll
¼ c. Dried Apricots		1 tsp. Margarine
¾ c. Mini Pretzels		½ c Melon Balls
⅓ c. Mixed Nuts		
12 oz. Diet Ginger Ale		

References

Obarzanek, E., Moore, T.J., Using feeding studies to test the efficacy of dietary interventions: Lessons from the Dietary Approaches to Stop Hypertension trial; Journal of the American Dietetic Association; 1999;99 (supplement); S9–S11.

Karanja, N.M., McCullough, M.L., Kumanyika, S.K., Pedula, K.L., Windhuaser, M.M., Obarzanek, E, Pao-Hwa, L., Champagne, C.M., Swain, J.F.; Pre-enrollment diets of Dietary Approaches to Stop Hypertension trial participants; Journal of the American Dietetic Association; 1999; 99 (supplement); S28–S34.

Harsha, D.W., Pao-Hwa, L., Obarzanek, E., Karanja, N.M., Moore, T.J., Caballero, B.: Dietary Approaches to Stop Hypertension: A summary of study results; Journal of the American Dietetic Association; 1999; 99 (supplement); S35–S39

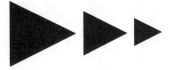 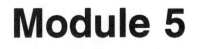

Module 5

Other Modification

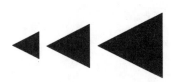

▶ DIETARY MANAGEMENT FOR LIVER DISEASE ◀

Description

Chronic liver disease and liver failure places great impact on the body's ability to metabolize protein, carbohydrate, vitamins, minerals, trace elements, and produce bile. Fat malabsorption and steatorrhea are common in fifty percent of patients with cirrhosis. Altered carbohydrate metabolism secondary to hormonal imbalances causes hyperglycemia and promotes a catabolic state. Hypoglycemia may be seen as glycogen stores are depleted and resist repletion. Altered hepatic vascular perfusion may result in ascites, edema, portal hypertension, and esophageal varices. High serum ammonia levels may result from ammonia produced in the gastrointestinal tract and as a byproduct of protein metabolism.

A 40 gram protein diet should be sent if physician orders diet as "Low Protein". Please refer to the 40–50 Gram Fat Diet.

Adequacy

Diets restricted to 60 grams of protein or less are inadequate in calcium, phosphorous, vitamins D and B_{12}, and may also be low in thiamin, riboflavin, niacin, folic acid, iron, and zinc. Since oral intake is usually poor and because the liver is the primary storage site for several vitamins and minerals, a multivitamin/mineral supplement is recommended. Depending on the patient's clinical picture, fat soluble vitamins may need to be given in a water-miscible form or intramuscularly.

Hepatitis

Objectives

1. Promote liver regeneration
2. Prevent or correct weight loss
3. Replenish glycogen stores
4. Prevent or alleviate hepatic coma

Principles

1. *Protein*—1.5–2.0 gm/kg IBW
2. *Carbohydrate*—high complex CHO, 300–400 gm/day to spare available protein and avoid hypo/hyperglycemia secondary to deranged CHO metabolism
3. *Calories*—35–45/kcal/kg IBW
4. *Fat*—to provide calories as needed

Additional Comments

Abstinence from alcohol for 4–6 months.
Small frequent meals may improve overall intake.
Monitor liver enzymes, serum proteins, and weight.
Vitamin mineral supplementation, especially B-complex vitamins.

Cirrhosis

Objectives

1. Promote liver regeneration
2. Correct nutritional deficiencies
3. Prevent fat stasis
4. Maintain or correct protein status
5. Provide supportive treatment for ascites, renal failure, and esophageal varices as needed.

Recommendations

1. **Protein**—1.5–2.0 gm/kg actual body weight, 75% HBV
2. **Carbohydrates**—300–350 gm/day to spare protein
3. **Fat**—moderate; may use MCT oil if tolerated better by patient
4. **Calories**—35–45 kcal/kg IBW
5. **Fluid and sodium** may need restriction if patient has ascites and/or edema.

Additional Comments

Abstinence from alcohol.
Encourage small frequent meals.
Soft textured foods if esophageal varices present.
Monitor liver enzymes, serum proteins, and ammonia levels to prevent impending encephalopic coma.
Monitor weight.
Vitamin-mineral supplementation.

Hepatic Encephalopathy/Coma

Objectives

1. Limit dietary protein to avoid excessive ammonia production.
2. Avoid hypoglycemia.
3. Avoid tissue catabolism.

Principles

1. **Protein**—0.5a–0.7 gm/kg IBW or less (75% HBV) depending on patient symptoms and serum ammonia levels. If encephalopathy improves, protein intake can be liberalized slowly by increments of 0.2 gm/kg per day to a final goal of 1.2 gm/kg.
   *Use of branched chain amino acid (BCAA) formulas as supplements to low protein diets or used alone in enteral or parenteral form remains controversial.
2. **Fat**—25–30% of total calories. May need to use MCT if fatty liver or steatorrhea are present.
3. **Calories**—35–45 gm/kg dry weight.
4. **Sodium**—250–2000 mg (10–43 mEq) depending on degree of ascites and/or edema.
5. **Fluid**—1000–1500 c.c.'s depending on degree of ascites and edema, electrolytes, and M.D.'s desired rate of diuresis.

Additional Comments

Encourage small frequent meals.
Soft textured foods if esophageal varices present.
Monitor ammonia level.
Monitor weight.
Vitamin/mineral supplementation, especially B complex.

Statement on Branched-Chain Amino Acids

Researchers have found that abnormal plasma amino acid profiles accompany hepatic insufficiency. Since the concentration of neuro-transmitters in the brain are controlled in part by plasma, the pattern of amino acids may play an important role in the pathogenesis of hepatic encephalopathy. Elevated levels of aromatic acids (phenylalanine, tyrosine, tryptophane, methionine) compete with decreased levels of branch-chain amino acids (leucine, isoleucine, valine) for entry across the blood brain barrier thus producing changes in the neurotransmitters. Normalization of the plasma amino acid pattern can be obtained with a special supplement high in branched-chain and low in aromatic amino acids. This may have a beneficial effect on encephalopathy as well as providing more appropriate nutritional support.

References

American Dietetic Association: *Manual of Clinical Dietetics*. Chicago: 1988.

Dallas–Fort Worth Hospital Council: *Dallas–Fort Worth Hospital Council Diet Manual:* Irving: 1992.

Kinney, J., Jeejeebhoy, K.N., Hill, G., Owen, O.: *Nutrition and Metabolism in Patient Care:* W.B. Saunders Co., 1988.

Mahan, K. and Arlin, M.: *Krause's Food, Nutrition and Diet Therapy,* 8th ed., Philadelphia: W.B. Saunders Co., 1992.

Pemberton, C., Moxness, K., German, M., Nelson, J., Gastineau, C.: *Mayo Clinic Diet Manual A Handbook of Dietary Practices,* 6th ed., Toronto: B.C. Decker, Inc., 1988.

Puckett, R.P. and Brown, S.M.: *Shands Hospital at the University of Florida Guide to Clinical Dietetics:* 5th ed., Dubuque: Kendall/Hunt Publishing Co., 1993.

Skipper, A., *Dietitians Handbook of Enteral and Parenteral Nutrition,* Aspen Publication, 1989.

Williams, S. Rodwell, *Nutrition and Diet Therapy,* 7th Edition, Mosby-Yearbook, Inc., 1993.

Suggested Meal Plans for Protein Restricted Diets*

Food Groups	Protein/ Serving	Number of Daily Serving					
		10 gm	20 gm	30 gm	40 gm	50 gm	60 gm
Milk	4 gm/svg.	—	2	2	2	2	2
Meats, Group I	6 gm/svg.	1	1	1	1	1	1
Meats, Group II	7 gm/svg.	—	—	1	2	3	4
Fruits, Group I & II	.5 gm/svg.	4	4	4	4	4	4
Vegetables, Group I & II	2 gm/svg.	1	2	2	2	2	2
Low Protein Starch	.2 gm/svg.	6	6	6	6	6	6
Starch, Group I & II	3 gm/svg.	—	—	1	2	3	4
Fats	trace/svg.	As Desired	As Desired	As Desired	As Desired	As Desired	As Desired
Beverages	trace/svg.	As Desired	As Desired	As Desired	As Desired	As Desired	As Desired
Free Foods	trace/svg.	As Desired	As Desired	As Desired	As Desired	As Desired	As Desired
Milk Substitute	.8 gm protein/½ c.	May be calculated into diet by dietitian as needed.					

*Refer to Renal Exchange Lists

Sample Menu—40 gram protein Diet

Breakfast	Lunch	Supper
½ c. Whole Milk	1 oz. Sliced Turkey	1 oz. Meatloaf
1 Scrambled Egg	1 Slice Bread	½ c. Rice
½ c. Sliced Peaches	Mayonnaise	½ c. Green Beans
2 Slices Low Protein Toast	1 Sliced Tomato	1 Slice Low Protein Toast
Margarine—1 Teaspoon	1 Slice Low Protein Toast	2 Teaspoons Margarine
Jelly—1 Teaspoon	1 Teaspoon Margarine	2 Low Protein Cookies
Coffee or Tea	1 Teaspoon Jelly	1¼ c. Watermelon
	½ c. Ice Cream	4 Canned Apricot Halves
	Tea	Tea

This sample menu provides approximately: 1642 Calories
782 mg Sodium
(if meats, starches, and vegetables are salt free, and there is no added salt)

Alcoholic Liver Disease

Malnutrition in chronic alcohol abuse occurs for several reasons. Alcohol replaces food in the diet. Ethanol provides approximately 7 kilocalories per gram with no significant amounts of protein, fat, vitamins, or minerals. Over a period of time this "empty" diet results in a depletion of nutritional stores and a deterioration of nutritional status.

Alcohol causes an inflammation of the stomach, pancreas, and intestine. This interferes with the normal digestive and absorptive processes resulting in malabsorption of nutrients. Poor dietary intake and malabsorption are the major factors contributing to vitamin deficiencies in alcoholism. Liver damage also plays a role with vitamin metabolism and storage. Thiamin deficiency is the most common vitamin deficiency seen with chronic alcoholism. Other vitamins commonly found to be deficient are vitamin B, folic acid, and ascorbic acid.

Alcohol and its conversion product, acetaldehyde, also interfere with the activation of vitamins by liver cells. Vitamin B_6, for instance, cannot be converted to its active forms by a diseased liver. Metabolism of vitamins A and D and folate are also affected.

Alcohol produces an increased need for the B vitamins which are required for alcohol metabolism. There is also an increased need for magnesium. Higher than normal levels of magnesium are excreted following alcohol consumption. This may precipitate magnesium deficiencies common in chronic alcoholism.

Malnutrition and alcoholism perpetuate a never ending circle. Malnutrition increases the destructive effects of alcohol on the liver while also causing gastrointestinal changes that contribute to the malabsorption problem and poor nutritional status already provoked by the alcohol.

Nutritional care, along with medical treatment, is of extreme importance for the alcoholic patient.

Cirrhosis: High Calorie (35–45 Kcal/Kg IBW)
High Carbohydrate (300–400 gm/day)
High Protein Diet (Protein—1.5–2.0 g./Kg./IBW)
Moderate Fat
Abundance of Vitamins, especially B-complex
Goal: To prevent further degeneration of liver cells and regenerate tissue that has not been irreparably damaged.
Ammonia Intoxication or Impending Hepatic Coma:
Low Protein Diet (HBV) (30g./day or 0.5 g./Kg.)
Sodium and Fluid restriction may be required.

References

Ester, N.J. and Heinemann, M.E.: *Alcoholism–Development, Consequences, and Interventions*. St. Louis: C.V. Mosby Company, 1977.

Mahan, K. and Arlin, M.: *Krause's Food, Nutrition and Diet Therapy*. 8th ed. Philadelphia: W.B. Saunders Co., 1992.

▶ DIETARY MANAGEMENT FOR ◀ COMPROMISED PULMONARY FUNCTION

Description

Chronic obstructive pulmonary disease or COPD, is the term used to describe a group of respiratory diseases. Characterized by chronic airflow obstruction, the group includes chronic bronchitis, asthmatic bronchitis, emphysema and alpha antritrypsin deficiency-related (AAT) emphysema. In many patients more than one of these diseases occur together, although there may be more symptoms of one than the other.

More than 16.4 million Americans have COPD. COPD is the 4th leading cause of death in the U.S., accounting for over 100,000 deaths in 1996. Cigarette smoking is the most important risk factor with 80%–90% of the cases due to smoking.

Depending on the severity of the disease, treatments may include bronchodilators which open up air passages in the lungs; antibiotics; and exercise to strengthen muscles. People with COPD may eventually require supplemental oxygen and may have to rely on mechanical respiratory assistance.

Malnutrition in chronic lung disease may include:

▶ anorexia
▶ GI disturbances
▶ malabsorption
▶ increased metabolic requirements
▶ dyspnea and fatigue

Some drugs may affect appetite and nutritional status. These drugs may include:

▶ Prednisone®   ▶ Theophyline®
▶ Albuterol®   ▶ Terbutaline®
▶ Metaproterenol®   ▶ Pirbuterol®
▶ Ipatropium Bromide®   ▶ Acetylcysteine

Depending on the drug(s) ordered, there may be drug to drug interaction and/or drug to nutrient interaction. If this becomes the case it may be necessary to:

▶ Increase K and Vitamin C
▶ Avoid caffeine
▶ Avoid charbroiled foods
▶ Limit xanthine intake
▶ May give with soft drink due to taste

The goals of nutrition screening and intervention are both preventive and therapeutic in nature. The link between malnutrition and COPD exacerbation is well described. Patients may fail to consume adequate energy for a variety of reasons; altered taste acuity is one possible factor. Because patients with COPD may need to consume up to an additional 1,000 kcal/day to maintain or gain weight, the sensory quality of the meal, especially taste, becomes important. Constant attention to the nutritional status of patients and maintenance of a reasonable weight has generally been associated with improved respiratory function.

Completion of a dietary assessment/screening is very necessary. The Basil Energy Expenditure (BEE) should be completed. A complete history needs to be done as well as anthropometrics, and check of physical finding and lab values.

Along with a caloric deficiency there usually is a protein deficiency. The protein requirement for a pulmonary compromised patient is:

Maintenance = 1.2 g–1.9 g of protein per kg of body weight
Repletion = 1.6 g–2.5 g of protein per kg of body weight

Micronutrients that may need to be supplemented in the diet regime include phosphorus, magnesium, calcium and potassium.

An increased intake of fluid is essential to keep mucus thin and easier to cough up. Unless the doctor advises otherwise, a consumption of three to four quarts of liquid per day is suggested.

If possible, the oral route to nutrition would be advised. If severe malnutrition occurs, a more invasive nutrition support therapy may be necessary. The critically ill on TPN should be given lipids infused with glucose solution to prevent excess CO_2 production.

The following are general guidelines suggested for a more optimum lifestyle.

▶ Eat foods from each of the basic four food groups.
▶ Limit salt intake. Too much sodium can cause fluids to be retained that may interfere with breathing.
▶ Limit intake of caffeinated beverage due to the caffeine may interfere with some medications and cause a feeling of nervousness.
▶ Avoid foods that produce gas and bloating.
▶ Try to eat the main meal at lunch to produce more energy to carry through the rest of the day.
▶ Choose easy to prepare foods to conserve on energy.
▶ Avoid foods that supply little or no nutritional value.
▶ Try eating six small meals a day instead of three large ones. This will keep from having a full stomach and causing a shortness of breath.
▶ Try to eat in a relaxed atmosphere, and make meals attractive and enjoyable.

For more information, the following association may be contacted.

American Association for Respiratory Care
11030 Ables Lane
Dallas, Texas 75229
(972) 243-2272
Fax (972) 484-2720
info@aarc.org

References

American Association for Respiratory Care, 11030 Ables Lane, Dallas, Texas, 75229; http://www.aarc.org/patient_resources/tips/copd.html.

Chapman-Novakofski, K, Brewer, S., Riskowski, J., Burkowski, C., Winter, L.; Alterations in taste thresholds in men with chronic obstructive pulmonary disease; Journal of the American Dietetic Association; December 1999, Volume 99, Number 12: pg 1536–1541.

University of Michigan, *Food and Nutrition Services, Guidelines for Nutritional Care,* Ann Arbor, Michigan, 1995.

▶ DIETARY MANAGEMENT FOR RENAL DISEASE* ◀

Description

When renal failure occurs, the kidneys are no longer able to excrete metabolic and toxic end products from the body. The patient with renal failure exhibits diminished urinary volume leading to elevated blood urea nitrogen and creatinine levels, acidosis, anemia, and anorexia. The nutritional management of patients with renal disease focuses on the intake of energy, protein, fluids, and electrolytes.

The major objectives of nutritional care are:

1. To decrease nitrogen retention with the use of protein restriction, while simultaneously providing adequate high biological value proteins to meet the body's essential amino acid needs.
2. To prevent edema and hypertension by restricting sodium and fluid intake.
3. To prevent hyperkalemia and life threatening cardiac arrythmias by restricting dietary potassium.
4. To provide adequate calorie intake to prevent body tissue catabolism and maintain desired body weight.
5. To regulate dietary phosphorous and assist phosphate-binding medications in controlling hyperphosphatemia and renal osteodystrophy.

In renal failure, the following factors predispose clients to malnutrition:
- ▶ Effects of uremia
- ▶ Poor appetite
- ▶ Nausea
- ▶ Vomiting
- ▶ Drug/nutrient interaction
- ▶ Effects of multi medications
- ▶ Metabolic alterations
- ▶ Numerous psychosocial issues

Adequacy

A protein restriction of 60 grams or less is inadequate in calcium, phosphorus, vitamin D, Vitamin B_{12}, and may also be low in thiamine, riboflavin, niacin, folic acid, iron, and zinc. The minimun recommended levels of essential amino acids, except methionine, can be obtained from one egg and ¾ cup of milk.

A restricted potassium diet of 1500 mg (38 mEq) or less is inadequate in ascorbic acid, thiamine, riboflavin, niacin, calcium, phosphorus, and vitamin D.

In addition to the decreased intake, vitamin losses are further aggravated by anorexia, nausea, vomiting, and dialysis. Supplementation of a multi-vitamin B complex preparation with at least 1 mg folic acid and 100 mg ascorbic acid is recommended with the use of all renal diets. Vitamin A levels should not be supplemented. With the threat of uremic osteomalacia to all renal patients, vitamin D, and calcium supplements are also recommended, but only after controlling the serum phosphorus.

Principles

The renal diet is complex and requires individual planning according to the patient's symptoms, laboratory tests, and nutritional status. Dietary changes must be made to concur with changes in the patient's medical condition.

*See ADA National Renal Diet: Professional Guide, Bradley PB, Cochran, C Hull A, Massiem Chicago, ILL The American Dietetic Assoc. 1993. This is a table which gives guidelines for nutrition recommendations for clients with renal disease.

	Predialysis GFR 4–10 ml/min	Hemodialysis	Peritoneal Dialysis
Energy (kcal/kg)	35–46 kcal	30–35 kcal	25–35 kcal
Protein (gm/kg)	.6–1.0 50–75% HBV	1.0–1.4 50–75% HBV	1.2–1.5 75% HBV
Fat	30–35%	30–35%	30–35%
Carbohydrate	55–65%	50–60%	45–50%
Fluid	Unrestricted until urine output decreases	1,000 cc/day + daily urine output	≥2000 cc
Sodium mg mEq	1000–3000 45–130	2000–3000 90–130	2000–4000 90–173
Potassium	Typically not Restricted	2.0–3.0 g/day	3.0–4.0 g/day
Phosphorous	10–12 mg/g dietary protein	12–15 mg/g dietary protein	12–15 mg/g dietary protein

Renal Diabetic Patient—Carbohydrate distribution 2/7-2/7-2/7-1/7.
Complex carbohydrate emphasized.

Calculation of Requirements

Nutritional requirements are generally based on the following parameters:
▶ Patient's height and weight
▶ Serum levels of albumin, potassium, sodium, calcium, phosphate, and blood urea nitrogen (BUN)
▶ Urine output
▶ Frequency of dialysis
▶ Other medical conditions

When calculating protein and/or energy requirements, base body weight on the patient's actual body weight (ABW), but if fluid-overloaded or obese, calculate the following manner.
▶ In the fluid-overloaded patient, calculate using a dry weight based on estimated usual weight.
▶ For the obese patient with 125% or more of ideal body weight (IBW), use the formula:

[(ABW − IBW × .25]
+ IBW
= adjusted body weight (kg)
(.25 represents the 25% of body fat tissue that is metabolically active)

Acute Renal Failure

Acute renal failure (ARF) is the sudden deterioration of glomerular filtration rate (GFR) or tubular function. A variety of causes can lead to ARF including decreased renal blood flow, exposure to nephrotoxic medications or diagnostic agents, and intrinsic renal disease. Depending unpon the form of ARF, many are reversible, but the mortality rate is high if the the patient requires any type of dialysis.

In the first phase of ARF, the blood urea nitrogen (BUN) and serum creatinine increase. With protein restriction during this time, the need for dialysis may be delayed. Often the next phase is the oliguric phase (urine output < 400 mL/day) in which fluid and sodium restriction is critical until dialysis is implemented. The following phase may be the diuretic phase during which the urine volume may double each day. The major concern during this phase is the excessive loss of fluid, sodium, and potassium. It is very important to closely monitor the daily loss of each and provide appropriate replacement. Refer to the chart of nutrient requirements. BUN may continue to increase causing a need for continued dialysis despite an improvement in fluid and electrolyte status.

If no permanent kidney damage has occurred, during the functional recovery stage, the BUN and creatinine will gradually return to normal. A diet that avoids excessive protein (0.8–1.0 g/kg) should be utilized due to this stage maybe being prolonged.

Objectives of nutritional care for ARF patients are to:

▶ Reduce uremic complications.
▶ Improve nutritional status.
▶ Decrease incidence of mortality.
▶ Plan adequate calories to prevent catabolism.
▶ Decrease protein for control of azotemia.
▶ Prevent fluid overload or dehydration.

The following guidelines are recommended for nutritional management of patients with ARF:

Energy: The goal is to achieve weight maintenance while recommending a caloric intake dependent on the nature and severity of the disease stage. A level of 35 Kcal/kg/day is suggested for weight maintenance without catabolism. Rapid increases in BUN may indicate catabolism and a need for increased calories. Uremia can result in the metabolic rate increasing by 20%.

Protein: Protein intakes of at least 1 g/kg actual body weight are usually necessary to achieve neutral or positive nitrogen balance, adjusted for obesity. If peritoneal dialysis is utilized, protein needs will increase to 1.2–1.5 g/kg as will major surgery, burns or abnormal losses. After dialysis treatments are discontinued, control catabolism and elevated BUN levels by adequate caloric intake and protein restriction.

During the oliguric phase of ARF, some patients may be unable to receive oral feedings due to vomiting and diarrhea. If this is the case, total parenteral nutrition (TPN) may be required to reduce protein catabolism. If TPN is utilized, use 1.0 to 1.5 g/kg of essential and non-essential amino acids in combination with dextrose and lipid administration until the patient can tolerate oral feedings again.

Sodium: Recommended sodium intakes are restricted according to the level of urinary excretion. During the oliguric phase, when urine output is very low, sodium intake is restricted to 1,000 to 2,000 mg per day. Sodium restriction is liberalized as sodium excretion increases during the diuretic phase.

Potassium: Recommended potassium intakes are restricted according to the level of urinary excretion. If the patient is consuming food, approximately 1 mEq of potassium is necessary for each gram of protein prescribed since all protein foods contain significant amounts of potassium. Hemodialysis and peritoneal dialysis baths can be adjusted for greater removal of potassium if necessary, but do not allow a potassium intake of greater than 70 mEq.

Fluids: In the oliguric and diuretic phases of ARF, fluid intake is extremely important and regulated according to the volume of urine excreted. Closely monitor intake and output of fluids, replacing output with intake and taking in account to add an amount for daily, insensible losses. Hemodialysis will allow an intake of 500–1000 cc of fluid more than the output. Peritoneal dialysis will allow a greater fluid intake if greater glucose concentrations of dialysate are utilized.

Adequacy

For the patient with ARF, it is difficult to comply with the energy and protein needs. When the patient is receiving renal replacement therapy, a supplementation of water-soluble vitamins is recommended.

Chronic Renal Failure

The kidney is the main organ for the excretion and regulation of body water, minerals and organic compounds. Chronic renal failure occurs when the kidney fails to accomplish the three basic functions it performs for the body. These functions are the excretory, regulatory and endocrine functions. To establish the degree of impairment, the glomerular filtration rate (GFR) is measured. Patients with a loss of 50% GFR will often continue to loose renal function, however, the rate of progression varies among individuals.

The goal of nutritional modification is to defer the need for dialytic therapy or transplantation by reducing uremic toxicity. The following guidelines are recommended for nutritional management of patients with CRF:

Energy: Patients with advanced renal failure often suffer from wasting or protein-calorie malnutrition. Adequate calories are required to prevent this. A caloric level of 35 Kcal/day is recommended for weight maintenance. Simple carbohydrates and fats should provide the non-protein calories and caloric supplements such as Polycose® or medium chain triglyceride oil may be required.

Protein: The recommended dietary protein intake is based on several factors, including the level of GFR and the type of dialysis utilized. When the GFR is reduced to 25% or less, usually a protein level of 0.8–1.0 g/kg/ day is an adequate restriction until the creatinine clearance is reduced to 10 ml/minute or less. Approximately 75% or consumed protein should be from high biological value sources to help ensure an adequate intake of essential amino acids while intaking a low-protein diet. Sources of these include milk, eggs, meat, fish and poultry. Negative nitrogen balance may occur if restrictions of less than 0.6 g/kg/day is consumed.

Sodium and Fluids: These levels must be individualized for each patient according to the patient's sodium excretion, urine output and GFR. The goal should be to have the sodium and fluid intake level at a maximum level tolerated by the patient, while preventing edema and hypertension.

Potassium: Unless the patient is hyperkalemic or oliguric, potassium is usually not restricted. If restriction is necessary, 50 mEq/day is usually adequate.

Phosphorus: Phosphorus should be moderately restricted in the patient's diet and phosphate-binding medication received with meals. Physicians usually prescribe antacids to reduce serum phosphorus. The antacids work as phosphate binders, binding the phosphorus in the gut so it is excreted in the feces and not absorbed into the bloodstream.

Diabetic patients with chronic renal failure should consume a high carbohydrate, moderate fat, low protein diet that is adequate in calories is required for the uremic diabetic patient. A similar, liberalized protein diet is recommended for the dialyzed diabetic patient. For patients on insulin or experiencing problems with gastroparesis benefit from consuming small, frequent meals and snacks.

Adequacy

A diet restricted in protein, phosphorus, sodium, potassium and fluid will be inadequate in calcium, iron, folate and the water-soluble vitamins, vitamin D and vitamin B_6.

Hemodialysis

Hemodialysis utilizes an artificial kidney (hemodialyzer) to remove metabolic waste products, excess electrolytes, and fluid out of the blood. Additionally, some essential nutrients are removed, including water-soluble vitamins, amino acids, and glucose. The treatments are usually administered 3 to 4 times per week and commonly last 3 to 4 hours. In hemodialysis, an opening into the blood vessels is required and is achieved either by using a central venous access or surgically constructing a fistula or vascular graft which joins an artery to a vein under the skin. Hemodialysis requires a stricter nutritional regimen than the other dialysis modalities, although all patients receiving dialysis need to be very careful about their dietary intake of protein, sodium, potassium, phosphorus, and fluid.

The nutritional intake for the hemodialysis patient needs to provide adequate calories and protein to prevent malnutrition. The prevention of electrolyte imbalance and excess fluid weight gain is a major concern. Phosphorus levels are closely monitored to prevent bone disease.

The following guidelines are recommended for nutritional management of patients on hemodialysis.

Energy: The average kilocalorie requirement for weight maintenance is 30–35 Kcal/kg/day. Increased kilocalorie intake may be necessary if anabolism occurs. To increase the kilocalories without increasing the protein level, simple carbohydrates and fats need to be increased.

Protein: The average protein requirement for the adult patient is 1.0–1.4 g/kg/day with 50–75% of the intake coming from sources of high biological value. The protein intake needs to be adequate to maintain positive nitrogen balance and must replace amino acids that are lost during dialysis.

Fat: The fat intake needs to be higher than ideal to provide an adequate caloric level. The level of fat should be between 30–35% of total ingested calories with no more than 10% coming from saturated fat sources.

Fluids: Fluid restriction for the patient is an important aspect of the diet. A restriction of 1,000 cc per day plus the daily urine output is adequate to control interdialytic weight gains.

Sodium: A restriction of 2,000 to 3,000 mg per day is important to control thirst and to prevent excessive fluid and weight gain. Diets lower than this level is usually unpalatable and the patient has difficulty following.

Potassium: A restriction of 2.0–3.0 g/day is essential because hyperkalemia can cause cardiac arrhythmias or even sudden death. The actual potassium level is based on laboratory values, residual renal function and potassium concentration of dialysate bath.

Phosphorous: Phosphorous restriction of 12–15 mg/g dietary protein is sufficient to control Hyperphosphatemia. A phosphorus binder must be taken with meals and snacks.

Vitamins: Due to poor dietary intake, dialytic procedure and altered metabolism, the hemodialysis patient loses water-soluble vitamins. A daily vitamin supplementation is highly recommended and should include:

▶ Thiamine—1.4 to 1.6 mg
▶ Riboflavin—1.6 to 2.0 mg
▶ Pyridoxine—10 mg
▶ Folic acid—1 mg
▶ Ascorbic acid—60 mg
▶ Pantothenic acid—5 to 20 mg

The hemodialysis diet needs to be individualized for each patient and closely monitored. A very thorough individualized diet instruction for each patient needs to be accomplished. This should include details on fluid guidelines, cooking procedures and a general reassurance that this diet is easy to implement in their home environment. Refer to the Renal Diet Exchange Lists for more instruction.

For further information about renal diets, refer to the following research: Beto, J.A., Which Diet for Which Renal Failure: Making Sense of the Options. *Journal of the American Dietetic Assoc.*, Vol 95 No. 8, pp. 898–903, August, 1995.

Sample Menu for Renal Disease

Breakfast	Lunch	Supper
½ c. Escalloped Apples	2 oz. Baked Chicken	3 oz. Tenderloin Steak
¾ c. Cornflakes	½ c. Rice	½ c. Noodles
1 Scrambled Egg	½ c. SF Green Beans	½ c. SF Spinach
1 Slice Low Protein Toast	1 Slice Low Protein Toast	1 Slice Low Protein Toast
3 tsp. Regular Oleo–Jelly	3 tsp. Regular Oleo–Jelly	3 tsp. Regular Oleo–Jelly
½ c. Milk	½ c. Fruit Cocktail with	¾ c. Blueberries and
1 c. Coffee	Cool Whip* Topping	Sugar Glaze
2 tsp. Sugar	Popsicle*	2 Low Protein Cookies
Pepper	1 c. Iced Tea–Lemon	1 c. Iced Tea–Lemon
	2 tsp. Sugar	2 tsp. Sugar
	Pepper	Pepper

Approximate Composition:
    65 gm protein
    917 mg sodium
    1898 mg potassium
    1767 kilocalories
    720 mg phosphorus

*Registered Trademark:
Brand names are used for clarification and do no constitute endorsement of that product.

Fluid Guidelines

Fluid restrictions are ususally ordered for individuals on dialysis and others with decreased urine output and/or fluid retention. Fluid includes items that are liquid at room temperature. Be sure to include jello, ice cream and soup in allowance. Glasses and bowls used in your facility may vary from these standards. Be sure to verify your facilities glass, bowl and coffee cup capacities.

It is understood that all food contains some fluid. However, fluid restrictions are ordered by M.D. with the understanding that fluid content in solid foods is NOT calculated. Fluids should include those fluids provided by both Nursing and Dietary departments.

▶ 1 cup = 8 ounces = 240 cc
▶ ¾ cup = 6 ounces = 180 cc
▶ ½ cup = 4 ounces = 120 cc
▶ ¼ cup = 2 ounces = 60 cc

Coffee Cup = 6 fluid oz. (180 cc)
Soup Bowl = 6 fluid oz. (180 cc)
Juice = 4 fluid oz. (120 cc)
    unless other portion indicated
Milk Carton = 8 fluid oz. (240 cc)
Nutritional Supplement = per facility policy

Creamer = ½ fluid oz. (15 cc)
Popsicles = 90 cc
Ice Cream/Sherbet = ½ cup or 120 cc
Gelatin = ½ cup or 120 cc
Ice Cube = 1 fluid oz. (30 cc)

Ideas for Controlling Thirst

► Drink beverages cold; they will be more thirst quenching.

► Follow the sodium restriction; high sodium foods and salt will increase thirst.

► Chew gum and eat hard candy between meals.

► Drink beverages at the end of the meal. Eat foods without drinking beverages at the same time.

► Take medication with jelly or applesauce whenever possible. Medication may be taken with the fluids on the meal tray if not contraindicated. (Some medication should not be taken with meals.)

► Rinse mouth with water, water flavored with lemon juice or mouthwash without swallowing.

References

Acceptable Protocol at a Renal Dialysis Unit, Gainesville, Florida.

Beto, J.A., Which diet for which renal failure: Making sense of the options. *Journal of the American Dietetic Association,* Vol. 95, Number 8, pp. 898–903, August, 1995.

Bradley P.B., Cochran, C., Hull A., Massie M. The American Dietitic Assoc. National Renal Diet: Professional Guide, Chicago, IL, 1993.

Niedert, K.C. ed. Nutrition Care of the Older Adult, Chicago, IL, The American Dietitic Assoc. 1998.

Puckett, R.P., and Brown, S.M.: *Shands Hospital at the University of Florida Guide to Clinical Dietetics.* 5th ed., Dubuque: Kendall/Hunt Publishing Co., 1993.

Spiegel, D.M., Burnier, M., Schrier, R.W., Acute renal failure: managing a devastating illness. *Postgrad Medical,* 1987; 82(4):96–105.

University of Michigan, *Food and Nutrition Services, Guidelines for Nutritional Care,* Ann Arbor, Michigan, 1995.

Renal Diet Exchange Lists

Milk or Equivalent List
Each exchange provides approximately:

    4 grams protein
    80 kilocalories (values may vary)
    60 mg sodium (2.6 mEq)
    180 mg potassium (4.6 mEq)
    120 mg phosphorus (8 mEq)

Milk: Fortified	**Amount in One Serving:**
Whole (3.5% fat)	½ cup
Lowfat (1.2% fat)	½ cup
Skim (non-fat)	½ cup
Powdered, Nonfat Dry (before adding liquid)	2 Tbsp.
Chocolate Milk, Skim	½ cup
Whole	½ cup
Sweetened, Condensed	2 Tbsp.
Evaporated	¼ cup

Cream:	
Half & Half (11.7% fat)	½ cup
Light (Coffee Cream)	½ cup
Sour Cream	½ cup

Dessert:	**Amount in One Serving:**
Custard	¼ cup
Ice Cream	½ cup
Ice Milk	½ cup
Pudding, homemade with cornstarch	½ cup
Sherbet	1 cup
Yogurt, Plain	½ cup

Foods to Avoid:

Buttermilk (Na)
Hot Chocolate, Cocoa (K)

Fruit and Juice List

Each exchange provides approximately:

trace of protein
80 calories
5 mg sodium
150 mg potassium (3.85 mEq)
15 mg phosphorus (1 mEq)

Fruit:	**Amount in One Serving:**
Apple	1 medium
Applesauce	½ cup
Apple Juice	½ cup
Blackberries	½ cup, 10 large
Cherries	½ cup, 10 large
Figs, canned	3 medium
Fruit Cocktail	½ cup
Grapes	10 large
Grape Juice	½ cup
Grapefruit	½
Lemon, raw	1 medium
Mango	½ cup
Papaya	½ cup
Peach Halves	2
Pear	1 medium or 2 halves
Pineapple	¾ cup
Pineapple Juice	½ cup
Plums	2 medium
Raspberries	½ cup
Strawberries	½ cup or 10 medium
Tangerine	1 large
Watermelon	½ cup

Foods to Avoid:

Bananas (K)
Kumquats (K)
All Dried Fruit

Bread, Cereal, and Starchy Foods

Each exchange provides approximately:

2.5 grams protein

70–120 kilocalories

200 mg sodium

30 mg potassium (0.77 mEq)

30 mg phosphorus (2 mEq)

Bread, Cereals, And Starch:	Amount in One Serving:
Bread, regular slice, all types	1 slice
English muffin	½
Cereal, cooked, not instant	½ cup
Bagel	½
Cereal, dry, unsalted	¾ cup
Matzos	1
Roll	1 small
Bun, hamburger	½
Pita bread, 6″ across	½
Melba toast	5 slices
Taco shells, 6″	2
Crackers, unsalted	6
Graham crackers	3
Rice, plain	½ cup
Pasta, macaroni	½ cup
Muffin, 2″	1
Biscuit, 2″	1
Waffle, 2″ × 2″	½
Pancake, plain 4″	1
Cornbread, 1½″ square	1 piece
Cake (angel or pound), 2″	1 slice
Pie (apple, cherry, blueberry, pineapple, strawberry, lemon lime), 3″	1 slice
Vanilla wafers	9
Oatmeal cookies	2 large
Shortbread cookies	3 small
Doughnut (cake or jelly)	1 medium

Foods to Avoid:

Cereals, Instant (Na, K)

Dry, such as Kellogg's Concentrate*, Life*,
      Grapenuts*, Product 19*, (protein, Na, K)
      Bran Cereals (K)

Commercial Mixes, such as:
      Waffle, Biscuit, Muffin Mixes (Na)
      Egg Rolls, Egg Buns (Protein)
      Flour, self-rising (Na)
      Pretzels, salted (Na)
      Popcorn, salted (Na)

Low Protein Starch List
Each exchange provides approximately:
.2 gm protein
80 kilocalories
10 mg sodium (.4 mEq)
12 mg potassium (.3 mEq)
5 mg phosphorus 0 mEq)

Low Protein Bread, ½″ Slice	1 slice
Low Protein Cereal (Porridge or Semolina)	1½ cup
Low Protein Cookies	2
Low Protein Pasta, Cooked:	
Low Protein Ribbed Macaroni (Rigatoni)	¾ cup
Low Protein Ring Macaroni	¾ cup
Low Protein Noodles (Tagliatelle)	¾ cup
Low Protein Rusk	2

Meat or Equivalent List
Each exchange provides approximately:
7 grams protein
75 kilocalories
30 mg sodium
100 mg potassium (2.56 mEq)
100 mg phosphorus (6.7 mEq)

Measure meats after cooking and trimming from bone.

Meat or Equivalent:	**Amount in One Serving**
Beef, pork, veal (preferably lean)	1 oz.
Chicken, hen, duck, turkey (no skin)	1 oz.
Chicken liver, calf liver	1 oz.
Fresh fish, crab, lobster	1 oz.
Tuna, salmon	¼ cup
Cottage cheese	¼ cup
Cheese (preferably low sodium)	1 oz.
Egg	1 large
Peanut butter, unsalted	2 Tablespoons

Foods to Avoid:

Salted Cheese and Cheese Spreads not listed (Na)
Salt-Cured Fish, Fowl and Meats not listed (Na)
Cold Cuts, Luncheon Meats, Salami (Na)
Liverwurst (Na)
Chipped Beef (Na)
TV Dinners (Na)
Ready-made Sandwich Fillings (Na)

Vegetable List

Each exchange provides approximately:

2 grams protein
50 kilocalories
20 mg sodium
150 mg potassium (3.85 mEq)
30 mg phosphorus (2 mEq)

Vegetables:	**Amount in One Serving:**
Asparagus	5 spears
Bean sprouts	⅓ cup
Beans (string or wax), boiled	½ cup
Brussels sprouts	5
Beets, boiled	½ cup
Broccoli, boiled	½ cup
Carrots, boiled	½ cup
Carrots, raw or cooked	1 medium
Corn, boiled	½ cup
Cucumber, raw	1 medium
Celery, raw or cooked	⅓ cup
Cabbage, raw or cooked	½ cup
Cauliflower, raw or cooked	½ cup
Eggplant	½ cup
Green Pepper	1 small
Greens (collard, beet, mustard, or turnip), boiled	⅓ cup
Green peas, boiled	⅓ cup
Lettuce, raw	½ cup
Okra, boiled	½ cup
Onions	½ cup
Rutabagas, boiled	½ cup
Squash, yellow or zucchini	½ cup
Tomatoes, stewed	⅓ cup
Tomatoes, raw	½ medium
Tomato, puree	3 Tablespoons
Turnip root, boiled	½ cup

Foods to Avoid:

Artichoke (K)
Avocado (K)
Dried Peas and Beans (K)
    Blackeyed Peas, Chickpeas, Cowpeas, Kidney Beans, Lima Beans (K)
Mushrooms, fresh (K)
Sauerkraut (Na)
Squash, Acorn and Butternut (K)
Tomato Paste (K)
Tomato Puree (K)
Tomato Juice (regular and low salt) (K)
V-8* Juice (regular and low salt) (K)

Fat List

Each exchange provides approximately:
Trace protein
45 kilocalories
50 mg sodium
Trace potassium
Trace phosphorus

Butter, salted	1 tsp.
Margarine, salted	1 tsp.
Mayonnaise, salted	2 tsp.

Unsalted Fats are in the "Free Foods Exchange"

Foods to Avoid:

Bacon Drippings (Na)
Salt Pork (Na)
Salad Dressings containing Eggs & Cheese (Protein, K)
Salted Nuts (Na, Protein, K)
Olives (Na)

Free Foods

The following foods and beverages contain negligible amount of protein, sodium and potassium:

Free Foods	Free Beverages +
Butter, Low Sodium	Alcoholic Beverages
Butter Balls	(Bourbon, Scotch, Rum, Vodka)
Candy Canes	use upon advice of physician
Candy Corn	Cal Power*
Chocolate Syrup (limit to	Controlyte*
1 Tbsp. per day)+	Cranberry Juice
Cool Whip+	Cream Soda
Corn Starch	Gingerale
Corn Syrup+	Grape Soda
Cotton Candy	Hawaiian Punch
Cranberry Sauce	Kool-Aid*
Dream Whip*+	Lemonade
Fondant, Plain	Mountain Dew*
French Dressing, Low Sodium+	Polycose*
Gumdrops	Root Beer
Hard Sugar Candy	Seven Up*
Honey (limit to 1 Tbsp. per day)+	Sprite*
Italian Dressing, Low Sodium+	Teem*
Jam	Wink*
Jelly	
Jelly Beans (not black licorice)	
Lard	
Life Savers*	
Lollipoops, Suckers	
Margarine, Low Sodium	
Marmalades	
Marshmallows	
Mayonnaise, Low Sodium	
Mints	
Oils+	

Popsicles+
Shortening, Solid Vegetable
Spices
Sourballs
Sugar, Granulated & Powdered
Sugar Substitute, Feather-Weight*, Sugar Twin*
Syrup, Maple and Cane
Tapioca
Vinegar+

Dialyzing Process for Vegetables (Method to Reduce Potassium in Some Vegetables)

1. Peel fresh vegetables and slice to ⅛″ thickness.
2. Soak at least 4 hours in warm water. Use 10 times the amount of water to the amount of vegetables. Drain.
3. Rinse in warm water.
4. Blanch vegetables for 5 minutes. Cook in 5 times the amount of water to the amount of vegetables.
5. Place serving portions in plastic bags and freeze.
6. Each serving may be cooked in variety.

Key

*Registered Trademark:
   Brand names are used for clarification and do not constitute endorsement of that product.
+ Count as Fluid
K—Potassium
Na—Sodium

High Potassium Diet 6000 MG (153 mEq)

Description

Potassium is a mineral that is essential to the human body. It is necessary for proper nerve stimulation, muscle contraction, and water balance. The high potassium diet may be prescribed when hypokalemia (plasma potassium less than 3.5 mEq/liter) is present. Hypokalemia can occur with prolonged use of diuretics or adrenal steroids, excessive diarrhea or vomiting, dehydration, diabetic acidosis, and renal disease.

Adequacy

This diet meets the 1989 Recommended Dietary Allowance for good nutrition as established by the Food and Nutrition Board of the National Research Council when the types of foods and amounts suggested are included daily.

Type of Foods	Foods to be Emphasized on a Regular Diet
Milk (3 or more cups daily)	Skim or lowfat yogurt with non-fat dry milk solids, chocolate milk, hot chocolate
Meat, Fish, Poultry and Meat Substitutes (8 ounces or more daily)	Cheese, peanut butter (1 Tbsp. = 1 oz. meat), dried beans, peas, and legumes (½ c. = 1 oz. meat)
Eggs or Egg Substitutes	Eggs, egg dishes made with cheese and milk
Fruits (2 or more servings; include ½ c. citrus daily)	Fresh apricots, avocados, bananas, berries, kiwi, melon, nectarines, oranges, peaches, pears, persimmons, plums, pomegranate, rhubarb, papaya; all dried fruit; fruit cocktail
Vegetables (include 2 or more servings of potatoes daily)	Artichokes, bamboo shoots, acorn and butternut squash, baked potatoes, french fries, instant mashed potatoes, sweet potatoes, pumpkin, yams, leeks, spinach, broccoli, mushrooms, tomatoes, turnips, tomato juice, vegetable juice
Bread, Cereal, Rice and Pasta (6 or more per day)	Enriched whole grain breads, cereals, and pasta; dark rye bread, pumpernickel, brown rice
Fats and Oil	Cream, half and half, salad dressings containing eggs and/or cheese, nuts
Soups	Any vegetable, cheese, or cream soup
Desserts	Those made with milk/milk products: ice milk, sherbet, ice cream, frozen yogurt, puddings, custard
Beverages	Gatorade*; juices, especially orange, prune, tomato, and vegetable
Miscellaneous	Chocolate, caramels, molasses, sunflower seeds

* Registered Trademark

Brand names are used for clarification and do not constitute endorsement of that product.

Note: Salt substitutes and other salt-free products made with potassium chloride are high in potassium.

▶ POTASSIUM CONTENT OF SALT SUBSTITUTE PRODUCTS ◀

Product	Potassium mEq per teaspoon	Potassium milligrams per teaspoon
Morton's Salt Substitute®	70	2730
No Salt® (Norcliff Thayer, Inc.)	68	2652
Diamond Crystal®	66	2574
Adolph's Salt Substitute®	65	2535
Nu-Salt® (Sugar Foods Corp.)	55	2145
Featherweight Garlic Salt Substitute®	53	2067
Morton's Seasoned Salt Substitute®	50	1950
Featherweight K Salt Substitute® (Chicago Dietetic Supply Inc.)	49	1911
Featherweight Seasoned Salt Substitute®	43	1677
Morton's Light Salt®	40	1560
Adolph's Seasoned Salt Substitute®	33	1287
Featherweight Poultry Seasoning®	16	624
Featherweight Meat Seasoning®	16	624
PaPa Dash–Salt Lover's	14	546
PaPa Dash–Lite, Lite, Lite	05	195

Sample Menu—6000 mg Potassium Diet

Breakfast	Lunch	Supper
½ c. Yogurt	4 oz. Roasted Chicken Breast	½ c. Cream of Mushroom Soup
½ Banana	½ c. Steamed Broccoli	4 oz. Roast Beef
½ c. Orange Juice	1 Large Baked Potato	1 Medium Sweet Potato
½ c. Bran Flakes	2 Tomato Slices	½ c. Spinach
2 Slices Rye Toast	2 Slices Rye Bread	¼ c. 3-Bean Salad
1 c. 2% Milk	1 tsp. Margarine	1 Bran Muffin
1 c. Coffee	1/2 c. Chocolate Pudding	1 tsp. Margarine
1 tsp. Margarine	1 c. 2% Milk	½ c. Fruit Cocktail
1 tsp. Jelly	1 c. Iced Tea	1 c. 2% Milk
		1 c. Iced Tea

This menu provides approximately 6000 mg Potassium and 2505 Calories

References

Mahan, K. and Arlin, M.: *Krause's Food, Nutrition and Diet Therapy.* 8th ed., Philadelphia: W.B. Saunders Company, 1992.

Dallas–Fort Worth Hospital Council: *Dallas–Fort Worth Hospital Council Diet Manual,* Irving: 1992.

The Food Processor® Nutrition and Fitness Program from ESHA Research, Salem, Oregon.

Low Potassium Diet

Description

Potassium (K+) is a mineral found in a wide veriety of foods. It plays an essential role in nerve stimulation and muscle contraction. High levels of potassium in the blood (hyperkalemia) can cause muscle twitching and irregularities of the heart. Hyperkalemia can be lethal when irregularities of the heart become severe.

These diets are designed for the person with hyperkalemia (above 5.0 mEq/liter) and/or for those who are unable to excrete potassium adequately. Most commonly, this is prescribed in cases of renal failure or obstruction. Other indications for the diets are acute dehydration, severe metabolic and diabetic acidosis, and adrenal insufficiency. The average intake of potassium in the American diet is 3–4 grams. When a physician orders "Low Potassium Diet" a 1500 mg diet usually is sent.

Adequacy

All levels of the diet tend to be low in fiber, ascorbic acid, thiamin, riboflavin, niacin, calcium, and vitamin D. In addition, the 1500 mg potassium diet is low in protein. The use of a multivitamin and mineral supplement is recommended with all potassium restricted diets.

Number of Servings

Food Groups	K+/serving	2500 mg (64 mEq)	2000 mg (51 mEq)	500 mg 38 mEq)
Milk	360 mg/1 cup	1 cup	1 cup	1 cup
Beverage	80 mg/1 cup	1 cup	1 cup	—
Meat, Fish, Poultry & Meat Substitutes	100 mg/oz.	7 ounces	7 ounces	4 ounces
Eggs	60 mg	1	1	1
Fruit I	100 mg	—	3	3
Fruit II	200 mg	3	—	—
Vegetables I	100 mg	—	2	2
Vegetables II	200 mg	2	—	—
Bread, Cereal Rice, and Pasta	50 mg	5	5	4
Desserts	50 mg	1	1	—
Fats	trace	As desired	As desired	As desired
Total mg Potassium		2500 mg	2000 mg	1520 mg

Type of Food	Foods Allowed	Foods Not Allowed
Milk (Limit all milk to 1 cup daily)	All milk	Condensed, malted and low sodium milk, chocolate milk, instant cocoa mixes, hot chocolate, Gatorade*, Postum*, and any sodas not listed
Meat, Fish, Poultry and Meat Substitutes (limit to amounts listed)	Any beef, cheese, chicken, duck, fish, ham, hot dogs, organ meats such as liver, kidney, and sweetbreads, pork, shellfish, turkey and veal; peanut butter (2 Tbsp. = 1 oz. meat)	
Eggs (limit to 1 daily)	Eggs	None
Fruits (limit to amounts listed)	*Group I* Acerola, 1 cup fresh Apple, fresh 2″–1 Applesauce, ½ cup Apricots, water-packed, 4 halves Blueberries, ¾ cup Cherries, canned, ½ cup Cherries, fresh, 10 Coconut, dried, shredded, sweetened, ½ cup Cranberries, ¼ cup Dates, 2 medium Figs, canned, 3	

Type of Food	Foods Allowed	Foods Not Allowed
Fruits (continued)	Fruit Cocktail, juice or water-packed, ½ cup Gooseberries, fresh, ½ cup Grapes, fresh, 1 cup Grapefruit Half, 4″ diameter Grapefruit, juice-packed, canned, ⅓ cup Lemon, 2″–1 Lime, 2″–1 Loganberries, frozen, ½ cup Peach, water-packed, ½ cup Pear, water-packed, ½2 cup Pineapple, fresh, ¾ cup Plums, canned, 3 medium Plums, fresh, 1 medium Raisins, 2 Tbsp. Raspberries, ½ cup Tangerine, 1 medium Apple Juice, ½ cup Apricot Nectar, ½ cup Grape Juice, ⅓ cup Lime Juice, ½ cup Peach Nectar, ½ cup Pear Nectar, ½ cup Pineapple–Orange Drink, ½ cup	

Fruits	*Group II:*
	Apricots, fresh, 2 medium
	Banana, ½ medium
	Blackberries, ¾ cup
	Boysenberries, 1 cup
	Cherries, fresh/frozen, 15
	Mango, fresh, ½ medium
	Melon:
	      Cantaloupe, ½ cup, pieces
	      Honeydew, ½ cup, pieces
	Nectarine, 1 medium
	Orange, fresh, 1 medium
	Papaya, ½ medium
	Peach, fresh, 1 medium
	Pear, fresh, 1 medium
	Persimmon, 2 medium
	Prunes, 3 medium, canned
	Strawberries, raw, 1¼ cup
	Strawberries, frozen, unsweetened, 1 cup
	Watermelon, 1¼ cup
	Grapefruit Juice, ½ cup
	Orange Juice, ½ cup
	Pineapple Juice, ½ cup
	Prune Juice, ⅓ cup
		All dried fruits

Vegetables (limit to amounts listed)	*Group I:* Bamboo Shoots, canned, ½ cup Brussel Sprouts, 3–4 cooked	Artichoke, avocado, fresh carrots, dried peas and beans, fresh greens, fresh

continued

Type of Food	Foods Allowed	Foods Not Allowed
Vegetables (continued)	Cabbage, raw, ½ cup 　　　cooked, ½ cup *Group I:* Cauliflower, cooked, ½ cup Corn, White, canned, 1½ cup Cucumber, ½ medium Eggplant, cooked, ½ cup Green Beans, cooked, ½ cup Lettuce, Iceberg, 1 cup Mixed Vegetables, ½ cup Onion, raw, ½ cup Pepper, Bell, small Rhubarb, cooked, ½ cup 　　　frozen, 1 cup Squash, Summer, cooked, ½ cup Turnip, cooked, ½ cup Turnip Greens, canned, ½ cup frozen, ⅜ cup Waxed Beans, cooked, ½ cup	mushrooms, squash (acorn and butternut), tomato puree, tomato paste, tomato juice, V-8 juice*, beet greens
Vegetables	*Group II:* Asparagus, cooked, ½ cup Beets, cooked, ½ cup Broccoli, frozen, ½ cup Carrots, cooked, ½ cup Cauliflower, raw, ½ cup Celery, fresh, ½ cup Collard Greens, cooked, ½ cup Corn, Cream Style, ½ cup 　　　Yellow, frozen, ½ cup 　　　On-the-Cob, 4″ ear Kale, cooked, ¾ cup Mustard Greens, cooked, ½ cup Okra, cut frozen, ½ cup 　　　cooked, 8–9 pods Potatoes (use dialyzing process for vegetables)**, mashed, ½ cup Pumpkin, canned, ⅓ cup Spinach, cooked ½ cup Squash: 　　　Zucchini, frozen, ½ cup 　　　Summer, raw, ½ cup 　　　Winter, baked, ½ cup Tomato, raw, 1 smallcanned, ½ cup Waxed Beans, frozen, ⅔ cup	Baked potatoes, instant potatoes, sweet potatoes
Bread, Cereal, Rice and Pasta (limit to amounts listed)	Limit to ½ cup portions: Rice, egg noodles, macaroni, spaghetti noodles Refined white bread, rolls, muffins, biscuits, bagels, english muffins; pancake, waffles, saltines, melba toast, pretzels, popcorn	Whole wheat and bran breads, muffins, biscuits, quick breads, and bread containing nuts

Type of Food	Foods Allowed	Foods Not Allowed
Bread, Cereal, Rice and Pasta (continued) (limit to amounts listed)	Cooked cereal ½ cup: Oatmeal, malt-o-meal, cream of wheat, cream of rice, grits and farina. Ready-to-Eat, ¾ cup: Corn Flakes*, Puffed Rice*, Puffed Wheat*, Rice Krispies*, Cherrios*, Alpha Bits*, Special K*, Chex*, Frosted Flakes*, Sugar Pops*, and Wheaties*	
Fats and Oil (as desired)	Oils, butter, margarine, shortening and lard. Limit serving size of mayonnaise and salad dressing to 1 Tbsp.	Nuts
Soups	Homemade or canned soups made with allowed vegetables, cream soups made with allowed milk	
Desserts (limit to amounts listed)	Angel food cake, ½th Sponge, 2 inch square Vanilla Wafers, 6 Graham Crackers, 3 Doughnut, 1 Pound Cake, 2″ square Shortcake, 2″ square Fruit Pie (made with allowed fruit), ⅛th Gelatin, ½ cup Cookies (2) such as: Butter, Lady Fingers, Coconut Macaroons, Shortbread, Sugar or Oatmeal As desired: Candy such as butterballs, candy canes, candy corn, cotton candy, hard sugar candy, jelly beans, sourballs, popsicles, lollipops, marshmallows, mints and Lifesavers*	Chocolate and cocoa containing desserts, candy bars, milk chocolate and any other desserts not listed
Beverages (limit to amounts listed)	Limit coffee, tea, and carbonated beverages to amounts listed As desired: Cranberry juice, gingerale, Kool-aid*, lemonade, limeade, Root Beer, Royal Crown Cola*, 7-Up*, Sprite*	Gatorade*, Postum*, and any sodas not listed
Miscellaneous	Salt, pepper, vinegar, spices in moderation, mustard, syrup, honey, jam, jelly, granulated and powdered sugar, lemon juice. Cool Whip*, Dream Whip*, cornstarch, corn syrup, tapioca, catsup (1 Tbsp.)	Salt free porducts such as S.F. mustard, salt substitutes; brown sugar, molasses, caramels, milk chocolate, chocolate syrup, and cocoa

*Registered Trademark: Brand names are used for clarification and do not constitute endorsement of that product.
**Dialyzing Vegetables (method to reduce potassium in some vegetables):
1. Peel fresh vegetables and slice to 1/8″ thickness.
2. Soak at least 4 hours in warm water. Use 10 times the amount of water to amount of vegetables. Drain.
3. Rinse in warm water.
4. Blanch vegetables for 5 minutes. Cook in 5 times the amount of water to the amount of vegetables.
5. Place one serving portion in plastic bags and freeze.
6. Each serving may be cooked in variety of ways: french fried, mashed, boiled, home-fried, etc.

Sample Menus of Potassium Restricted Diets 1500 mg (38 mEq) K

Breakfast	Lunch	Supper
Cranberry Juice	Kool Aid*	Lemonade
½ c. Applesauce	2 oz. Baked Chicken	2 oz. Tenderloin Steak
1 Scrambled Egg	½ c. Buttered Green Beans	½ c. Buttered Noodles
1 Slice Toast	½ c. Canned Peaches	½ c. Buttered Cooked Carrots
Margarine–Jelly	with Cool Whip*	½ c. Canned Pears
1 cup Milk	1 Roll	1 Slice Bread
Salt, Pepper, Sugar	Margarine–Jelly	Margarine–Jelly
	Gingerale	1 Popsicle
	Salt, Pepper, Sugar	1 cup Sprite*
		Salt, Pepper, Sugar

2000 mg (51 mEq) K

Breakfast	Lunch	Supper
Cranberry Juice	Kool Aid*	Lemonade
½ c. Grapefruit Sections	3 oz. Baked Chicken	4 oz. Tenderloin Steak
¾ Corn Flakes	½ c. Rice	½ c. Noodles
1 Scrambled Egg	½ c. Green Beans	½ c. Cooked Carrots
1 Slice Toast	½ c. Canned Peaches	½ c. Canned Pears
Margarine–Jelly	with Cool Whip*	1 Slice Bread
1 cup Milk	1 Roll	Margarine–Jelly
1 cup Coffee	Margarine–Jelly	2 Sugar Cookies
Salt, Pepper, Sugar	1 cup Gingerale	1 cup Sprite*
	Salt, Pepper, Sugar	Salt, Pepper, Sugar

2500 mg (64 mEq) K

Breakfast	Lunch	Supper
Cranberry Juice	Kool Aid*	Lemonade
½ c. Grapefruit Sections	3 oz. Baked Chicken	4 oz. Tenderloin Steak
¾ c. Corn Flakes	½ c. Rice	½ c. Noodles
1 Slice Toast	Tomato Slices with 1 Tbsp.	½ c. Broccoli
Margarine–Jelly	French Dressing	½ c. Canned Pears
1 cup Milk	1 slice Angel Food Cake	1 Slice Bread
1 cup Coffee	with ¾ c. Blueberries	Margarine–Jelly
Salt, Pepper, Sugar	and Cool Whip*	1 cup Sprite*
	1 Roll	Salt, Pepper, Sugar
	Margarine–Jelly	
	1 cup Gingerale	
	Salt, Pepper, Sugar	

References

Adams, C.: *Nutrition Value of American Foods, Handbook 456,* Washington D.C.: U.S. Dept. of Agriculture, 1975.

American Dietetic Association: *Handbook of Clinical Dietetics,* New Haven, Conn.: Yale University Press, 1981.

Goodhart, R. and Shils, M.: *Modern Nutrition in Health and Disease,* 6th ed. Philadelphia: Lea & Feibger, 1980.

Pennington, A.T.: *Bowes and Church's Food Values of Portions Commonly Used,* 16th ed., Philadelphia: J.B. Lippincott, 1994.

Margie, J.D., Anderson, C., Nelson, R.A., and Hunt, J.C.: *The Mayo Clinic Renal Diet Cookbook.* New York: Golden Press, 1974.

 STATEMENT ON LOW CALCIUM DIETS ◀

In normal persons, urinary calcium has little correlation with calcium consumption since intestinal absorption of calcium decreases when dietary intake is excessive. Use of a low calcium diet is not indicated for use as a diagnostic tool for hypercalciuria.

Use of calcium-restricted diets for hypercalciuria (greater than 200 mg calcium in a 24 hour urine collection) is controversial. The type of hypercalciuria must first be determined in order to prescribe effective treatment.

For patients with absorptive hypercalciuria type II, a dietary restriction of 400–600 mg per day may be indicated. Restricting calcium to less than 400 mg yields no additional benefit and may result in negative calcium balance. A restriction of dietary oxalates would also be indicated for this treatment therapy. The goal is to prevent recurrance of calcium oxalate renal stones.

Patients with absorptive hypercalciuria type I and renal hypercalciuria should consume 800–1200 mg of calcium daily. This is equivalent to the Recommended Dietary Allowances. A low calcium diet for the patient with renal hypercalciuria could actually be detrimental.

If thiazide diuretics are utilized to decrease urinary calcium, a moderate dietary sodium restriction (90–100 mEq/day) is in order. The sodium restriction reduces the saturation of calcium salts in the urine.

A high fiber diet (30 grams of more per day) may also be beneficial in decreasing urinary calcium because phytic acid in fiber combines with dietary calcium in the intestine to form calcium phytate which is then excreted.

References

Dallas–Fort Worth Hospital Council: *Dallas–Fort Worth Hospital Council Diet Manual.* Irving: 1992.

Puckett, R.P. and Brown, S.M.: *Shands Hospital at the University of Florida Guide to Clinical Dietetics,* 5th ed. Dubuque: Kendall/Hunt Publishing Co., 1993.

Mahan, K. and Arlin, M.: *Krause's Food, Nutrition and Diet Therapy,* 8th ed. Philadelphia: W.B. Saunders Company, 1992.

Massey, C., Roman-Smith, H., Sutton, R.: Effect of Dietary Oxalate and Calcium on Urinary Oxalate and Risk of Formation of Calcium and Oxalate Kidney Stones. *Journal of the American Dietetic Association,* Vol. 93, No. 8, August 1993.

Pemberton, C., Moxness, K., German, M., Nelson, J., and Gastineau, C.: *Mayo Clinic Diet Manual A Handbook of Dietary Practices.* 6th ed. Toronto: B.C. Decker, Inc., 1988.

FDA Diet Manual, 1988.

Calcium Restricted Diet

Description

This diet provides 400–500 milligrams calcium and may be used with a low oxalate diet to reduce formation of renal calculi in known stone forming patients. A calcium restricted diet in itself is generally not indicated for correction of hypercalcemia and hypercalciuria.

Adequacy

This diet does not meet the 1989 Recommended Dietary Allowances for iron, calcium, thiamin, riboflavin, and vitamin D for women of child-bearing age, according to the Food and Nutrition Board of the National Research Council.

Type of Foods	Foods Allowed	Foods Not Allowed
Milk (Limit to ½ c. or ½ c. equivalent daily)	½ c. whole, lowfat or skim milk, lactaid milk, cream or the equivalent ¼ c. evaporated milk, ½ c. yogurt, ½ c. cottage cheese, 1 oz. Camembert or Bleu cheese, ½ c. ice cream or sherbet, ½ c. custard or pudding	Milk and milk products in excess of ½ cup per day. All other cheeses
Meat, Poultry, Fish and Meat Substitutes (Limit to 6 ounces daily)	Beef, fish, chicken, turkey, pork, lamb, veal, bacon, peanut butter	Salmon, sardines, soybean curd (tofu), shellfish, bass, tripe, oysters, herring, and cheeses (except those allowed under milk group), legumes
Eggs (Limit to 1 per day)	Whole eggs, whites, yolks, or egg substitutes, prepared with allowed ingredients	Eggs or egg dishes prepared with foods omitted
Fruits (2 or more servings daily–include citrus daily)	Fresh, frozen, and canned fruits and fruit juices except those omitted. Limit orange juice to ½ c. daily or 1 medium orange	Dates, figs, prunes, kumquats, raisins, calcium fortified juices
Vegetables (3 or more servings daily)	All fresh, frozen, or canned, except those omitted	Broccoli, cabbage, chard, collards, dandelion greens, kale, mustard greens, okra, spinach, turnip greens, rhubarb; all au gratin, scalloped or creamed vegetables, hominy
Bread, Cereal, Rice and Pasta (6 or more servings daily)	All enriched white, whole wheat, rye and pumpernickle breads and rolls; plain crackers such as saltines and graham; all ready-to-eat cereals; all enriched regular cooked cereals; rusk and rice cakes	Pancakes, waffles, french toast; bread, rice, crackers or pasta prepared with cheese or cheese flavoring; granola, instant hot cereals
Fats and Oil	Margarine, butter, cooking and salad oils, non-dairy cream substitutes	Except in allowed amount (see milk section), sour cream
Soup	Bouillon, broth based soups made with allowed foods	Cream or milk based soups; those containing cheese or other foods omitted

Type of Foods	Foods Allowed	Foods Not Allowed
Desserts	Angel, pound and sponge cakes, cookies; fruit pies, gelatin desserts; pudding, ice cream or frozen yogurt with daily milk allowance; gum drops, hard handy, jelly beans, marshmallows	Chiffon, custard or cream pies; cakes, cookies, pies made with milk products; caramels, chocolate candy
Beverages	Coffee, instant tea, cereal beverages, carbonated drinks, fruit flavored drinks	Brewed tea, hot chocolate, cocoa mixes and other beverages made with milk products
Miscellaneous	Salt, pepper, spices, mustard, catsup, soy sauce, vinegar, sugar, corn syrup, honey, jellies, jams, sugar substitutes in moderation, imitation maple syrup	Molasses, maple syrup, dark brown sugar, vitamin supplements with vitamin D or calcium, or bone meal; Brewers yeast, meat tenderizer

Sample Menu

Breakfast	Lunch	Supper
½ c. Orange Juice	2 Tbsp. Peanut Butter	3 oz. Steak
1 Hard Boiled Egg	2 Slices Whole Wheat Bread	Baked Potato
¾ c. Cornflakes	Fresh Pear	½ c. Green Beans
2 Slices Toast	Sliced Tomato with	Lettuce Salad with
½ c. Milk	Italian Dressing	French Dressing
Margarine	Jelly	Dinner Roll
Jelly	Instant Iced Tea	Margarine
Sugar	Sugar	Angel Food Cake
Coffee		Lemonade

References

Dallas–Fort Worth Hospital Council: *Dallas–Fort Worth Hospital Council Diet Manual.* Irving: 1992.

Florida Dietetic Association Diet Manual, 1988.

Pemberton, C., Moxness, K., German, M., Nelson, J., and Gastineau, C.: *Mayo Clinic Diet Manual A Handbook of Dietary Practices.* 6th ed. Toronto: B.C. Decker, Inc., 1988.

Pennington, J.; *Bowes and Church's Food Values of Portions Commonly Used.* 16th Edition, J.B. Lippincott Co., 1994.

Osteoporosis and Increased Calcium Diet

Description

Osteoporosis is a reduction in quality of bone, ultimately resulting in "porous bones". With the disease, bone strength decreases because bones slowly lose mineral content and their internal supporting structure. Eventually, bones can become so weak they easily fracture and lead to potential disability.

Bone loss is natural in the aging process, yet it's only when bones become thin and brittle that osteoporosis symptoms occur. These symptoms include leg and foot cramps; loss of height; lower back pain; hip, wrist and spine fractures; and dowager's hump which is the forward bending of the spine in the upper back.

An estimated seven to eight million people in the United States have osteoporosis and another 17 million are at high risk as a result of low bone density. Caucasian and Asian women often risk getting the disease because their bones are less dense then the bones of women of other ethnicities. A healthy diet and regular exercise may help prevent or even reverse the illness.

The risk factors include:

▶ a family history of osteoporosis
▶ having an early or surgically induced menopause before the age of 45 (both ovaries removed)
▶ hormonal change–post menopausal women
▶ being physically inactive and lacking weight bearing exercise
▶ smoking cigarettes
▶ excessive alcohol intake
▶ a diet habit that is low in calcium sources (dairy products and some vegetables like broccoli)
▶ individuals who take high doses of cortisone-like drugs (therapies used in asthma, arthritis, or cancer) or taking high doses of thyroid medication

An adequate calcium intake during childhood through age 24 is important in the achievement of peak bone mass that lends to the prevention of osteoporosis later in life. The Recommended Dietary Allowance (RDA) for adults is set at 800 mg/day, with increases to 1200 mg/day during pregnancy and lactation. The RDA for adults is based on an estimated loss of 200–250 mg/day obligatory loss and estimated absorption of 30–40%. The recommendation for infants is 400–600 mg/day, for children 1–10 yrs., 800 mg/day, and for ages 11–24, 1200 mg/day. The current calcium requirement for post-menopausal women is 1500 mg/day and 1000 mg/day for pre-menopausal. Calcium citrate and calcium citrate-malate are preferred over calcium carbonate, which the body doesn't digest well. Take supplements with meals, when they're better digested.

Calcium rich foods include low-fat dairy products like milk, cheese and yogurt; green leafy vegetables such as spinach, collard greens, turnip greens and broccoli; fish, especially canned sardines and salmon with bones; and calcium fortified products such as orange juice, breads, cereals and cottage cheese. Lactose intolerance limits the sources of calcium in the diet. It is very difficult to meet these increased requirements without milk in the diet. Lactose enzyme treated milk and milk products are available and are especially important for the elderly population.

Vitamin D is necessary for calcium absorption and elderly people who do not receive exposure to sunlight may be deficient. Vitamin D alone is not an effective treatment for osteoporosis. The RDA for vitamin D for adults over 24 years is 5 ug/day or 200 IU. The older population falls into the recommended range of 400 IU to 800 IU daily.

Physical activity can slow mineral loss, help maintain posture and improve overall fitness to reduce the risk of falls. A combination of activities is often recommended to help prevent or treat osteoporosis. Excercises typically include:

▶ Weight-bearing activities that include walking, jogging and stair climbing are beneficial. These activities you do on your feet with your bones supporting your weight. These work directly on bones in your legs, hips and lower spine to slow mineral loss. For a patient with diagnosed osteoporosis, walking, at least a mile a day, is usually the best weight-bearing exercise because it minimizes jarring to your bones.
▶ Weightlifting is a strength and resistance training that can help strenghten muscles and bones in the arms and upper spine. Caution should be used if the patient is diagnosed with osteoporosis before performing this activity. A consultation with a physical therapist and/or physician is necessary to design a program that includes proper lifting techniques.
▶ Back strengthening exercises work on muscles rather than bone. Studies suggest that strengthening back muscles may maintain or improve posture.

Hormone replacement therapy is the most effective therapy available to reduce the rate of bone loss and protect against fractures. The maximum results are seen when estrogen therapy is initiated within 4 to 6 years of menopause.

Adequacy

This diet is adequate for all nutrients according to the 1989 National Research Council's Recommended Dietary Allowances provided a balanced diet of all food groups is followed.

References

Puckett, R.P., and Brown, S.M.; Shands Hospital at the University of Florida Guide to Clinical Dietetics, 5th ed. Dubuque: Kendall/Hunt Publishing Co., 1993.

Mayo Clinic Health Oasis Wed Site; http://www.mayohealth.org/mayo/9808/htm/exe_osteo.htm.

University of Michigan Hospitals, Food and Nutrition Services, Guidelines for Nutritional Care, Ann Arbor, Michigan, 1995.

▶ STATEMENT ON OXALATE RESTRICTED DIETS ◀

Dietary restriction of oxalate may be used as therapy to reduce recurrance of calcium-oxalate kidney stones. Hyperoxaluria can be caused by fat malabsorption secondary to gastrointestinal disease or bypass, a high oxalate diet, or excessive vitamin C intake.

Initial dietary restriction for calcium-oxalate stone forming patients can be limited to foods definitely known to increase urinary oxalate. To date, eight foods have been shown to increase oxalate excretion: spinach, nuts, tea, chocolate, beets, rhubarb, strawberries, and wheat bran. More extensive restriction of foods containing oxalate may be appropriate if deletion of the items listed above is not effective in preventing stone formation.

A low calcium low oxalate diet may be indicated for known stone-formers with type II hypercalciuria. (See statement on calcium restricted diets.)

A low fat oxalate restricted diet may be indicated for patients with significant steatorrhea secondary to small bowel disease, intestinal bypass surgery, or pancreatic insufficiency. In malabsorptive states, fatty acids bind with calcium so that oxalate is more available for absorption. Calcium restriction is contraindicated under these circumstances because of the mechanisms on increased oxalate absorption. Calcium supplementation of up to 1000 mg per day may be warranted.

The effects of oxalate restricted diets should be evaluated by means of laboratory analysis or urine composition. Dietary effectiveness should be evaluated and restrictions should be tailored to meet individual needs.

References

Dallas–Fort Worth Hospital Council: Dallas–Fort Worth Hospital council Diet Manual. Irving: 1992.

Mahan, K. and Arlin, M.: Krause's Food, Nutrition and Diet Therapy, 8th ed. Philadelphia: W.B. Saunders Company, 1992.

Massey, C., Roman-Smith, H., Sutton, R.: Effect of Dietary Oxalate and Calcium on Urinary Oxalate and Risk of Formation of Calcium and Oxalate Kidney Stones. Journal of the American Dietetic Association, Vol. 93, No. 8, August 1993.

Pemberton, C., Moxness, K., German, M., Nelson, J., and Gastineau, C.: Mayo Clinic Diet Manual A Handbook of Dietary Practices. 6th ed. Toronto: B.C. Decker, Inc., 1988.

Puckett, R.P. and Brown, S.M.: Shands Hospital at the University of Florida Guide to Clinical Dietetics, 5th ed. Dubuque: Kendall/Hunt Publishing Co., 1993.

Oxalate Restricted Diet

Description

This diet reduces oxalates in the diet and is used for the prevention of calcium-oxalate stones associated with gastrointestinal disorders and steatorrhea. This may occur with ileal bypass or re-section, Crohn's disease, celiac sprue, or pancreatic insufficiency. This diet also limits vitamin C intake which is metabolized to oxalates.

Adequacy

This diet meets the 1989 Recommended Dietary Allowances for good nutrition as established by the Food and Nutrition Board of the National Research Council when the types and amounts of foods listed in the "Regular" diet are consumed.

The following foods contain more than 10 mg/serving and should be omitted from the Regular diet:

Type of Foods	Foods Not Allowed
Meat, Fish, Poultry, Cheese	Peanut butter, soybean curd (tofu), peanuts, almonds, pecans, cashews, and walnuts
**Fruits (Limit Vitamin C rich fruits to 1 serving per day)	Blackberries, blueberries, dewberries, gooseberries, fruit cocktail, raspberries and strawberries; concord grapes, tangerines, juices made from any of the fruits listed above, citrus peels and red currants
**Vegetables	Beans: green, waxed, dried and baked Greens: collard, mustard, beet, dandelion; kale, leeks, spinach, escarole, pokeweed, watercress, parsley, swiss chard; beet tops and roots, celery, chives, eggplant, sweet potatoes, okra, green pepper, summer squash, rhubarb and rutabaga
Bread, Cereal, Rice and Pasta	Grits, white corn, soybean crackers, and wheat germ
Soups	Soups made with foods omitted; tomato soup
Desserts	Fruitcakes or any dessert made with foods omitted
Beverages	Drinks containing chocolate or cocoa; Ovaltine*, tea, and draft beers. Vitamin C fortified drink mixes
Miscellaneous	Marmalade, Vitamin C supplements, chocolate, cocoa, pepper (in excess of 1 tsp. daily)

*Registered Trademark: Brand names are used for clarification and do not constitute endorsement of that product.
**There is a wide seasonal variation in the oxalate content of foods. Variations may also exist associated with the age of the plant, the part of the plant, the climate, and the soil conditions.

Sample Menu

Breakfast	Lunch	Supper
½ c. Orange Juice	3 oz. Sliced Turkey	3 oz. Steak
Oatmeal	2 Slices Bread	Baked Potato
2 Slices Toast	Sliced Cucumber	½ c. Carrots
Hard Boiled Egg	with Italian Dressing	Lettuce Salad
1 c. Milk	Fresh Pear	with French Dressing
Margarine	Mayonnaise	Dinner Roll
Jelly	Sugar	Margarine
Sugar	Instant Tea	Angel Food Cake
Coffee		1 c. Milk

References

Mahan, K. and Arlin, M.: *Krause's Food, Nutrition and Diet Therapy,* 8th ed. Philadelphia: W.B. Saunders Company, 1992.

Massey, C., Roman-Smith, H., Sutton, R.: Effect of Dietary Oxalate and Calcium on Urinary Oxalate and Risk of Formation of Calcium and Oxalate Kidney Stones. *Journal of the American Dietetic Association,* Vol. 93, No. 8, August 1993.

Pemberton, C., Moxness, K., German, M., Nelson, J., and Gastineau, C.: *Mayo Clinic Diet Manual A Handbook of Dietary Practices.* 6th ed. Toronto: B.C. Decker, Inc., 1988.

Calcium Restricted Oxalate Restricted Diet

Description

This diet is used when it is necessary to restrict the dietary calcium to such a degree that an increased absorption of oxalates may occur. It provides approximately 400 mg calcium per day, eliminates foods with greater than 10 mg oxalate per serving, and restricts vitamin C intake.

Adequacy

This diet does not meet the 1989 Recommended Dietary Allowances for calcium, thiamin, riboflavin, and vitamin D as established by the Food and Nutrition Board of the National Research Council.

Type of Foods	Foods Allowed	Foods Not Allowed
Milk (Limit to ½ c. daily)	No more than ½ c. whole milk, lowfat, or skim milk or the equivalent: ¼ c. evaporated milk, ½ c. yogurt, ½ c. cottage cheese, 1 oz. camembert or bleu cheese, ½ c. ice cream or sherbet, ½ c. custard or pudding	Milk and milk products in excess of ½ cup per day.\n\nAll other cheeses
Meat, Poultry, Fish and Meat Substitutes (Limit to 6 ounces daily)	Beef, fish, chicken, turkey, pork, lamb, and veal	Salmon, sardines, shellfish, bass, tripe, oysters, herring, legumes, cheeses, peanut butter, and soybean curd (tofu)

Type of Foods	Foods Allowed	Foods Not Allowed
Eggs (Limit to 1 per day)	Eggs, including egg substitutes, prepared with allowed ingredients	Those prepared with cheese or other foods omitted
Fruits (2 or more servings daily)	Fresh, frozen and canned fruits and fruit juices except those omitted Limit Vitamin C rich fruits to 1 serving per day	Blackberries, blueberries, dewberries, gooseberries, raspberries, strawberries; cantaloupe, citrus peel, cranberries and juice; concord grapes, dates, figs, prunes, red currants, dried fruits; raisins, kumquats, calcium fortified juices; fruit cocktail; juices made from any of the fruits listed above
Vegetables (3 or more servings daily)	All fresh, frozen or canned, vegetables except those listed to avoid	All beans; greens: collard, mustard, beet, spinach, turnip, dandelion, beet roots, chard, chives, celery, cabbage, broccoli, eggplant, kale, leeks, escarole, pokeweed, parsley, green pepper, summer squash, rutabaga, sweet potatoes, swiss chard, watercress, okra, hominy; any vegetable made with milk or cream sauce
Bread, Cereal, Rice and Pasta (6 or more servings daily)	All enriched white, rye, whole wheat, pumpernickle, breads and rolls, plain crackers such as saltines, soda crackers, graham crackers, rice cakes; All ready-to-eat cereals, enriched regular cereals, white or brown rice, egg noodles	Soybean crackers, wheat germ, grits, white corn chips or tortillas; any breads, pasta or crackers made with milk, cheese or cheese flavoring; granola, instant cereals, French toast, pancakes, waffles
Fats and Oil	Margarine, butter, cooking and salad oils, non-dairy cream substitutes	Cream except in allowed amount (see milk allowance), sour cream, almonds, cashews, peanuts, pecans, walnuts
Soup	Bouillon, broth based soups made with allowed foods	Cream or milk based soups; those containing cheese or other foods omitted; tomato soup
Desserts	Angel, pound and sponge cakes, cookies, fruit pies, gelatin desserts; pudding, ice cream, sherbet, frozen yogurt within milk allowance; hard candy, gum drops, jelly beans, marshmallows	Fruit cakes, chiffon, custard, or cream pies; cakes, cookies, pies made with milk; all chocolate, chocolate candies, and caramels

Type of Foods	Foods Allowed	Foods Not Allowed
Beverages	Coffee, instant tea, cereal beverages, carbonated drinks, fruit flavored drinks (avoid those fortified with vitamin C)	Brewed tea, hot chocolate, cocoa mixes and other beverages made with milk products
Miscellaneous	Salt, pepper (not to exceed 1 tsp/day), spices, catsup, mustard, soy sauce, worchestershire, vinegar, sugar, corn syrup, honey, jelly, jam, imitation maple syrup, sugar substitutes in moderation	Maple syrup, meat tenderizers, pepper in excess of 1 tsp/day), supplements containing calcium, bone meal or Vitamin C or D; molasses, dark brown sugar, or Brewers yeast

Note: There is wide seasonal variation in the oxalate content of foods. Variations may also be associated with age of the plant, the part of the plant, climate, and the soil conditions.

Sample Menu

Breakfast	Lunch	Supper
1 Hard Boiled Egg	2 oz. Sliced Turkey	3 oz. Steak
¾ c. Cornflakes	2 Slices Whole Wheat Bread	Baked Potato
2 Slices Toast	Sliced Cucumbers with	½ c. Carrots
½ c. Milk	Italian Dressing	Lettuce Salad with
½ c. Orange Juice	Fresh Pear	French Dressing
Margarine	Sugar, Mayonnaise	Dinner Roll
Jelly, Sugar	Instant Tea	Angel Food Cake
Coffee		Margarine
		Lemonade

References

Dallas–Fort Worth Hospital Council: *Dallas–Fort Worth Hospital Council Diet Manual*. Irving: 1992.

Florida Dietetic Association Diet Manual, 1988 edition.

Massey, C., Roman-Smith, H., Sutton, R.: Effect of Dietary Oxalate and Calcium on Urinary Oxalate and Risk of Formation of Calcium and Oxalate Kidney Stones. *Journal of the American Dietetic Association*, Vol. 93, No. 8, August 1993.

Pemberton, C., Moxness, K., German, M., Nelson, J., and Gastineau, C.: *Mayo Clinic Diet Manual A Handbook of Dietary Practices*. 6th ed. Toronto: B.C. Decker, Inc., 1988.

Pennington, J.: *Bowes and Churches Food Values of Portions Commonly Used*: 16th ed., J.B. Lippincott, Co. 1994.

▶ STATEMENT ON LOW PURINE DIETS ◀

Purines are precursors of uric acid. In the body, uric acid is synthesized primarily from endogenous sources and secondarily from exogenous sources. Dietary restrictions have very little influence on uric acid formation. Medication is the most effective method of treatment. Dietary restrictions are indicated only when blood uric acid levels can not be controlled by drug therapy alone.

References

Dallas–Fort Worth Hospital Council: *Dallas–Fort Worth Hospital Council Diet Manual.* Irving, 1992.

Mahan, L.K., Arlin, M.: *Krause's Food, Nutrition and Diet Therapy.* 8th ed. Philadelphia: W.B. Saunders Company, 1992.

Moderately Restricted Purine Diet

Description

This diet is used to assist in the reduction of uric acid production in the body. The diet may be used in the treatment of gout, gouty arthritis, or other instances when it is desirable to reduce the dietary intake of purine nitrogen and drug therapy is not tolerated. Since fat may prevent excretion of uric acid from the kidney, the diet is also moderately low in fat. Fluid intake of two or more quarts per day is recommended.

Adequacy

With proper selection, this diet meets the 1989 Recommended Dietary Allowance for good nutrition as established by the Food and Nutrition Board of the National Research Council when the types of foods and amounts suggested are included daily.

Type of Foods	Foods Allowed	Foods Not Allowed
Milk (2 or more cups daily)	Lowfat or skim milk, cocoa made with skim milk	Whole milk, 2% milk
Meat, Poultry, Fish and Meat Substitutes	Limit to 2–3 ounces per day: beef, pork, lamb, veal, chicken, turkey and fish except those omitted Two or more servings: Peanut butter (1 Tbsp. = 1 serving), and skim milk cheeses	Liver, heart, kidney, brains, sweetbreads, goose, partridge, mackeral, herring, mussels, anchovies, sardines, and scallops
Eggs	As desired; prepared any way except fried	Fried eggs
Fruits (2 or more servings daily–include citrus daily)	All fresh, frozen or canned fruits, or juices	None
Vegetables (3 or more servings daily–include a dark green leafy or deep yellow vegetable 3–4 times weekly)	Limit to 5 servings weekly: asparagus, dried peas or beans, mushrooms, celery, spinach, soybeans, and green peas; all others as desired	Fried potatoes, potato chips, mashed potatoes made with cream or whole milk
Bread, Cereal, Rice and Pasta (6 or more servings daily)	All whole grain or enriched breads and cereal products, noodles, rice, macaroni, spaghetti, and other pastas Limit to 2 servings weekly: bran, oatmeal and wheat germ	Corn chips
Fats and Oil (3 servings daily—1 tsp. = 1 serving)	Butter, margarine, oil, salad dressings, and nuts	Cream, meat extracts, and gravy

Type of Foods	Foods Allowed	Foods Not Allowed
Soups	Cream soups made with allowed vegetables and skim milk	Broth, bouillon, consomme, and meat stock soups
Desserts	All made from allowed foods; i.e.–ice milk, lowfat frozen yogurt, gelatin, graham crackers, vanilla wafers	Mincemeat pie if made with meat; rich desserts high in fat, i.e.–pastries, doughnuts, cream pies, cakes, cookies
Beverages	Regular and decaffeinated coffee, tea, and carbonated beverages	Alcoholic beverages
Miscellaneous	Condiments, herbs, spices, salt, pepper, vinegar, sugar, jam, jelly, honey, syrup, candy, and marshmallows	Bakers and brewer's yeast

Sample Menu

Breakfast	Lunch	Supper
½ c. Grapefruit Juice	2 oz. Roast Beef	1 c. Macaroni & Cheese
½ c. Cream of Wheat	1 Baked Potato	½ c. Green Beans
1 Scrambled Egg	½ c. Beets	1 c. Tossed Salad with
1 Slice Toast	2 Slices Bread	French Dressing
1 tsp. Margarine	1 tsp. Margarine	2 Slices Bread
Jelly	1 Slice Angel Food Cake	1 tsp. Margarine
1 C. Skim Milk	Hot Tea–Sugar	½ c. Peach Halves
Coffee–Sugar		1 c. Skim Milk
		Coffee–Sugar

References

American Dietetic Association: *Manual of Clinical Dietetics*. Chicago: 1988.

Dallas–Fort Worth Hospital Council: *Dallas–Fort Worth Hospital Council Diet Manual*. Irving: 1992.

▶ DIETARY MANAGEMENT FOR PANCREATIC DISEASE ◀

Description

The patient's clinical condition indicates the form of nutrition support used in the management of pancreatic disease. The two stages of pancreatitis are the acute stage and the chronic state.

Acute pancreatitis warrants oral nutrition to be completely withheld and total parenteral nutrition (TPN) should provide nutrition support until the acute inflammation has settled and oral intake can resume again. While the patient is on TPN and waiting to resume an oral diet, enteral nutrition may be required to ease back into oral intake (see chapter on Parenteral and Enteral Nutrition). Oral intake is usually initiated with a clear liquid or formula diet and advances slowly to solid foods of six small meals. The small meals should be comprised of low-fat, high carbohydrate, high protein foods (see chapter on Gallbladder Diseases for the low-fat diet).

All alcoholic beverages should be avoided. The patient with acute pancreatitis must have nutritional therapy goals to include:

 Rest the pancreas

▶ Until eating can be resumed, nutritional depletion must be prevented

Chronic pancreatitis usually is indicated by impaired secretion of pancreatic enzymes leading to maldigestion and malabsorption. Loss of 90% of the pancreatic tissue causes pancreatic insufficiency, with weight loss and steatorrhea. Replacement pancreatic enzymes, taken orally with meals, may be used if the patient has pain, steatorrhea, diarrhea, or overt malnutrition (weight loss). With this stage of pancreatitis, a diet low in fat where fat comprises less that 25% of total calories, and high in protein and carbohydrate is helpful to the patient. This diet can be supplemented with medium chain triglycerides (MCT). Adequate amounts of vitamins, minerals and trace elements should be consumed. The patient with steatorrhea may need fat-soluble vitamin and mineral suplementation.

If there is an extensive amount of pancreatic disease, the insulin-secreting capacity may be diminished leading to glucose intolerance and indicating a diet to be used that is used for diabetes mellitus management. An alternative to this diet would be the implementation of elemental formula diets which have been used with success.

The patient with chronic pancreatitis must have nutritional therapy goals to include:

▶ Help prevent maldigestion and malabsorption
▶ Replete tissue deficits
▶ Control blood glucose if and when glucose intolerance occurs

Adequacy

To ensure the diet intake has adequate calories, protein, vitamins, minerals and fluids, individual assessment of the patient's nutritional status, nutritional requirements and clinical condition must be obtained. The physician should order a nutrition consultation, specifying the acute and/or chronic condition.

References

Puckett, R.P., and Brown, S.M.: *Shands Hospital at the University of Florida Guide to Clinical Dietetics.* 5th ed. Dubuque: Kendall/Hunt Publishing Co., 1993.

Zeman, F.J., *Clinical Nutrition and Dietetics,* Macmillan Publishing Company, New York, 1983.

▶ DIETARY MANAGEMENT FOR GALLBLADDER DISEASE ◀

Description

The main goal of nutritional therapy for the patient with diseases of the gallbladder and bile ducts should be to provide symptomatic relief. This nutritional therapy is prescribed as a low-fat diet of 40–50 grams of fat or 20 grams of fat in more severe cases. If the patient is obese, weight reduction is suggested.

A low-fat diet can provide relief in the treatment of cholelithiasis, choledocholithiasis, cholecystitis, and biliary dyskinesia due to fats stimulating gallbladder secretion and sphincter of Oddi action. Fat tolerance varies greatly patient to patient so the diet needs to be individualized. No differentiation has been made between saturated and unsaturated fat in the diet, but in keeping with more healthy trends, unsaturated fats should be consumed in a greater quantity.

If an acute attack occurs, which is usually caused by bile duct obstruction, a clear liquid diet should be implemented temporarily. Protein from the diet can be supplied by skim milk and carbohydrate is supplied by fruit juices, gelatins and fruit ices. Only as tolerated should solid foods be reintroduced to the diet.

Adequacy

The low-fat diet meets the 1989 Recommended Dietary Allowances in all nutrients if a proper amount and variety of foods are consumed.

References

Krause, M.V., Mahan, L.K., *Food, Nutrition and Diet Therapy,* (6th ed.), W.B. Saunders Co., Philadelphia, 1979.

Puckett, R.P., and Brown, S.M.: *Shands Hospital at the University of Florida Guide to Clinical Dietetics.* 5th ed. Dubuque: Kendall/Hunt Publishing Co., 1993.

40–50 Gram Fat Diet

Description

This diet is prescribed for the person with diseases of the liver, gallbladder, or pancreas in which disturbances of digestion and absorption of fat may occur. The fat content is limited to 40–50 grams daily. If a diet is ordered as "Low Fat", a 40–50 gram fat diet usually is sent.

Adequacy

This diet meets the 1989 Recommended Dietary Allowance for good nutrition as established by the Food and Nutrition Board of the National Research Council when the types of food and amounts suggested are included daily.

Type of Foods	Foods Allowed	Foods Not Allowed
Milk (2 or more cups daily)	Skim milk, cocoa made from skim milk, buttermilk or evaporated milk made from skim milk, 1% milk, powdered skim milk	Whole milk, 2% milk, milk drinks, chocolate milk, eggnogs, alcohol and milkshakes, evaporated milk and condensed milk
Meat, Fish, Poultry and Meat Substitutes (4–6 ounces daily. No more than 3 gm fat/oz.) Recommended preparation methods are broiling, roasting, (on rack), grilling or boiling	Poultry (without skin): cornish hen, chicken, turkeyVeal (all cuts); Beef: USDA good or choice cuts (i.e., round, sirloin, flank, steak, tenderloin, and chopped beef) Roast (rib, chuck, rump) Steak (cubed, Porterhouse T-bone) Fresh ham, canned, cured, or boiled ham, Canadian bacon, tenderloin, chops, loin roast, Boston butt, cutlets Lean lamb: chops, leg, roast All fresh and frozen fish: fresh, frozen or canned in water: crab, lobster, scallops, shrimp, clams, oysters Tuna (canned in water) Herring (uncreamed or smoked) Sardines (canned, drained) Salmon (canned in water) 95–98% Fat-free luncheon meat Tofu Tempeh Natto	Any fried, fatty, or heavily marbled meat, fish, or poultry: most USDA prime cuts of beef ribs, or corned beef; ground pork, sausage, ham hocks, pig's feet, chitterlings, ground lamb, duck, goose, tuna (packed in oil), and salmon (packed in oil). Sausage: Polish, Italian, Knockwurst, smoked bratwurst, frankfurter. Luncheon meats: bologna, salami, and pimento loaf

Type of Foods	Foods Allowed	Foods Not Allowed
Meat, Fish, Poultry and Meat Substitutes (4–6 ounces daily. No more than 3 gm fat/oz.)— **Continued**	Cottage cheese (dry curd, 1% fat) Skim Farmer's Cheese, part skim mozzarella or ricotta, diet cheeses (with less than 55 kcal/oz.)	High fat cheeses–cheddar, American, blue cheese, brie, edam, limburger, romano, monterey, provolone, swiss, muenster, roquefort, brick colby, gouda, pimento cheese
Eggs	Limit to 1 whole egg per day, egg whites as desired, egg substitute without fat as desired	Fried egg
Fruits (2 or more servings daily–	All fruit juices, fresh, frozen, canned, or dried	None
Vegetables (3 or more servings daily–include 1 green or yellow daily)	All fresh, frozen or canned. Potatoes	Buttered, au gratin, creamed or fried unless made with allowed fat; potato chips
Bread, Cereal, Rice and Pasta (6 or more servings daily)	Enriched white and whole grain bread; hamburger buns, hard rolls, saltine crackers, graham crackers, melba toast, corn tortillas, air-popped popcorn	Quick breads, biscuits, cornbread, sweet rolls, waffles, pancakes, fritters, donuts, muffins, popcorn prepared with fat, snack crackers, popovers
	All cereals except those containing foods not allowed; spaghetti, noodles, macaroni, rice	Granola cereals, cereals containing nuts or coconut; corn chips, fried rice
Fats and Oil (3–5 servings daily)	1 Tbsp. peanut butter 1 tsp. fortified margarine or butter 1 tsp. oil or shortening 1 tsp. mayonnaise 1 Tbsp. salad dressing or cream cheese 1 strip of bacon ⅛ of 4′ diameter avocado 2 Tbsp. light cream 1 Tbsp. heavy cream 6 small nuts 5 small olives	All others. Any in excess of prescribed amounts
Soups (As desired)	Fat-free broth Fat-free vegetable soup Cream soup make with skim milk Packaged dehydrated soups made with allowed ingredients	All others
Desserts	Angel food cake, sherbet made with skim milk, gelatin, ices, popsicles, fruit whips made with skim milk, sorbet, gelatin popsicles, lowfat frozen yogurt, fruit and juice bars, vanilla wafers, graham crackers, lady fingers, arrowroot cookies, fat-free cakes, cookies, and ice cream	Cake pie, ice cream, ice milk, cookies, pastry and desserts containing chocolate, cream, coconut, nuts, shortening or fat (unless calculated as part of fat allowance) most commercial desserts

Type of Foods	Foods Allowed	Foods Not Allowed
Beverages	All coffee, tea, and carbonated beverages	None
Miscellaneous	Salt, sugar, jelly, jam, marmalade, syrup, honey, hard sugar candy, herbs, spices, flavoring, cocoa powder, catsup, vinegar, lemon juice, pickles, white sauce made with skim milk	Cream sauces

Sample Menu

Breakfast	Lunch	Supper
Orange Juice	Apple Juice	Grape Juice
Oatmeal	3 oz. Roast Pork	3 oz. Broiled Chicken (no skin)
1 Hard Cooked Egg	Diced Potato	Steamed Rice
Toast	Green Beans	Carrots
1 tsp. Margarine	Sliced Tomato Salad	Fruit Gelatin Salad
Jelly	Angel Food Cake	Orange Sherbet
Skim Milk	Bread	Bread
Coffee	1 tsp. Margarine	1 tsp. Margarine
Sugar	Jelly	Jelly
	Skim Milk	Iced Tea–Sugar
	Iced Tea–Sugar	

References

American Dietetic Association: *Manual of Clinical Dietetics.* Chicago: 1988.

Dallas–Fort Worth Hospital Council: *Dallas–Fort Worth Hospital Council Diet Manual.* Irving: 1992.

Puckett, R.P. and Brown, S.M.: *Shands Hospital at the University of Florida Guide to Clinical Dietetics,* 5th ed., Dubuque: Kendall/Hunt Publishing Co., 1993.

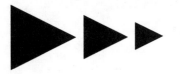 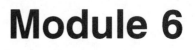

Module 6

Modification for Special Needs

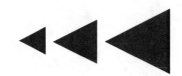

▶ TRANSPLANTATIONS ◀

Objective of Nutrition Care

Nutritional therapy goals before and after all transplantations should be to delivery the patient in optimal nutritional status capable for the clinical condition and maintain status. The following are general guidelines **before transplantation:**

▶ Obtain diet history
▶ Assess nutritional status
▶ Achieve and maintain optimal nutritional status
   After transplantation—
▶ Promote wound healing
▶ Achieve adequate protein status
▶ Achieve and maintain desirable body weight
▶ Minimize drug-induced metabolic changes and side effects Vitamin and/or mineral supplementation is suggested

Various medications prescribed for the patient may interfere with initial nutritional management goals and need to be closely monitored.

The diet protocol varies among facilities according to guideline philosophies established by the medical support team within each facility. Prior to obtaining or establishing the nutritional protocol at your facility the following diet parameters can serve as an established successful protocol.

Cardiac Transplant

The goal of pretransplant nutritional management is to condition the patient for surgery at optimal nutritional status to reduce the risk of posttransplant morbidity and mortality. For most patients this is a repletion phase, but for others, weight reduction may be desirable. A nutritional assessment needs to be determined to obtain the patient's clinical condition. Patients exhibiting cardiac cachexia may need the addition of supplements, tube feedings or hyperalimentation to facilitate delivery of adequate nutrition.

When ventilatory support is discontinued and bowel sounds are adequate postoperatively, the diet is progressed as follows:

▶ Clear Liquid
▶ Full Liquid (low cholesterol, 2 to 4 gram sodium)
▶ AHA Step-2 Diet
      200 mg cholesterol
      Low-fat, low saturated fat
      2 to 4 gram sodium
      High fiber
      Limited concentrated sweets

Adequacy

This diet is adequate in all nutrients if a proper amount and variety of foods are consumed by the patient, except the postoperative clear liquid. Vitamin and/or mineral supplementation is recommended.

Liver Transplant

An essential part of pre-operative care is nutritional assessment and repletion. Protein-energy malnutrition is common in this group of individuals secondary to the high catabolic state, malabsorption, and poor dietary intake to anorexia and severe dietary restrictions. Nutritional therapy for liver transplant patients varies depending on the function of the transplanted liver, post-transplant medical complications, length of time from transplantation, and the side effects of immunosuppressive drugs. It is essential to periodically re-evaluate modifications in energy, protein, carbohydrate, fluid, sodium, potassium, calcium, vitamins and minerals.

Candidates for liver transplants may need aggressive nutritional repletion, such as tube feedings or parenteral nutrition. Aggressive preoperative nutritional support results in an increased positive outcome following transplantation.

Parenteral nutrition can progress with the first 3 days following surgery. The patient is NPO until the bowel sounds return. The patient may be fed by tube feeding if enteral intake does not progress sufficiently.

Typical diet protocol is:
- ▶ Clear liquids
- ▶ Soft solids
- ▶ 4 gram sodium diet with no potassium containing salt substitutes
      Protein—1.5 to 2.0 gram/kg/day
      Calories—BEE + (30% to 50% above BEE)

Adequacy

Actual nutrient intake depends upon the individual's appetite, food preferences and ability to eat. Provided the individual consumes a wide variety of foods in adequate amounts, the diet will meet the Recommended Dietary Allowances. Vitamin and mineral supplementation may be indicated.

Kidney Transplant

Kidney transplantation provides a viable option for individuals with end-stage chronic renal failure. Pre-operatively an extensive physical evaluation is required. Optimal nutritional status must be achieved prior to surgery for desired results. The obese individual needs consultation to be on a pre-operative weight reduction regimen.

Standard protocol for diet therapy post-operatively is:

Calories—28–30 kcal/kg actual body weight
Protein—1.5 gram/kg ideal body weight
No concentrated sweets
Cholesterol—300 mg/day or less
2 to 4 gram sodium with no potassium containing salt substitute

Adequacy

Actual nutrient intake depends upon the individual's appetite, food preferences and ability to eat. Provided the individual consumes a wide variety of foods in adequate amounts, the diet will meet the Recommended Dietary Allowances. Minerals such as calcium and phosphorus may be depleted due to drug therapy. A vitamin and mineral supplement is routinely recommended. If hypercalcemia is present from pre-existing secondary hyperparathyroidism, supplementation of vitamin D and calcium is avoided.

References

Fischer, J.E., Branched-chained enriched amino acids solutions in patients with liver failure: An early example of nutritional pharmacology, *Journal of Parenteral and Enteral Nutrition,* 14(6), Supplement, pp. 249S–256S, 1990.

Puckett, R.P. and Brown, S.M.: *Shands Hospital at the University of Florida Guide to Clinical Dietetics.* 5th ed. Dubuque: Kendall/Hunt Publishing Co., 1993.

Ragsdale, D., Nutritional program for heart transplantation, *The Journal of Heart Transplantation*, 6(4), pp. 228–232, 1987.

University of Michigan Hospitals, *Food and Nutrition Services, Guidelines for Nutritional Care*, Ann Arbor, Michigan, 1995.

▶ BONE MARROW TRANSPLANTATION ◀

The type of nutritional support for the patient in bone marrow transplantation (BMT) depends upon the phase of care and the individual's needs. After the decision has been made to proceed with the transplantation, the patient's nutritional status is evaluated, and a diet history is completed.

At the **pretransplant** evaluation, individuals are seen to identify nutritional risk factors, to determine baseline values for nutritional assessment parameters to establish nutritional support goals and to explain the posttransplant diet and use of TPN. The majority of BMT patients are found to be well-nourished prior to transplantation and the goal of nutritional support is maintenance rather than repletion of lean body mass. Knowing the patient's food preferences and dislikes serves as a reference in the post-transplant phase when oral feeding is resumed.

The nutritional complications of the pre-transplant phase (several days of high-dose chemotherapy and total body irradiation) may include nausea, vomiting, esophagitis, mucositis, xerostomia, thick viscous saliva, anorexia, dysgeusia, early satiety, diarrhea and steatorrhea. Due to a greatly decreased oral intake, total parenteral nutrition (TPN) is usually progressed after the last dose of chemotherapy to minimize tissue loss. The pretransplant phase may also result in the loss of immune competence and of the body's ability to deal with infection.

Since much of the medical care of the immunocompromised patient is designed to prevent or treat infection, anything that comes in contact with the patient must have low counts of microorganisms. Consequently, when oral feeding is possible, a low bacteria diet is initiated.

The low bacteria diet restricts foods that contain gram-negative bacteria, molds and yeasts. The diet includes well-cooked foods and fresh fruits and vegetables that potentially may be contaminated. Food-handling and preparation techniques that greatly minimize bacterial contamination must be followed. The patient receiving a discharge diet consultation must be taught the proper food preparation/serving techniques to be used at home. These include:

▶ Take-out food, fast food and restaurant food is not recommended.
▶ **Wash hands prior to handling food.**
▶ Clean food preparation surfaces and wooden cutting boards with a 10% bleach solution (Mix 1 part bleach with 9 parts water). Allow surface to air dry. Rubber or plastic cutting boards can be washed in the same manner as dishes.
▶ Wash dishes, pots and utensils including the can opener with very hot soapy water. Rinse with running hot water and allow to air dry (do not use dish towels). The automatic dishwasher may also be used.
▶ Do not use a microwave oven to cook or reheat foods other than canned foods which are already sterile.
▶ Do not use a barbecue grill to cook food.

As the patient's oral intake increases, TPN is tapered off so that the parenteral and oral intake together meets the individual's nutritional requirements. The effects of medications used in the treatment of bone marrow transplant complications on the gastrointestinal system may require various dietary modifications and changes in food consistency and texture to improve oral intake.

If enteral feeding are prescribed, as appropriate, certain precautions to reduce bacterial contamination of tube feedings must be followed. These include;

▶ Administration of only commercially sterile products
▶ Aseptic handling of formulas during mixing (when necessary) and administration
▶ Use of closed systems
▶ Use of sterile water to reconstitute or dilute formulas
▶ Limiting hang time to eight hours (or the recommendation of your facility Infection Control Department) regular bacteriologic surveillance of enteral formulas and their delivery

Frequent assessment of nutritional status during the immediate **posttransplant** period is required as the greatest risk for serious infection or gastrointestinal graft-versus-host disease (GVHD) occurs during this time. Symptoms of GVHD include nausea, vomiting, anorexia, abdominal cramping, secretory diarrhea, bloody stools, malabsorption, altered intestinal motility and ileus. Twenty-four hour intake and output should be closely monitored, especially for stool and emesis volume, as increases may be indicative of GVHD. Serum zinc and copper levels may need to be monitored with excessive gastrointestinal tract losses. Some medications given for infection and GVHD may result in severe wasting of magnesium and potassium. A diet sufficient in calories, rich in protein, and limited in fat is recommended.

Upon discharge form the hospital, the individual is followed for several months as the risk for developing numerous complications still persists until at least 100 days postransplant. Nutritional status is usually stable by this time, although nutrition problems associated with infections, drug toxicities, and chronic GVHD may be detected.

The physician should order a nutrition consult for bone marrow transplantation upon admission. The diet order should indicate the low bacteria diet to be implemented upon admission if oral food intake is indicated.

Adequacy

The low bacteria diet meets the 1989 Recommended Dietary Allowances for all nutrients unless the patient is consuming 1,200 kilocalories or less, or the patient's food aversions of intolerances greatly limit the variety of food selections. It is recommended for those patients to supplement their diet with a daily multiple vitamin which provides nutrients at a level equivalent to the RDA.

▶ Low Bacteria Diet ◀

Type of Food	Foods Allowed	Foods Not Allowed
Beverages	Coffee, instant coffee, tea, instant tea, fruit-flavored powdered drink mix, carbonated beverages, canned fruit drinks, pasteurized beer, bottled seltzer water, sterile water and ice	Non-pasteurized beer, wine, bottled and distilled water
Dairy products	Instant hot cocoa mix, single serving cartons of pasteurized milk, commercial milkshake products, canned milk, half-and-half creamer, American cheese, cream cheese in individual packets, powdered instant breakfast drinks, canned puddings, commercially prepared single serving refrigerated puddings, single serving containers of ice cream and sherbet	Non-pasteurized milk and milk products, bulk milk and milk products, buttermilk, yogurt, cheese (except American), cottage cheese, sour cream, whipped cream, non-dairy whipped topping

Low Bacteria Diet—(continued)

Type of Food	Foods Allowed	Foods Not Allowed
Meat, meat substitutes	All hot, well-cooked beef, pork, poultry, and fish; canned meats, fish, and shellfish; hot dogs, well cooked; **well-cooked eggs;** spaghetti sauce; frozen commercial mixed entrees, heated thoroughly, including chicken and beef pot pies, macaroni and cheese, beef stroganoff, spaghetti with meat sauce; smooth peanut butter; canned beans, legumes, refried beans; baby food in jars	Deli meats, processed luncheon meats, raw eggs, dried meats (beef jerky), rare and medium cooked meats and seafood, lasagna, pizza
Breads, cereals, starches	All breads, English muffins, bagels (except onion), hamburger and hot dog buns, dinner rolls, tortillas, hot and cold cereals except as noted, pancakes, waffles, french toast, blueberry and plain muffins, donuts except as noted, cooked white or sweet potatoes, yams, french fries, hash brown potatoes, instant mashed potatoes; cooked rice, pasta, and noodles; chow mein noodles, snack chips in single serving bags (pretzels, corn, tortilla, and potato chips), crackers popcorn	All raisin and nut containing cereals, breads, cinnamon rolls, and sweet rolls, donuts with cream fillings, onion bagels, raw potatoes, au gratin potatoes, potato salad, macaroni salad
Vegetables	All canned vegetables and juice, canned bean salad, frozen vegetables (well cooked), baked fresh squash	Fresh vegetables, onion rings
Fruits	Canned fruit, canned and bottled fruit juices, baked apples	Fresh fruits and juices, raisins, all other dried fruits
Desserts, sweets	Pound and angel food cakes, cookies, cupcakes, fruit pies, popsicles, jello, homemade custard, candy (hard candies, jelly beans, gum drops, orange slices, gummy bears, lemon drops, marshmallows, peanut butter cups, plain chocolate disc candies), chewing gum	All varieties of nuts and dried fruits, Crackerjacks®; cakes, cookies, pies, and pastries made with nuts, dried fruits, cream, or cheese; candy bars
Fats	Margarine, vegetable oil, fat for deep-fat frying, shortening, mayonnaise, tartar sauce from individual packets, canned gravy and sauces	Butter, homemade gravy, hollandaise sauce, tartar sauce and mayonnaise from multi-serving containers, cream sauces
Soups	All hot canned and dehydrated packaged soups, broths, and bouillons	Homemade soups, commercial refrigerated and frozen soups, cold soups

Low Bacteria Diet—(continued)

Type of Food	Foods Allowed	Foods Not Allowed
Miscellaneous	Individually packaged mustard, ketchup, taco sauce, lemon juice, salad dressing, jam, jelly, cranberry sauce, honey, and syrup; seasonings, spices, and pepper added before cooking; sugars, salt, canned chocolate syrup, dill pickles, canned black olives, glucose polymers, powdered supplements reconstituted with sterile water, all canned supplements, canned dips	Condiments from multi-serving containers, Bleu cheese and Roquefort dressing, green olives, sweet pickle relish; seasonings, spices, and pepper added after cooking

References

Aker, S.N., Lenssen, P., Darbinian, J., Cheney, C.L., Cunningham, B., Nutritional assessment in the marrow transplant patient, *Nutr Supp Serv.,* 1983; 3 (10):22–26.

Lennsen, P., Aker, S.N., *Nutritional Assessment and Management During Marrow Transplantation: A Resource Manual,* Seattle, WA: Fred Hutchinson Cancer Research Center, 1985.

Puckett, R.P. and Brown, S.M.: *Shands Hospital at the University of Florida Guide to Clinical Dietetics.* 5th ed., Dubuque: Kendall/Hunt Publishing Co., 1993.

Pemberton, C.M., Moxness, K.E., German, M.J., Nelson, J.K., Gastineau, C.F., *Rochester Methodist Hospital and Saint Marys Hospital, Mayo Clinic Diet Manual: A Handbook of Dietary Practices,* (6th ed), B.C. Decker, Inc., Toronto, pp. 195–196, 225–227, 1988.

Szeluga, D.J., Stuart, R.K., Brookmeyer, R., Utermohlen, V., Santos, G.W., Energy requirements of parenterally fed bone marrow transplant recipients. *Journal Parenteral and Enteral Nutrition,* 1985;9:139–143.

University of Michigan Hospitals, Food and Nutrition Services, *Guidelines for Nutritional Care,* Ann Arbor, Michigan, 1995.

 ## NUTRITIONAL CARE OF BURN PATIENTS ◀

Description

Severe burns present a challenge in nutritional therapy because of the quantity of nutrients required, catabolic changes, gastrointestinal dysfunction, increased insensible water loss, increased heat loss, and anorexia. Nitrogen excretion following major burns depends upon the extent and depth of the burn. The nitrogen loss becomes even greater if infection develops. In order for protein to function primarily for building and repairing body tissues, a sufficient amount of non-protein calories are needed to meet energy requirements.

In addition to protein loss, fluid and electrolytes are lost through exudation. Adequate fluid and electrolytes are required to maintain circulatory volume and prevent acute renal failure. Treating the burns with silver nitrate soaks causes electrolytes to be leached out thus requiring continuous fluid and electrolyte replacement.

Adequate nutritional support may be accomplished by using an oral diet with commercial supplements in patients with small, relatively uncomplicated burns. However, enteral tube feedings, in addition to an oral diet, may be necessary in patients with burns over more than 40% of body surface area and in those who cannot consume sufficient calories and protein to meet the heightened metabolic demands of the burn injury. Enteral nutrition is the method of choice for nutritional support because of the beneficial effect on gastrointestinal (GI) mucosal mass and because of decreased risk of infection. Parenteral nutrition should be reserved for those instances when GI tract function is absent or when caloric needs cannot be met by enteral feedings alone.

The following formula may be used to calculate the nutritional requirements of the burn patient. (Children > 3 years of age to adults):

Calories	=	25 × actual body weight (kg) + 40 × percent of body surface area burned.
Protein	=	1 gm/kg IBW + 3 gm protein × percent of body surface area burned.
Carbohydrate	=	45–55% of total calories
Fat	=	30–40% of total calories

Initial protein needs for children with burns should be based on g protein/kg admission or preburn weight. For the child < 1 year of age, 2.5–3.5 g protein/kg body weight is prescribed since excessive protein loads may compromise infants' immature kidneys. Children > 1 year of age receive 2–3 g protein/kg body weight or 20% of total kilocalories from protein. For pediatric trauma patients with mild to moderate stress, the RDA for protein according to age and weight is used. However, in cases of severe stress, ie. closed head injury or spinal cord injury, 1–2 times the RDA should be provided.

No specific recommendation has been set for vitamin and mineral allowances in burn patients. Therapeutic levels of iron may be needed if anemia develops. Patients are usually unable to eat sufficient quantities of food to correct an iron deficiency. Therapeutic doses of ascorbic acid and zinc supplementation have been shown to improve wound healing.

Adequacy

Actual nutrient intake depends on the individual's appetite and ability to eat. Provided that the individual consumes a wide variety of foods in adequate amounts, the diet will meet the Recommended Dietary Allowances of 1989. When individuals are under stressful conditions, the 1989 Recommended Dietary Allowances may not be adequate to meet nutrient needs.

References

Gottschlich, Michele M., *Nutrition Support Dietitions,* ASPEN, 1993.

Mahan, K. and Arlin, M.: *Krause's Food, Nutrition and Diet Therapy.* 8th ed. Philadelphia: W.B. Saunders Co., 1992.

Puckett, R.P. and Brown, S.M.: *Shands Hospital at the University of Florida Guide to Clinical Dietetics.* 5th ed., Dubuque: Kendall/Hunt Publishing Co., 1993.

Schneider, H.A., Anderson, C.E. and Coursin, D.B.: *Nutritional Support of Medical Practice.* Hagerstown: Harper and Row, 1977.

University of Michigan Hospitals, Food and Nutrition Services, *Guidelines for Nutritional Care,* Ann Arbor, 1995.

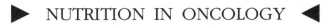

▶ NUTRITION IN ONCOLOGY ◀

The progressive growth of cancer leads to striking alterations of structure and function in the host organ. All too often, cachexia is the result. This syndrome is characterized by anorexia, weakness, and nutritional depletion. Cachexia results from local structural changes due to tumor growth, decreased food intake, maldigestion, malabsorption, and altered metabolism.

Weight loss is one of the common manifestations of cancer. Anorexia is unquestionably one of the common causes of weight loss. Weight loss in cancer patients is associated with loss of body fat and protein.

Oral feeding, enteral nutrition by tube, and parenteral nutrition are all potentially useful in the nutritional management of the cancer patient. Treatment of anorexia and improvement in the patient's nutritional state often lead to an increased sense of well being and enhance the likelihood of positive response to therapy.

Guidelines for Designing a Diet and Feeding the Cancer Patient

Nutritional support of the cancer patient must be individualized according to the treatment and his/her own needs. All patients should be counseled regarding the importance of nutrition for disease management.

1. A detailed diet history should be obtained to determine past and present food preferences and eating habits, calorie and protein intake, specific food intolerances, taste abnormalities of altered taste sensations and distribution of feedings throughout the day.

2. The following may be used to calculate protein needs of adult patients with cancer. See the section in this chapter, Nutritional Assessment of the Patient, to calculate weight and calorie parameters.

	Protein gm/kg IBW
Nonambulatory, Sedentary	1.0
Slightly Hypermetabolic: for weight gain/anabolism	Normal Maintenance, Increased Protein Demands (i.e., protein-losing enteropathy, hypermetabolism, extreme wasting)
Hypermetabolic or Severely Stressed: Malabsorption	1.5–2.5

3. If the patient has been losing weight, the first realistic goal of nutritional intervention may be to prevent further loss of weight.

4. Encourage oral food intake gently, but persistently.

5. Encourage six smaller meals instead of three regular meals if the patient needs more calories, has complaints of nausea and vomiting, early satiety or anorexia. Snacks should be available during the day.

6. Encourage high calorie, high quality protein drinks between meals instead of low calorie beverages. Supplements should be encouraged early to prevent weight loss (milkshakes and commercial supplements).

7. Head and neck surgery or radiation may cause difficulties in chewing or swallowing. A patient may do better with thick-consistency liquids (i.e. milkshakes) or semi-solid foods (i.e. mashed potatoes). Addition of commercial food thickeners may be beneficial. Gravies and cream sauces may aid in swallowing. The chin should point slightly down toward the chest in order to ensure that the windpipe is closed off during swallowing. If saliva production is decreased, lemon drops may help to stimulate saliva production.

8. Pain and nausea can interfere with eating. Pain and/or anti-nausea medications could be timed to be given one-half hour prior to meals.

9. Aroma, color, and pleasing service of food are especially important for individuals with cancer in which "taste blindness" (loss of taste) has occurred. Special attention to the aesthetics in food service is vital to eating.

10. Encouraging some exercise, such as a short walk (with physician's approval), one-half hour prior to a meal may help stimulate the appetite.

11. If a person is not able to consume adequate calories orally, alternate routes of administering nutrition may have to be considered:
    a.) Enteral hyperalimentation (tube feeding)—use the gastrointestinal tract if functional.
    b.) Central hyperalimentation (TPN).
    c.) Peripheral hyperalimentation (PPN).

For further information about nutrition in oncology, refer to the following research:

Bass, F.B., Cox, R.H., The need for dietary counseling of cancer patients as indicated by nutrient and supplement intake. *Journal of the American Dietetic Association,* Vol. 95, Number 11, pp. 1319–1321, November, 1995.

Nutritional Assessment of the Patient

Weight Parameters

1. Calculations of Ideal Body Weight (IBW):
    Females: 100 lbs per 5 feet + 5 lbs per inch > 5 feet
    Males: 106 lbs per 5 feet + 6 lbs per inch > 5 feet
    + or − 10% for small or large frame sizes. Height and weight tables are not normally used.
2. Actual weight as a percentage of usual body weight (UBW). UBW is the preferred reference for oncology patients.
    % UBW = Actual Weight divided by UBW × 100
    UBW standards:
    Normal   >95% UBW
    Mild depletion   85–95% UBW
    Moderate depletion   75–85% UBW
    Severe depletion   <75% UBW
3. Weight loss/time standards parameters are expressed as weight change divided by time standard:
    Significant weight loss = 1–2% per one week; 5% per one month; 7.5% per three months; 10% per six months
    Sever weight loss = >2% per one week; >5% per one month; >7.5% per three months; 10% per six months

Calorie Parameters

1. Basal energy expenditure (BEE):
    Harris Benedict Equation including out of bed/activity factor of 1.3 and cancer "correction factor" of 1.6 for hypermetabolic state. If patient is febrile, 12% of BEE is added per degree Centigrade above 37 degrees, 7% of BEE per degree Fahrenheit above 98.6 degrees. The Harris Benedict formula for basal energy expenditure (BEE):
    • Females: 655.10 + 9.56 × weight (kg) + 1.85 × height (cm) − 4.68 × age (years) = BEE
    • Males: 66.47 + 13.75 × weight (kg) + 5.00 × height (cm) − 6.76 × age (years) = BEE
2. 30–35 Kcal/Kg weight/day for maintenance
    >35–45 Kcal/Kg weight/day for anabolism
    For the patient on total parenteral nutrition the caloric requirement may be calculated as 40–45 Kcal/Kg weight/day. See chapter on parenteral enteral nutrition.

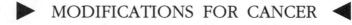

▶ MODIFICATIONS FOR CANCER ◀

Description

Nutritional support of the cancer patient presents complex problems. The cancer patient is often anorexic and malnourished. The diet must be individualized for each patient in order to improve or maintain adequate nutritional status.

Radiation Therapy

Nutritional problems may develop depending on the location and extent of the area treated. It is important for the dietitian to begin working with the patient when therapy begins, stressing good nutritional habits, and emphasizing the importance of weight maintenance while receiving treatment with radiation.

Area Treated	Effect Upon Nutrition	Suggested Treatment
I. Head and Neck	1. Thickened saliva and dry mouth due to suppression of salivary glands.	Foods prepared with sauces, gravies or additional liquid (may have to use artificial saliva).
		Sucking sugar-free mints or chewing sugar-free gum to aid dry mouth.
	2. Loss of Appetite.	Small frequent meals.
	3. Loss of or change in taste.	Provide individual food preferences.
	4. Mucositis beginning in the second to third week of treatment resulting in sore irritated mouth, tongue, and throat.	High protein, high calorie soft diet. Supplementary feedings such as milkshakes. Use of a straw to drink liquids when mucositis is present. Avoid extremely hot or cold foods, highly seasoned foods, acidic foods, sharp or rough foods such as pretzels or potato chips.
	5. Dental deterioration with loss of teeth.	Avoid sweets that may leave sugar coating on teeth.
II. Tonsilor Region, Palate, Tongue, Nasopharynx	1. Painful burning throat to tart or acid foods.	Bland, soft, puree or liquid diet as required with high protein and high calorie nourishments. Avoid tart or acid foods.
	2. Soreness of mouth.	Same as above.
	3. Loss of appetite and taste.	Small, frequent meals; Exercise 5–10 minutes prior to meal; Provide individual preferences.
III. Whole Abdomen	1. Small bowel enteritis causing diarrhea and malabsorption.	Use low residue diet. If diarrhea persists, use elemental diets. Increase fluids, especially water.
	2. Nausea when radiation field is over stomach.	Small, frequent feedings. Bland foods or cold, non-aromatic foods when nausea is present.

Area Treated	Effect Upon Nutrition	Suggested Treatment
IV. Pelvic (Uterine, Cervix or Ovaries)	1. Diarrhea.	Low residue diet. Small, frequent feedings. Eliminate raw vegetables, fruits and whole grain products.
Surgery **I. Oropharyngeal Area**	1. May require tube feeding.	Place on tube feeding if required. Progress to liquids, puree or soft as tolerated.
II. Esophagus	1. Gastric Stasis. 2. Malabsorption. 3. Fistulas.	Liquid, puree, soft, bland, tube feeding or elemental diet, depending on patient's tolerance Frequent feedings.
III. Stomach: Gasterctomy	1. Dumping Syndrome. 2. Steatorrhea. 3. Loss of intrinsic factor.	Gastrectomy "Anti-Dumping" diet. Individualized diet.
IV. Intestines (Colostomy or Ileostomy)	1. Malabsorption. 2. Diarrhea. 3. Electrolyte and water imbalance.	Conventional foods if tolerated. May need liquids; progress to low residue and regular diets. Avoid any troublesome foods.

Gas Producing Foods—To be avoided, depending upon individual tolerances.

Apple, Raw
Asparagus
Dried Peas and Beans
Cabbage Family
(Broccoli, Brussel Sprouts,
Cabbage and Cauliflower)
Sweet Potatoes
Onions/Leeks
Corn

Fish
Certain Cheeses
(Roquefort, Brie and
other strong cheeses)
Milk
Melon
Nuts
Highly Seasoned Foods
Eggs

Peppers
Turnips
Sauerkraut
Rutabagas
Cucumbers

High Fiber Foods—When introducing new foods, add no more than one per day.
Foods with seeds, hard to digest kernels or cellulose
Raw Fruits (Oranges, Apples, Strawberries)
Cooked Vegetables (Spinach, Corn)
Popcorn
Nuts
Coconut
Tomatoes
Note: Highly seasoned foods to be introduced in the same manner.

Foods That May Contribute To Diarrhea—Avoid when diarrhea is present.
   Green Leafy Vegetables
   Broccoli
   Dried Beans
   Raw Fruits Except Bananas
   Highly Seasoned Foods

Foods That May Help Diarrhea
   Bananas
   Applesauce
   Rice
   Tapioca
   Creamy Peanut Butter

Foods That Reduce Fecal Odor
   Cranberry Juice
   Yogurt
   Buttermilk

Foods That May Produce Strong Fecal Odor
   Fish
   Chicken
   Fried Eggs

General Considerations For Mild Constipation
   Increase Fluids to 2 quarts per day
   Increase Fruit Juices
   Increase Cooked Fruits
   Increase Cooked Vegetables
   Increase Whole Grain Breads and Cereals
   Add Wheat Bran

Chemotherapy

The nutritional goals for the patient receiving chemotherapy are weight maintenance and adequate nutrient intake. During treatment these goals may be difficult to meet due to the possible side effects. Chemotherapeutic agents may produce many side effects that can affect the nutritional status of the patient. Each patient's diet should be individualized according to his needs and wants.

Associated Problems	Suggested Treatment
I. Loss of Appetite	Encourage patient to eat even when they do not feel like eating. Approach eating as an important part of therapy. Frequent, small meals and snacks.
II. Nausea and Vomiting	Avoid eating several hours before therapy. Carbonated beverages such as Coke, Sprite or Gingerale help curb nausea. Use small frequent meals to prevent prolonged empty stomach. After periods of sleep or rest, dry crackers or toast eaten before activity begins to help curb nausea. Tart foods such as pickles (dill or sour) and lemon may help. Popsicles and gelatin desserts increase fluid intake and are satisfying. Sense of smell

Associated Problems	Suggested Treatment
	is often altered or heightened during chemotherapy. Cold meat plates, sandwiches, fruit plates, cottage cheese, and other cold foods offer good nutrition without having an overpowering aroma that may cause nausea. Medications can easily alter the sense of taste, making foods that are normally favorites taste differently. Select foods that are appealing and, if the taste is not as expected or is undesirable, try another food. Relax and chew foods well to prevent and/or minimize anxiety and a tense stomach.
III. Sore and/or Ulcerated Mouth or Throat	Soft or bland diet as tolerated. Frequent, small meals served cold or at room temperature. Elimination of citrus and tomatoes.
IV. Taste Alterations Aversion to Sweets	Try: tart foods as lemon juice or dill pickles; milkshakes made with buttermilk or add coffee flavoring; using more seasonings, such as salt.
Aversion to Red Meats	Try: non-meat protein sources such as dairy products, soy products, legumes, nuts or commercial protein supplements; cold protein sources such as cheeses, eggs, luncheon meats, or beef jerky; fish or poultry marinated in fruit juice or wine.

Additional Comments

For patients receiving:

1. Radium implants for cervical cancer — Try: a fiber restricted diet during treatment to minimize intestinal mobility which can move the implant from its proper position.
2. Steroid treatment — Try: a temporary diabetic diet if glucose tolerance is significantly reduced by the treatment. Reduction of sodium intake may also be indicated.

Immunosuppression can occur during cancer therapy. An important food safety issue that should be emphasized with individuals is avoiding the use of raw eggs or uncooked egg products as a source of protein. To reduce the risk of food-borne illness by *Salmonella*, eggs and egg products should be cooked to 145°F and or use pasteurized eggs.

Just about all the chemotherapeutic agents affect dietary intake. Nausea and vomiting can occur quite frequently with all agents. The drug dosage, length of treatment, metabolic rate of the patient, and susceptibility to the side effects influence the degree to which the patient is effected.

The following table lists the expected side effects to chemotherapy.

► Nutritional Related Effects of Chemotherapy ◄

Drug	Nausea and Vomiting	Altered Taste or Smell	Mucositis (M) Stomatitis (S)	Diarrhea (D) Constipation (C)
Alkylating Agents				
Alkeran	mod to sev		mod to sev	(D) mod
Busulfan	mild	mod		
Cormustine	mild	mod		
Chlorambucil	mild		mild	
Cisplatin	mild	mod		
Cyclophosphamide	mod	mod	mild to mod	(D) mild
Dacarkozine	mild to mod		mod	rare
Mechlorethamine	sev			(D) milk

Drug	Nausea and Vomiting	Altered Taste or Smell	Mucositis (M) Stomatitis (S)	Diarrhea (D) Constipation (C)
Antibiotics				
Bleomycin	mild	anorexia	(S)	
Dactinomycin	sev	mod	(S)	(D)
Daunorubicen	mod		(M)	(D)
Doxorubicien	mod		(S)	
Anti-Metabolites				
Cytarbine	mild	mod	mod	(D)
Methotrexate	mild to sev	mod	(S)	(D)
Hormones				
Etoposide	mild to mod	mod	(S)	(D)
Miscellaneous				
Asparagenase	mod	anorexia		(D)
Hydroxyurea	mild	mod	mod	(D) (C)
Procarbozine*		mod	(S)	(D)
Vinblastine	mild			
Vincristine	mild	mod	mod	(D)

mod = moderate

sev = severe

*Avoid foods high in tyramine

References

Diet Manual; The University of Texas System Cancer Center, Houston: 1981.

Gottschlich, Michele M., *Nutrition Support Dietetics,* ASPEN, 1993.

Guide to Normal Nutrition and Diet Modification Manual. 2nd ed., Gainesville: Shands Teaching Hospital and Clinics, 1977.

Hart, B.E., RD,CD, *Clinical Diet Manual* (9th ed.), Food and Nutrition Management Services, Inc., 1993.

Mahan, K. and Arlin, M.: *Krause's Food, Nutrition and Diet Therapy,* 8th ed., Philadelphia, W.B. Saunders, Co., 1992.

Puckett, R.P., and Brown, S.M.: *Shands Hospital at the University of Florida Guide to Clinical Dietetics.* 5th ed., Dubuque: Kendall/Hunt Publishing Co., 1993.

Renneker, M. and Leib, S.: *Understanding Cancer.* 2nd ed., Palo Alto: Bull Publishing Co., 1979.

Rosenbaum, E., Stitt, C., Drapin, H., and Rosenbaum, I.: *Nutrition for the Cancer Patient.* Palo Alto: Bull Publishing Co., 1980.

Winch, M.: *Nutrition and Cancer.* New York: John Wiley & Sons, 1977.

 PRESSURE ULCERS ◀

Description

A growing concern for the elderly population (over 65 years) in long term care facilities or home care settings is the development of pressure sores (decubitus ulcer, bedsore). Body sites that are more prone to sores include the sacrum, shoulder blades, heels, elbows, and the back of the head. An inappropriate dietary intake, disease and disability increases the risk of malnutrition and pressure sores. Poor nutrition with accompanying weight loss seems to contribute directly to the formation of pressure sores. The patient's nutritional status plays a major role in whether the sores heal.

Insufficient food intake leading to slower healing is often the result of ill-fitting dentures, broken teeth, no teeth, swallowing problems, impaired vision, depression, diabetes and dysphagia.

The following classification system is used frequently to designate the severity of skin breakdown.

▶ **Stage 1:** Area reddened with no breakdown of epidermis.

▶ **Stage 2:** Blister or tissue loss involving the epidermis or dermis. The ulcer is superficial and appears clinically as an abrasion, blister, or shallow crater.

▶ **Stage 3:** Tissue loss involving the subcutaneous tissue. The ulcer appears clinically as a deep crater with or without undermining of adjacent tissue.

▶ **Stage 4:** Full thickness skin loss with widespread destruction involving muscle, bone, or tendon.

A nutritional assessment of nutritional status and estimation of energy and nutritional needs for each patient should be initially implemented. Food preferences should be noted and the food acceptance and fluid intake closely monitored. An evaluation of feeding skills, chewing and swallowing abilities is important to obtain and this could be done by an evaluation of a specialist in swallowing problems.

The first priority of the dietary protocol is a sufficient caloric intake by the patient. Calorie requirements range from 2,200 to 3,500 Kcal per day (30–35 Kcal/Kg body weight/day). Increased protein intake of 1.2–1.5 grams of protein per kilogram of actual body weight is recommended. Stage 3 and 4 pressure sores may require even more protein. Increased vitamin C intake of 120 mg or more is recommended. If a malnutrition status is concluded, a vitamin supplement should be prescribed. A patient being monitored for food intake and is consuming less than 75% of estimated caloric intake, may be considered a recipient for a medical nutritional supplement.

Zinc is important to promote wound healing and zinc intake may be low in the elderly population. A zinc supplement of between 15 to 25 mg/day may be required, but only for a short-term due to long-term zinc supplementation could lead to copper deficiency. Increase the vitamin C intake to 1–2 g.

Supplementation such as nutrition support may be ordered.

If patient is NPO and or maintained on clear liquids or IV for more than 5 days a tube feeding or TPN is recommended.

For further information about nutrition for pressure sores, refer to the following research:

Gilmore, S.A., Robinson, G., Posthauer, M.E., Raymond, J., Clinical indicators associated with unintentional weight loss and pressure ulcers in elderly residents of nursing facilities. Journal of the American Dietetic Association, Vol. 95, Number 9, pp. 984–992, September, 1995.

Adequacy

The actual nutrient intake depends upon the individual's appetite, preferences and ability to eat. The diet will meet the 1989 Recommended Dietary Allowances if a variety of foods are consumed.

References

Gilmore, S.A., Robinson, G., Posthauer, M.E., Raymond, J., Clinical indicators associated with unintentional weight loss and pressure ulcers in elderly residents of nursing facilities. *Journal of the American Dietetic Association,* Vol. 95, Number 9, pp. 984–992, September, 1995.

Maklebust, J., Pressure ulcer incidence in high risk patients managed on a three-layered air cushion. *Decubitus,* 1988; 1(4):30–40.

Omnibus Budget Reconciliation Act 1987. Nursing Home Reform Legislation, 1987. Interpretive Guidelines: Transmittal #274 **State Operations** Manual, 1995.

Ringsdorf, W.M., Cheraskin, E., Vitamin C and human wound healing. *Oral Surg Oral Med Oral Path.* 1982;53(3):231–236.

Puckett, R.P., and Brown, S.M.: *Shands Hospital at the University of Florida Guide to Clinical Dietetics*. 5th ed. Dubuque: Kendall/Hunt Publishing Co., 1993.

Pressure Ulcers in Adults: Prediction and Prevention. Washington, DC: Agency for Health Care Policy and Research; 1992. Publication 92-0047.

Mead Johnson Enteral Nutritionals, Preventing Pressure Sores, Study Guide, Bristol-Myers Squibb Company, Evansville, Indiana, pp. 7–8, 22–30, 1989.

Pressure Ulcer Treatment Clinical Practice Guidelines. US Dept of Health & Human Svs., Public Health Svs., Agency for Health Care Policy & Research AHCPR Publication No 95-0650, Dec. 1994.

▶ DETERMINATION OF CALORIC REQUIREMENTS FOR ADULTS ◀

The determination of an individual caloric needs can only be approximated. Basal energy expenditure (BEE) is best estimated by the Harris-Benedict Equation.

Total energy requirement is estimated as:

BEE × activity factor × injury factor = Total energy requirement (kcals)

Harris-Benedict Equation

Males: $BEE = 66 + (6.3 \times lbs.) + (12.9 \times in.) - (6.8 \times yrs.)$

Females: $BEE = 655 + (4.3 \times lbs.) + (4.7 \times in.) - (4.7 \times yrs.)$

lb. = weight in pounds

in. = height in inches

yrs. = age in years

Activity Factor:

Very Sedentary—	1.2
Sedentary (most people)	1.3
Ambulatory—	1.6

Injury factor:

Surgery Minor—	1.1
Surgery Major—	1.2
Infection—	1.2–1.5
Trauma:	
Skeletal—	1.35
Head/Multiple—	1.60
Burn—	1.5
Cancer—	1.2–1.5

Example:

The patient is a 25 year old male, height 5'10", weight 160 lbs. He is confined to bed following major surgery.

$BEE (kcals) = 66 + (6.3 \times 160\ lbs.) + 12.9 \times 70\ in.) - (6.8 \times 25\ yrs.) = 1678\ kcals$

Total Energy Expenditure (kcals) = 1678 kcals × 1.2 × 1.2

= 2416 kcals

▶ Determination of Ideal Body Weight (IBW) ◀

Body Frame Size	Women	Men
Medium	Allow 100 lbs for the first 5 feet of height and add 5 lbs for each additional inch	Allow 106 lbs. for the first 5 feet of height and add 6 lbs for each additional inch
Small	Subtract 10 percent	Subtract 10 percent
Large	Add 10 percent	Add 10 percent

References

Harris, J.A., Benedict, F.G.: A Biometric Study of Basal metabolism in Man. Carnegie Institution of Washington D.C., 1919, Pub. N. 279.

Long, C.L., Schaffel, N., Geiger, J.W., Schiller, W.R., et al: Metabolic Response to Injury and Illness: Estimation of Energy and Protein Needs from Indirect Calorimetry and Nitrogen Balance. *JPEN,* 3:452–456, 1979.

Mahan, K. and Arlin, M.: *Krause's Food, Nutrition and Diet Therapy.* 8th ed., Philadelphia: W.B. Saunders Company, 1992.

▶ NUTRITION AND ACQUIRED IMMUNODEFICIENCY ◀ SYNDROME (AIDS)

Introduction

The World Health Organization (WHO) estimates that 10–14 million people world wide have been infected with Human Immunodeficiency Virus (HIV), the causative factor of Acquired Immunodeficiency Syndrome (AIDS). The Center for Disease Control (CDC) estimates from 1.2–1.7 million people in the United States are presently infected with HIV, including males, females and children. Infection with HIV is a major Public Health problem in the United States. It is estimated that 0.5–3 million individuals are infected with the virus but have no clinical symptoms. The number of children infected with AIDS continues to increase and by the year 2000 it is estimated that children will represent a quarter of the 10 million Americans with AIDS. The CDC reported that in 1994, that the rate of AIDS in the general population was 0.9 per 1,000. AIDS is among the top five leading causes of death in the United States. AIDS is the most severe form of HIV and was first defined by the CDC in 1982 with the first reported case in 1981.

AIDS causes severe alteration in the immune system due to the presence of certain opportunistic infections or life threatening tumors, in a progressive sequence that depletes the CD4 T-cells, that subsequently impair the immune system. AIDS is a multi-system disease which may cause disturbances to the gastrointestinal, pulmonary, renal, and central nervous system, as well as systemic infections. Examples of infections and tumors occurring are:

Pneumocystis carinii Pneumonia (PCP)
Cytomegalovirus
Non-Hodgkins lymphoma
Kaposi's sarcoma KS
Chronic entercolitis
Candidiasis of the esophagus
Various other nontypical microbial infections and neoplasm's

Once a person tests HIV positive they can remain asymptomatic for months or years. During this time they may still transmit the virus to others. The progression of HIV to AIDS may be influenced by the following factors:

Age
Nutritional statue
Genetic make-up
Type of exposure to HIV
Presence of other immunosuppressive infections

In addition to suppression of the immune system, there are a number of clinical systems associated with HIV infection. The usual disease progression is: acute flu-like illness→through an asymptomatic state➝possible persistent generalized lymphadenopathy➝to AIDS Related Complex (ARC) which includes the signs and symptoms of fatigue, seborrhea, eczema, fevers, diarrhea, muscle pain, night sweats, weight loss, oral candidacies, herpes zoster and other opportunistic infections that are not life threatening and finally➝to life threatening AIDS.

Pediatric AIDS

The CDC has classified the diagnosis of pediatric HIV infection to children under 13 years of age. The clinical manifestations of HIV infection are similar to those in adults although the disease can progress very rapidly in infants. In addition to the symptoms seen in adults, children with HIV infection may exhibit failure-to-thrive and developmental disabilities. Otitis media is a common bacterial opportunistic disease. Children with HIV infection may also exhibit chronic enlargement of their parotid and salivary glands, another feature uncommon to the adult pattern of disease.

Food-borne Illness and AIDS

Persons with HIV infection are particularly susceptible to developing clinical diseases through the consumption of food or water borne pathogens. Strict precautions with regard to food safety should be observed as food borne illnesses can cause diarrhea, nausea and vomiting all of which can make it difficult to eat and can lead to more weight loss. To decrease the possibility of ingesting foodborne pathogens the following guidelines should be followed:

▶ Adhere to good personal hygienic habits, such as washing hands with warm water (115°), a disinfectant soap, especially after handling raw fruits, vegetables and meats and before handling cooked foods.

▶ Maintain a sanitary environment for the storage and preparation of food and keep work area and equipment clean and in good repair.

▶ Be sure that cutting boards are sanitized after each use. For best results use one teaspoon of bleach to one gallon of water, soak for ten to fifteen minutes, rinse and air dry. If dishes have chips or cracks they need to be sanitized in hot (minimum of 145° F water and detergent) or if crack or chip is large discard.

▶ Other tips include

• Check the dates on all food purchases, **don't** purchase or use any foods past the "sell by" or "use by" date on the package label

• Avoid unpasteurized milk and dairy products, avoid cheese that contains mold

• Wash, peel all raw fruits and vegetables, do not use foods that contain mold, soft spots, breaks in peel, or brown spots

• Store all refrigerated food at 40 degrees F or lower, and frozen foods at 0 degree or lower. (It may be a wise idea to purchase a refrigerator thermometer, place in the refrigerator, monitor.)

• Thaw food in a refrigerator and or microwave oven, **never** at room temperature

• Completely cook foods to proper internal temperatures, keep foods hot/cold, avoid cross contamination of cooked and raw foods, reheat all left-overs to an internal temperature of 165 degrees F for at least 15 seconds; refrigerate leftover food immediately after eating, label, date and use within 1–3 days.

• Purchase and use meat thermometers for the preparation of meat

• **Do not eat raw meat, poultry or fish of any kind, don't use cracked eggs, nor eat eggs that are not fully cooked, unless pasteurized eggs are used.**

• Employ a pest control service to control cockroaches, flies, and rodents. Check with a veterinarian if you have pets, especially if litter boxes are used. Follow their guidelines/recommendations.

• The sanitary preparation of infant formula is a must. Older infants and small children should not be fed directly from baby food jars. Nursing mothers who are HIV positive should not breastfeed their infants as the virus can be transmitted in breast milk. Use sterile, nutritionally adequate commercial formulas that are available.

• When eating out avoid salad bars, meats that are not cooked to the well done stage, and check all utensils and glassware for cleanliness.

Nutrition and AIDS

Complications associated with AIDS may occur at any time **after** infection with HIV and in most cases puts patients at nutritional risk. Concurrent medical problems, in addition to the viral infection, contribute to alterations in nutritional status. Maintaining nutritional status may be difficult yet is an essential competent of the care plan. In addition to an individualized nutrition care plan, chemotherapy, radiation and drug therapy may be a part of the overall care plan. These therapeutic options may also contribute to nutritional problems.

The major nutritional concerns include:

1. weight loss
2. dysphagia
3. diarrhea
4. malabsorption
5. dysgeusia
6. nausea and vomiting
7. depression, anxiety, organic brain disease, dementia, (neurological manifestations)
8. low-grade temperature, high temperature spikes
9. mineral and vitamin abnormalities
10. pressure ulcers
11. respiratory complications
12. renal failure

1. Weight loss is a critical problem for patients with AIDS. Decreased weight loss may result from a decreased food intake, malabsorption, increased metabolic demands associated with fever, and neoplastic complications of AIDS. Loss of lean body mass, a lowering body potassium content, and loss of body water have been described in conjunction with HIV infection wasting. A relative increase in total body water and extracellular water volume tend to mask the loss in body weight and body cell mass. It has been reported that patients may lose as much as 50% of body cell mass prior to death.

To lessen weight loss the individual should be encouraged to eat and follow the suggestions listed below.

▶ Keep easy to prepare foods on hand such as, canned fruits, soups, and frozen meals. Keep favorite foods on hand. Limit foods with strong odors.

▶ Don't drink liquids before meal time and drink only small amounts during meal time.

▶ Keep carry out numbers handy, sign up for Meal-on-Wheels program.

▶ Have a friend join you for meals, enjoy your favorite foods, in pleasant surroundings.

▶ Keep liquid supplements, frozen milkshakes, puddings, other high protein, high calorie foods on hand. Eat whenever you want.

▶ Eating at regular times is important but it is more important to eat when you feel like it and to eat the foods you enjoy. Strive for balance

2. Dysphagia in individuals with HIV infection may be caused by tumors, neurological changes and, herpes simplex. *Candida* infection which appears to be common with HIV infection can cause difficulty in swallowing, due to lesions in the oral cavity and/or esophagus. Dysphagia can make eating and swallowing difficult and painful. Special attention should be paid to the teeth and gums as well as observation for choking or gagging, poor chewing ability, and oral leaking or drooling. Suggestions to help with sore mouth, swallowing, dry mouth can be found Section 2, Module 2, Dysphagia diets, as well as Section 2, Modification for Oncology.

3. Diarrhea is a common complication of HIV infection and may be caused by a number of factors such as medication, therapy, opportunistic infections, malabsorption, gastrointestinal pathogens, stress and hypoalbuminemia. The intake of fluids is important to avoid dehydration however caffeine and alcohol should be avoided as caffeine stimulates the intestine and alcohol can cause more dehydration. Other suggestions include:

▶ Drink "slushy" beverage, eat jello, popsicles, and sherbet.

▶ The loss of fluids may also cause a loss of the potassium, which may cause leg cramps and fatigue. Replace with sports drinks (e.g. GATORAID), bananas, orange juice.

▶ Avoid gassy foods, foods high in fiber, and if milk or milk products are a problem use one of the commercial available products to reduce the discomfort.

▶ On the advice of the medical team, antidiarrheal medications may be used.

4. Malabsorption is common in individuals who have chronic diarrhea. Malabsorption may also be the result of long standing increased losses related to vomiting, astrointestinal blood loss, and enteric protein loss. Nutrient absorption problems include fat, lactose, sucrose, and Vitamin B12 malabsorption. Fluid, electrolyte, and mineral status must be monitored closely with those individuals with high-volume diarrheal output. (3–10 bowel movements per day)

5. Dygeusia is a change in taste which may affect the nutritional status of the patient with HIV infection. Medications often used in the treatment produce taste alterations. Some medicines affecting taste changes include:

zidovudine (commonly known as AZT), used for AIDS
acyclovir, used for **herpes simplex**
amphotericin B, used for **Crytococcal meningitis**
pentamidine, used for *Pneumocystis carinii* pneumonia
nystatin, used for **candidiasis**
bleomycin and vinblastine sulfates, used for Kaposi's
(See end of text for new test/trial drugs)

6. Nausea and vomiting may cause the individual to limit their food intake, some individuals may refuse to eat, and others avoid certain foods altogether. Nausea and vomiting may be experienced due to medications, chemotherapy and certain drugs. The most common drugs to cause a problem include trimethoprim-sulfamethoxazole (TMP-SMX) and pentamidine. Lesions in the oropharyngral and oral-esophageal areas caused by Kaposi's sarcoma may also be a caustic agent. To assist in controlling nausea and vomiting:

▶ Eat small frequent meals.

▶ When feeling nauseated, eat dry toast or salty crackers.

▶ Cold foods such as yogurt, jello, puddings seem to soothe.

▶ When cooking order becomes bothersome, order out or have a friend prepare your food at their home.

▶ Avoid strong odor foods, such as members of the cabbage family.

▶ Spicy foods may be bothersome; avoid them.

▶ Avoid overly sweet or fried foods.

▶ Drink clear, cool liquids between meals.

▶ Remain in a sitting or standing position for at least two hours after eating.

7. Depression and anxiety are common reactions of an individual who has been diagnosed with a terminal illness. Loss and support of friends and family, worries over financial obligations are additional factors. Organic brain disease and dementia may be common in some AIDS patients. These problems may limit shopping, meal preparation and make it difficult to maintain high sanitary and hygienic conditions. These conditions may also impair self-feeding, regular meal times and decreased food intake. Economic and financial concerns over loss of job, insurance and the inability to purchase food and medication and provide for care providers add stress and anxiety to the existing problem.

8. Low-grade temperature elevations and/or high temperature spikes are common in individuals with AIDS. Persistent fever is associate with *Pneumocystis carinii* pneumonia (PCP), *cryptosporidium enteritis* and *Mycobacterium avium-intracellulare* (MAI). Other infections, as well as drug reactions, may also cause fevers. If fevers or night sweats occur the intake of fluids needs to be increased.

9. A number of alterations in mineral and vitamin status have been observed with HIV infection. Some medical professionals suggest the use of mineral/vitamin supplements that contain 100–200% of the RDA for vitamin and minerals. There are studies available that show blood levels of selenium are significantly diminished in individuals with AIDS. Zinc level have been shown to be decreased when compared to healthy subjects. (Physicians should prescribe additional minerals as appropriate to each individual.) Mineral and vitamin supplements to do not replace eating a balanced diet. When supplements are used they should be taken with meals. The use of mega vitamins and minerals is common practice for individuals with AIDS. Using megadoses of nutrients and unconventional nutritional therapies may cause additional problems such as diarrhea, nausea, loss of appetite and in some cases can do damage to the liver and kidneys. Dietitians and other members of the interdisciplinary team should be consulted to provide supportive counseling.

10. Pressure ulcers may become a problem when an individual has to spend most of their time in bed. The individual should get out of bed as much as possible. The skin should be kept healthy, and linens should be kept dry and free of wrinkles. See Section II, Modification for Special Needs for nutrition therapy for pressure ulcers.

11. Respiratory complications are seen in many individuals with HIV/AIDS. Those individuals may have increased energy and caloric requirements. Oral intake may be poor.

12. Renal failure is a complication of AIDS in some individuals and is caused by complications of sepsis and the development of glomerular lesions. Hemodialysis and continuous ambulatory peritoneal dialysis (CAPD) may be indicated. See Section II Modification for Renal Disease.

Nutritional Guidelines

The goals of nutritional management are:
▶ preserve lean body mass for age and sex
▶ maintain appropriate hydration status and electrolytes within normal range
▶ minimize malabsorption
▶ provide adequate levels of all nutrients
▶ provide aid/counseling for drug-related nutritional problems
▶ individualize the care plan
▶ seek input from individual/family
▶ enhance quality of life through sensory and social attributes of food

As with all patients, nutrition intervention and counseling are a component of the total care plan. The individual with HIV will need to receive a:
▶ nutritional screening
▶ nutritional assessment
▶ diet history
▶ review of biochemical data
▶ medication record
▶ anthropometrics (See Section 1 Module 3)

After a complete assessment the nutrition care team will need to determine the BEE adjusted for stress and activity. (See end of chapter for calculation formula). Calories will need to be increased by 7–10%, protein requirements may be as high as 2.0–2.5 g/kg of body weight. Fluid requirements should be assessed, especially for those patients where fevers, vomiting or diarrhea are present. The fat intake should be closely monitored and not be higher than 20% of calories due to the adverse effect on the immune system. Vitamins and minerals should be supplemented to meet 100% of the RDAs (see Appendix for RDA).

To alleviate malabsorption and/or diarrhea associated with lactose-intolerance, the use of special products maybe useful. (See Module on Special Needs).

Mechanical soft and/or soft diets may be needed for patients who have *Candida* infection or ulceration, and/or partial esophageal obstruction. See Section 2 modification of Regular diet. Patients who have mouth and esophageal problems should avoid extremes in temperature of foods/liquids. Strong odor foods may increase nausea/vomiting and refusal to eat.

For infants and children with AIDS the use of the RDAs for age should meet their needs except in failure-to-thrive cases where an increase in protein is needed. Pediatric formulas may need to be modified (with additional protein, carbohydrates, fats and/or vitamins). Formulas will need to be individualized for age, health status, and lactose tolerance.

Other Considerations

The use of caffeine may need to be reduced to treat diarrhea. Alcohol intake will need to be monitored since certain drugs in the treatment plan may be adversely affected by alcohol. The use of spices may need to be reduced especially for those patients who have mouth and/or esophageal pain, experience nausea or vomiting or have esophageal obstruction. Citrus fruits and acidic foods and juices may need to be restricted if the patient has mouth or esophageal pain or lesions. Fiber restriction may be indicated for diarrhea associated with bowel disease. See Section 2 modification for texture and consistency. Gluten free diets may be needed for patients with enteropathy. See Section 2 Modification for Special Needs. Other modifications may be necessary depending on the needs of the individual patient and the location and type of infection/tumors.

Parenteral and Enteral Nutrition

Enteral and/or parenteral nutrition may need to be ordered when there is an absence of normal gut functions, for individuals who are experiencing intractable diarrhea/malabsorption, and when there is a need for calorie, protein supplementation and/or texture modification. When oral intake and/or tube feedings are inadequate or contraindicated, parenteral nutrition should be ordered. See Module 1 Section 3.

Nutritional Adequacy

The diet is adequate and will meet all the 1989 RDAs when the individual consumes the variety of food served and in the quantities specified. In those cases where the individual is under extreme stress, has excessive diarrhea, nausea/vomiting and malabsorption the diet may be inadequate.

Physicians Order

Registered dietitian consult for assessment and recommendation.
Regular diet, if no complications.
RD to recommend diet modifications, based on assessments.
As applicable, oral supplementations, enteral and/or parenteral nutrition may be ordered.

New Medications

New medications for the treatment of HIV are continually being tested. The interdisciplinary team will need to be knowledgeable concerning the medications the individuals are taking as there is always a possibility of side effects.

Some of the newest medications that are being tested are listed below:

▶ SPV-30 (study) is a boxwood tree extract and is suppose to decrease the viral load and increase the CD8 count.

▶ Famciclovir is a new herpes drug and has shown to lower the rate of the virus shedding. Herpes virus is more serious in people with AIDS.

▶ Thaliodomide (Synovir) is available to treat AIDS wasting.

▶ Interfron is available as a secondary treatment for patients with malignant melanoma. Interfron A, has been used to treat Kaposi's cancer, *condylomata acuminata,* and chronic hepatitis B and C.

▶ Delavirdine is a member of the new antiretroviral class called non-nucleoside reverse transcriptase inhibitors. Delavirdine in combination with AZT or ddl produces a greater reduction in viral blood.

▶ itazoxanide is in trial status for the treatment of *cryptosporidiosis.*

▶ DaunoXome (daunorubicin citrate liposome injection) for the primary treatment of advanced Kaposi's sarcoma.

▶ ddl (Videx) as a primary therapy for HIV, especially for children.

There are other studies being conducted. As of this date there is no medication or therapies available on the market that will cure an individual with HIV.

Product Manufacturers: (Listing of products does not imply endorsement; the list is for information only.)

Mead Johnson
Nutritional Division
2400 Pennsylvania Street
Evansville, In 47721
(812) 429-5000

Norwich Eaton Pharmaceuticals, Inc.
17 Eaton Avenue
Norwich, NY 13815-0232
(607) 335-2111

Clintec Nutrition Company
Three Parkway North
Suite 500
P.O. Box 760
Deerfield, IL 60015-0760
(800) 422-ASK2 (2752)

Lactaid, Inc.
P.O. Box 111
Pleasantville, NJ 08232
(800) 257-8850

Clintec Nutrition Company
Three Parkway North
Suite 500 P.O. Box 760
Deerfield, IL 60015-0760
(800) 422-ASK2 (2752)

Sandoz Nutrition
Clinical Products Division
5320 West 23rd Street
P.O. Box 370
Minneapolis, MN 55440
(800) 369-3000

Sherwood Medical
Cheesebrough-Ponds, Inc.
Hospital Products Division
33 Benedict Place
Greenwich, CT 06830
(203) 661-2000

Ross Laboratories
625 Cleveland Avenue
Columbus, OH 43216
(614) 227-3333

Vitamite
Consumer Service Dept.
Delhi Specialties International
24 North Clinton Street
Defiance, OH 43512-1899
(888) 443-3930

References

AIDS Program, Center for Infectious Disease, Center for Disease Control, Revision of the CDC Surveillance Case Definition for Acquired Immunodeficiency Syndrome, *Morbidity and Mortality Weekly Report,* 36(IS), pp. 35–155, 1987.

Bristol-Myers Squibb Company, *Nutritional Care of the Patient with AIDS,* Bristol-Myers Squibb Company, Evansville, IN, 1990.

Dietary Modifications in HIV Disease, Ross Laboratories, Columbus, Ohio, 1992, pp. 1–23.

Keithley, J.K., Kohn, C.L., Managing nutritional problems in people with AIDS, *Oncology Nurs Forum*, 17(1), pp. 23–27, 1990.

McEvoy, G.K. (ED) *AHFS Drug Information 91,* American Hospital Formulary Service, Bethesda, MD, pp. 401–410, 1991.

National Cancer Institute *Eating Hints: Recipes and Tips for Better Nutrition During Cancer Treatment,* Bethesda, MD, NIH, Publication No. 91-2079, 1990.

National Institutes of Health, National Institute of Allergy and Infectious Diseases *Testing for HIV: How to Help Yourself,* Bethesda, MD, NIH Publication No. 92-2061, Sept. 1992.

Osmond, D., Growth of the epidemic in the US: Rates for incidences and mortality, *The AIDS Knowledge Base,* The Medical Publishing Group, Waltham, Massachusetts

Positively Aware, The Journal of Test Positive Aware Network, Vol. 7 No. 3, May/June, 1996.

Puckett, R.P., and Brown, S.M., *Guide to Clinical Dietetics* (5th ed), Kendall/Hunt Publishing Co., Dubuque, IA, pp. 113–121, 1993.

Puckett, R.P. and Norton, L.C., *HACCP, The Future Challenge* (2nd ed), The Norton Group, Inc. Publishers, Missouri City, TX, pp. 10–15, 1996.

Raiten, D.J., *Nutrition and HIV Infection: A Review and Evaluation of the Extant Knowledge of the Relationship Between Nutrition and HIV Infection,* Life Sciences Research Office, Federation of American Societies of Experimental Biology, 1990.

Salomon, S.B., Davis, M., and Gardner, C.F. *Living Well with HIV and AIDS: A Guide to Healthy Eating,* The American Dietetic Assoc., Chicago, IL. 1993.

Sandoz Nutrition Corporation, *Nutrition for Persons with AIDS or AIDS-Related Complex,* Minneapolis, MN, 1990, pp. 1–13.

Schreiner, J.E., *Nutrition Handbook for AIDS,* (2nd ed), Carrot Top Nutrition Resources, Aurora, Colorado, 1990.

Surgeon General's Report on Acquired Immune Deficiency Syndrome, US Department of Health and Human Services; Report No. HEI. 2:AC7/2, Washington, DC, 1987.

Task Force on Nutrition Support in AIDS, Guidelines for Nutrition Support in AIDS, *Nutrition,* 1989–5, pp. 39–46.

University of Michigan Medical Center, *Guidelines for Nutritional Care,* Ann Harbor, MI., pp. 21–21.8, 1995.

US Department of Health and Human Services, Public Health Service, Food and Drug Administration, *Eating Defensively: Food Safety Advice for Persons with AIDS,* DHHS Publication No. (FDA) 90-2232, May 1990.

US Department of Health and Human Services, Public Health Service, Centers for Disease Control and Prevention, *Caring for Someone with AIDS at Home: A Guide,* Bethesda, MD HIV/DHAP/9-95-052, CDC NAC No. D187, 1995.

A special acknowledgment is given to Ray M. Davis, Program Manager, Alachua County Chapter of the American Red Cross, Gainesville, FL for providing information for the lay person. For copies and information on how to order, check with your local chapter of the American Red Cross. The following list does not contain all the information available.

Information for the workplace:

HIV/AIDS Education, Reaching Out, Order number ARC 6012

Hispanic HIV/AIDS Program: Information Packet ARC 6013 (6/94)

A variety of posters are available—329595.

Don't Listen to Rumors, 329510

Workplace HIV/AIDS Program (English and Spanish), includes marketing kit, guide for training, posters and a video

Your Job and HIV: Are there Risk?

General Public, Adult Audience:

Women, Sex, and HIV, 329537
Children, Parents, and AIDS, 329540
School Systems and HIV: Information for Teachers and School Officials, 329541
Guide for Homecare for Persons living with AIDS, 329542
Testing for HIV Infection, 32447
Living with HIV Infection, 329548
HIV and AIDS, 329560

A special acknowledgment is given to the North Central Florida AIDS Network, Inc. Gainsville, FL for providing information. If there is an AIDS Network in your community contact them for advice, information and assistance.

If more information is needed about food and nutrition related to HIV disease call the American Dietetic Assoc. at 800-366-1655 to secure the name of a Registered Dietitian in your area.

A special acknowledgment is given to Judy Perkin Dr. PH, Dean Health Professions, University of Texas, Pan American Campus, McAllen, TX for information and encouragement.

WEB-SITE (Information from *The Journal of Test Positive Aware Network,* May/June, Vol. 7, No. 3, 1996)

The Internet contains information concerning HIV/AIDS. The American Medical Assoc. as well as individual living with HIV have set up web pages. If you use the web verify the information that it contains. Rely on information from established publications such as *JAMA* and CDC. The following WEB pages contain information that will be beneficial to the healthcare team.

Abbot Labs: http://www.pond.com/ritonavir (information on ritonavir) 800-414-AIDS CDC National AIDS Clearinghouse: http://cdcnac.asemsys.com.72/ (offers AIDS Daily Summary, general AIDS information, workplace issues, prevention, information, treatment information, living with AIDS)

*JAMA*HIV/AIDS Information Center: http://www.ama-assn.org (set up by the *Journal of the American Medical Assoc.* Contains peer-reviewed HIV/AIDS information and other resources for health care professional and the public)

MED HELP International: http://medhelp.netusa.net (on-line searchable medical library offering text written in a nontechnical manner)

NewsFile: http://www.newsfile.com (health new posted every Monday; **link to Web/Med available.**

Be aware of information overload!!

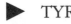 ► TYRAMINE RESTRICTED DIET ◄

Description

Patients receiving monoamine oxidase inhibitors (MAOI) are unable to metabolize tyramine. When tyramine builds up, symptoms of severe hypertension, headaches, nausea, and tachycardia may occur. A tyramine restricted diet helps prevent these symptoms. Diet counseling should be prior to and at initiation of drug therapy. The diet should be followed for four weeks beyond drug therapy.

Adequacy

This diet meets the 1989 Recommended Dietary Allowance for good nutrition as established by the Food and Nutrition Board of the National Research Council when the types of foods and amounts suggested are included daily. Females ages 11–50 should include a good source of iron daily.

Type of Food	Foods Allowed	Foods Not Allowed
Milk (2 or more cups daily)	Whole and lowfat milk	Chocolate milk
Meat, Poultry, Fish and Meat Substitutes (6 or more ounces daily)	All except those omitted, cream cheese or cottage cheese	Aged and processed cheese, caviar, pickled or dried herring, liver, sausage: dry, summer, pepperoni, hard salami, bologna
Eggs	Eggs	None
Fruits (2 or more servings daily—include citrus daily)	All except those omitted, **plums, **ripe bananas	None
Vegetables (2 or more servings daily—include a dark green leafy or deep yellow vegetable 3–4 times weekly)	All except those omitted, **eggplant, **spinach, **tomatoes	Brown bean pods (English beans and Chinese pea pods); lentils, lima beans, soy beans, sauerkraut
Bread, Cereal, Rice and Pasta (6 or more servings daily)	All; baked products raised with yeast are allowed	Yeast extracts
	All cereals	None
Fat and Oils	All except those omitted. Limit peanuts to 1/2 c. daily	Sour cream
Soups	All except those omitted	Packaged soup
Desserts	All except those containing chocolate	Chocolate and products made with chocolate
Beverages	Coffee, tea, carbonated beverages	Alcoholic beverages
Miscellaneous	All except those omitted	Chocolate, soy sauce

** Limit to two ½ cup servings daily

▶ Sample Menu ◀

Breakfast	Lunch	Supper
Orange Juice Grits Scrambled Egg Toast–Margarine Jelly Milk Coffee–Sugar	Cottage Cheese Sliced Tomato on Lettuce with Mayonnaise Crackers Canned Peaches Angel Food Cake Milk Tea–Sugar	Beef Sirloin Baked Potato Green Beans Tossed Salad French Dressing Bread–Margarine Sherbet Tea–Sugar

Questions have been raised concerning the following list of foods with the use of MAO inhibitors. These foods are unlikely to cause problems unless consumed in large quantities:

Ripe Avocado
Ripe Fresh Banana

There is insufficient evidence to support exclusion of the following foods:

Figs
Raisins
Meat Tenderizers

Medications to avoid:

Cold Medications (includes cough syrup)
Nasal Decongestants (tablets, drops or spray)
Hay Fever Medications
Sinus Tablets
Weight Reducing Preparations, Pep Pills
Anti-Appetite Medicines
Asthma Inhalants
Some Local Anesthetics

References

American Dietetic Association: *Manual of Clinical Dietetics.* Chicago: 1988.

Dallas–Fort Worth Hospital Council: *Dallas–Fort Worth Hospital Council Diet Manual.* Irving: 1992.

▶ STATEMENT ON ACID-ASH AND ALKALINE-ASH DIETS ◀

Altering the pH value of urine is thought to be helpful in the prevention and/or treatment of some urinary tract stones and infections. The primary method of changing the pH value of urine is medication. Dietary management may slightly alter urine acidity levels.

The description of foods as either "acid-ash" or "alkaline-ash" refers to the reaction of the ash that remains after the combustion of foods under laboratory conditions. Acid-ash foods tend to promote more acidic urine, while alkaline-ash foods cause more alkaline urine. There is a great deal of variation in test results; therefore, the exact relation between diet and urine pH values is somewhat questionable.

An acid-ash or alkaline-ash diet is considered to be supplemental to acidifying or alkalinizing medications. Restricting the diet without use of medication is thought to be of little use. For either diet, avoiding excessive use of any one food is the most advisable dietary treatment.

Reference

Pemberton, C., Moxness, K., German, M., Nelson J., and Gastineau, C.: *Mayo Clinic Diet Manual A Handbook of Dietary Practices,* 6th ed. Toronto: B.C. Decker, Inc., 1988.

▶ INFANTS AND CHILDREN WITH METABOLIC DISORDERS ◀

There are numerous metabolic abnormality conditions that inflect the pediatric population. The nutritional management of these disorders is essential so the child can enjoy the quality of life that they can be comfortable with. There is a need to provide ongoing nutrition education and counseling for both caregivers and children so that as the children reach adolescence they are able to manage their own diets.

Some of these metabolic disorders include:
▶ Maple Syrup Urine Disease
▶ Tyrosinemia

▶ Organic Acidemias
▶ Galactosemia
▶ Glycogen Storage Diseases
▶ Prader-Willi Syndrome
▶ Wilson's Disease

For additional information about these disorders, refer to the following diet manuals:

Puckett, R.P., and Brown, S.M.: *Shands Hospital at the University of Florida Guide to Clinical Dietetics.* 5th ed. Dubuque: Kendall/Hunt Publishing Co., 1993.

University of Michigan Hospitals, Food and Nutrition Services, *Guidelines for Nutritional Care,* Ann Arbor, Michigan, 1995.

Hart, B.E., *Clinical Diet Manual* (9th ed.), Food and Nutrition Management Services, Inc., 1993.

Pemberton, C.M., Moxness, K.E., German, M.J. , Nelson, J.K., Gastineau, C.F., *Rochester Methodist Hospital and Saint Marys Hospital, Mayo Clinic Diet Manual: A Handbook of Dietary Practices,* (6th ed.), B.C. Decker, Inc., Toronto, 1988.

MCT Ketogenic Diet

Description

The ketogenic diet is a calculated diet used to reduce or prevent seizure disorders who have not responded to drug therapy or who have complications associated with drug toxicity. A state of ketosis is maintained by using a high fat, low carbohydrate diet. Medium chain triglyceride (MCT) oil is used as the main source of fat and calories since it is rapidly absorbed into the gastrointestinal tract. The MCT diet uses the exchange list prepared by the American Dietetic Association and the American Diabetes Association. Household measures are used in measuring foods. The diet is most effective in children less than 10 years old.

Adequacy

This diet does not meet the Recommended Dietary Allowance for vitamin D, B-complex vitamins, zinc, calcium, and iron for the child Birth–10 years of age as established by the Food and Nutrition Board of the National Research Council. Supplementation to provide the RDA is recommended for calcium and a multivitamin with iron. The high fat content of the diet may cause elevations in serum cholesterol.

Method of Calculation

Energy:	Energy need is established according to the Recommended Dietary Allowances using age, weight, and height.
MCT Oil:	The amount of MCT oil to be given is determined by the amount needed to induce ketosis (usually 50–70 percent of the total calories). MCT oil = 8.3 kcal/g
Protein:	The protein allowance is approximately 0% of total calories.
Carbohydrate:	The carbohydrate allowance is approximately 19 percent of the total calories. Maximum calories for protein and carbohydrate combined are 29 percent of total.
Dietary Fat:	At least 11 percent of total calories should be in the form of dietary fat (fat other than MCT oil).
NOTE:	Linoleic acid should supply 1 to 2 percent of total calories. Sources of linoleic acid include corn and safflower oil.

General Guidelines of Diet

1. The MCT ketogenic diet, like the traditional ketogenic diet, must be implemented gradually to increase tolerance and avoid abdominal pain, diarrhea, and vomiting. Any abrupt changes in the ketogenic diet may cause nausea or vomiting. The ratio of ketogenic to antiketogenic substances (K;rsAK) should be altered over a 3 to 4 day period. The diet progression should follow the following steps:

   Day 1: Give the child only water or artificially sweetened beverages with no calories, caffeine, or aspartam for 24 hours.

   Day 2: Provide one-third of the diet (20% Kcal as MCT).

   Day 3: Provide two-thirds of the diet (40% Kcal as MCT).

   Day 4: Provide full ketogenic diet (50% to 70% Kcal as MCT).

2. Only the calculated meals and snacks are allowed in addition to zero calorie drinks in the ketogenic diet. No substitutions should be given unless approved by the dietitian. The child should be encouraged to finish the entire meal or snack, but if resistence is encountered, foods from one meal may be eaten later but before the next meal or snack.

3. If food intake is inadequate, MCT oil and protein foods should be consumed first. However, if this procedure is not possible, the oil should be distributed throughout the meal to avoid gastrointestinal upset.

4. It is important that all medications or preparations containing carbohydrates (sugar, sorbitol, mannitol or alcohol) be avoided or given in a sugarless form, including toothpaste and mouthwash. Some medications with carbohydrate may be permitted if there are no suitable substitutes.

5. At least 9 to 21 days are needed for the effects of the diet to become apparent. For the best results, the diet should be allowed to continue for at least six months.

6. MCT oil may be used in cooking as well as taken directly as MCT milk (skim milk blended with MCT oil). When taken as a drink, sip slowly to avoid gastrointestinal upset.

Guidelines for the Types of Foods Allowed

1. Fruits and fruit juices—fresh, frozen, or canned without sugar added. Dried fruits contain a large amount of sugar and therefore must not be used.

2. Vegetables are to be plain—fresh, frozen, or canned. They may be cooked in water with allowed seasoning, sauteed in the allowed fat, or used to prepare soups. Measure after cooking.

3. Meat, fish, and poultry are weighed after cooking and should be baked, broiled, roasted, or stewed. Meats should be free of flour, bread crumbs, visible fat, or skin. Sauces and gravies are allowed if accounted for in the meal plan using the appropriate exchanges. Weigh after cooking.

4. Skim milk is recommended to allow other dietary fats in the diet to increase palatability.

5. At least an 1/8 teaspoon iodized salt is needed daily to meet the RDA for iodine.

6. The following may be used in moderation without weighing:

Fat-free Broth or Bouillon
  (dilute to half strength)
Juice of ½ Lemon or Lime
Vinegar
Chicory, Endive, Lettuce
  (½ cup chopped),
Parsley, Watercress
1 inch slice of Whole Sour
  Dill Pickle
1 to 2 small Radishes

Few drops Vanilla, Peppermint,
  Almond, Walnut, Lemon
  Flavorings
Onion Juice or Powder
Garlic Powder or Fresh
Salt
Pepper
Artificial Sweeteners:
  Saccharine, Aspartame
3 Ripe Olives

1 English Walnut
1 Brazil Nut
2 Butternuts
2 Pecans
3 Filberts
Cocoa
Sugar Free Drinks
Sugar-Free Gelatin
Celery
Cucumbers

Mustard
Basil
Paprika
Chives
Cinnamon
Dill
Curry
Lemon Pepper
Oregano

▶ Sample Meal Plan and Sample Menu ◀

Breakfast	¼ c. Skim Milk Exchange	2 oz. Skim Milk
	2 Tbsp. MCT Oil	2 Tbsp. MCT Oil
	½ Fruit Exchange	¼ c. Unsweetened Orange Juice
	1 Bread Exchange	½ c. Cooked Oatmeal
Lunch	⅛ Skim Milk Exchange	1 oz. Skim Milk
	1 Tbsp. MCT Oil	1 Tbsp. MCT Oil
	½ Fruit Exchange	½ Small Apple
	½ Bread Exchange	½ Slice Bread
	1 Meat Exchange	1 oz. Lean Chicken
	1 Fat Exchange	1 tsp. Margarine
Mid-Afternoon	⅛ Skim Milk Exchange	1 oz. Skim Milk
	1 Tbsp. MCT Oil	1 Tbsp. MCT Oil
	½ Fruit Exchange	¼ c. Unsweetened Applesauce
Supper	¼ Skim Milk Exchange	2 oz. Skim Milk
	2 Tbsp. MCT Oil	2 Tbsp. MCT Oil
	1 Vegetable Exchange	½ c. Green Beans
	½ Bread Exchange	¼ c. Mashed Potatoes
	2 Meat Exchanges	2 oz. Lean Roast Beef
	1 Fat Exchange	1 tsp. Margarine
		⅛ tsp. Iodized Salt
Night	⅛ Skim Milk Exchange	1 oz. Skim Milk
Nourishment	1 Tbsp. + 1 tsp. MCT Oil	1 Tbsp. + 1 tsp. MCT Oil
	½ Fruit Exchange	1 small water-packed Peach Half

For additional information about the Ketogenic Diet, refer to the following diet manuals:

Puckett, R.P. and Brown, S.M.: *Shands Hospital at the University of Florida Guide to Clinical Dietetics.* 5th ed. Dubuque: Kendall/Hunt Publishing Co., 1993.

University of Michigan Hospitals, Food and Nutrition Services, Guidelines for Nutritional Care, Ann Arbor, Michigan, 1995. Additional material includes a new book entitled *The Epilepsy Diet Treatment, An Introduction to the Ketogenic Diet,* written by Dr. John Freeman, Millicent T. Kelly, RD,LD and Jennifer Freeman. The book is available through Demos Publications, 386 Park Avenue South, New York, New York, 10016 or by calling 1-800-532-8663.

More information, including a video, may be ordered from:
Jim & Nancy Abrahams
Founders of the Charlie Foundation
To Help Cure Pediatric Epilepsy
1223 Wilshire Blvd., #815
Santa Monica, CA 90403
1-800-367-5386

Centers that practice the Ketogenic Diet are located nationally and are listed at the end of this section.

References

American Dietetic Association: *Manual of Clinical Dietetics.* Chicago: 1988.

Carroll, J., Koenigsberger, D.; The Ketogenic Diet: A practical guide for caregivers; Journal of the American Dietetic Association; March 1998:98:316–321.

Dallas–Fort Worth Hospital Council: *Dallas–Fort Worth Hospital Council Diet Manual.* Irving: 1992.

Puckett, R.P. and Brown, S.M.: *Shands Hospital at the University of Florida Guide to Clinical Dietetics.* 5th ed., Dubuque: Kendall/Hunt Publishing Co., 1993.

University of Michigan Hospitals, Food and Nutrition Services, *Guidelines for Nutritional Care*, Ann Arbor, Michigan, 1995.

Centers that Practice the Ketogenic Diet

CALIFORNIA
CHILDREN'S HOSPITAL
OAKLAND
Dept. of Neurology
74752 52nd Street
Oakland, CA 94609
Phone: 510-428-3590
Doctor: Dr. Donald Olson
  Dr. Robin Shannahan

CALIFORNIA
EPILEPSY AND BRAIN
MAPPING CENTER
1245 Wilshire Blvd., Ste. 810
Los Angeles, CA 90017
Phone: 213-481-1777
Doctor: Dr. William Sutherling
Nurse: Jeri Sutherling
Dietitian: Danine Hayes,
  Cherrill Rimba

CALIFORNIA
STANDFORD UNIVERSITY
MEDICAL CENTER
Dept. of Neurology H3160
Lucile Salter Packard Children's
Hospital at Stanford
Stanford, CA 94305
Phone: 415-498-5175
Doctor: Dr. John Matthew Sum
Nurse: Terry Crowley, RN, PNP
Dietitian: Margie Schaff, RD

CALIFORNIA
UCLA SCHOOL OF MEDICINE
Los Angeles, CA 90024
Phone: 310-825-6196
Doctor: Dr. Donald Shields
Nurse: Diana Kinnon,
Diana Sahakian, Sue Yodovin

DELAWARE
AL DUPONT INSTITUTE
Dept. of Pediatric Neurology
1600 Rockland Road
Wilmington, Delaware 19803
Phone: 302-651-4000
Doctor: Dr. Winslow Borkowski
Nurse: Joan Blair
Dietitian: Pat Moore

FLORIDA
SHANDS HOSPTIAL AT THE
UNIVERSITY OF FLORIDA
1600 SW Archer Road
Box 100325
Gainesville, FL 32610
Phone: 352-395-0403
Dietitian: Christina McClernan,
MS, RD
Nurse: Debbie Ringdahl, ARNP,
MSN

GEORGIA
CHILD NEUROLOGY ASSOC.
5455 Meridian Mark Road, #530
Atlanta, GA 30342
Phone: 404-256-3535
Doctor: Dr. Trevathan
Nurse: Ruth Neil, Linda Scott

GEORGIA
EMORY UNIVERSITY
Div. of Child Neurology
2040 Ridgewood Drive, NE
Atlanta, GA 30322
Phone: 404-727-5756
Doctor: Dr. Philip Holt

ILLINOIS
LAKE FOREST HOSPITAL
900 N. Westmoreland, #123
Lake Forest, IL 60045
Phone: 708-735-0300
Doctor: Dr. Michael Chez
Nurse: Jamie Kessler
Debbie Balasco
Dietitian: Edye Wagner

INDIANA
270 E. Day Street, Ste 230
Mishawska, IN 46545
Phone: 219-272-0092
Doctor: Dr. Shuman
Nurse: Rhonda Hammond

MARYLAND
JOHNS HOPKINS UNIVERSITY
Pediatric Epilepsy Center
Meyer 2, Room 130
600 N. Wolfe Street
Baltimore, MD 21287
Phone: 410-955-9100
Doctor: Dr. John Freeman
Nurse: Kathy Parks

MARYLAND
MT. WASHINGTON HOSPITAL
1708 West Rogers Avenue
Baltimore, MD 21209
Phone: 410-955-6145
Doctor: Dr. Sills, Dr. Freeman
Nurse: Sandra Nagy
Dietitian: Paulette McMillan

MASSACHUSETTS
CHILDREN'S HOSPITAL, H2
300 Longwood
Boston, MA 02115
Phone: 617-735-8461
Doctor: Dr. Holmes
Nurse: Joan Anderson

NEW YORK
MONTEFIORE MEDICAL
CENTER
111 E. 210th Street
Bronx, NY 10467
Phone: 718-920-4378
Doctor: Dr. Karen Ballban-Gill
Nurse: Christine O'Dell

OHIO
CLEVELAND CLINIC
9500 Euclid Avenue
Cleveland, OH 44106
Phone: 216-444-5514
Doctor: Dr. Green, Dr. Rothner
Dr. Weinstock

OHIO
CHILDREN'S HOSPITAL
700 Children's Drive
Columbus, OH 43205-2696
Phone: 614-722-4625
Doctor: Dr. Chang Yong-Tsao
Dr. Warren Lo, Dr. Anne Joseph
Nurse: Carole Garrard
Judy Gibeaut
Dietitian: Carol Williams
Cindy Jensen

OREGON
OR HEALTH SCIENCES UNIV.
3181 SW Sam Jackson Park Road
Portland, OR 97201-3098
Phone: 503-494-5692
Doctor: Dr. Jeffrey Buchhalter
Nurse: Kristine Healy

PENNSYLVANIA
THE CHILDREN'S HOSPITAL
OF PHILADELPHIA
324 S. 34th Street
Philadelphia, PA 19104-9786
Phone: 215-590-1719
Doctor: Dr. Brown
Nurse: Claire M. Chee

PENNSYLVANIA
UNIV OF PITTSBURGH
University of Pittsburgh
125 DeSoto St.
Pittsburgh, PA 15213
Phone: 412-692-5525
Doctor: Dr. Patricia K. Crumrine

TEXAS
8440 Walnut Hill Lane #510
Dallas, TX 75231
Phone: 214-750-8881
Doctor: Dr. David Sperry

TEXAS
UNIV OF TX MEDICAL
SCHOOL, Dept. of Neurology
POB 20708
Houston, TX 77025
Phone: 713-792-5780
Doctor: Dr. Wheless
Nurse: Wendy Weisenfluh

TEXAS
EPILEPSY ASSOC OF
SAN ANTONIO/SOUTH TX
5430 Fredericksburg Rd, Ste 508
San Antonio, TX 78229
Doctor: Dr. Jorge A. Saravia
Nurse: Nancy Elling
Dietitian: Mary Susan Spears

NOVA SCOTIA/CANADA
IW KILLAM HOSP FOR CHILD
POB 3070
Halifax, NS B3J3G6
Phone: 902-428-8479
Doctor: Dr. Camfield
Nurse: Edyth Smith

Phenylketonuria (PKU)

Description

Individuals with phenylketonuria (PKU) have an autosomal recessive disorder caused by a deficiency of the hepatic enzyme, phenylalanine hydroxylase (PAH). This enzyme is responsible for converting phenylalanine to tyrosine. In PKU, the plasma phenylalanine is increased and plasma tyrosine is decreased which will ultimately affect the central nervous system neurotransmitter synthesis. For the untreated individual with PKU, clinical symptoms start to appear at 3 to 6 months of age and include irreversible severe development delay, eczema, microcephaly, musty body odor, and hyperactivity. If treatment with a low phenylalanine, tyrosine-supplemented diet is begun at an early stage in life, preferably before 3 weeks of age, these symptoms are eliminated.

There are three clinical classification categories of individuals with PKU. The first category is classic PKU which is comprised of individuals of all ages with plasma phenylalanine levels of ;eg20 mg/dL on an unrestricted diet. The dietary phenylalanine intake would be less than 450 mg/day to maintain the appropriate plasma phenylalanine levels.

Mild atypical PKU is the second classification where the individual would have plasma phenylalanine levels > 10 to < 20 mg/dL on an unrestricted diet. The dietary phenylalanine intake would be greater than 450 mg/day, but no more that 1000 mg/day which is still well below that of an unrestricted diet.

Benign hyperphenylalaninemia is the third clinical classification which characterizes individuals with a plasma phenylalanine level of ≤ 10 mg/dL on an unrestricted diet. These individuals do not require diet restriction except possible for women during pregnancy.

The incidence of all classifications of PKU is estimated in the Unites States to be approximately 1 in 11,000 births, with equal numbers of affected males and females. The incidence varies among different ethnic populations.

Early dietary intervention is essential in the diagnosed newborn for normal intelligence. Untreated PKU individuals results in developmental delay and retardation. Infants that remain untreated are very irritable and often have myoclonic seizures.

Maternal PKU (MPKU) refers to the risk for the fetus to be gestationally exposed to elevated blood phenylalanine levels. There is a chance for both the non-PKU and PKU fetus of a PKU mother. Possible symptoms for the newborn of a MPKU mother include mental retardation, microcephaly, congenital heart disease and low birth weight. The nutritional management includes careful control of the plasma phenylalanine level to remain in the range of 2 to 6 mg/dL. Weekly plasma phenylalanine levels with dietary adjustments are recommended. Suggested protein and energy intake are based on age and ideal weight for height and should be adjusted if weight gain is not appropriate, plasma amino acids are low, or pregnancies are spaced less than a year apart.

The goals for nutritional intervention in the management of diagnosed PKU individuals are to:
▶ Maintain 2 to 4 hour postprandial plasma phenylalanine between 2 to 10 mg/dl with normal plasma tyrosine values.
▶ Monitor weight gain and growth, which may be delayed if phenylalanine is over restricted.
▶ Good nutritional status is achieved.
▶ Provide repeated nutritional education to both the child and caregivers so that the child feels in control of their own diet when they reach adolescence.

After the infant has been diagnosed with PKU, where the plasma phenylalanine (phe) level is > 10 mg/dL and normal plasma tyrosine, it is very important to lower the plasma phe as soon as possible. If the infant is hospitalized, a normal dilution of a low phe formula or medical food (see table on Medical Foods Used in the Treatment of Phenylketonuria) is fed until the plasma phe drops to the treatment goal of 2 to 10 mg/dL. If the infant is not hospitalized, then a normal dilution low phe formula is fed for 24 to 48 hours followed by a mixture of phe restricted formula and an infant formula to provide the recommended phe, protein, energy and fluid intake.

The recommended daily nutrient intake is individualized for each patient with the appropriate levels established after the appropriate plasma phe and tyrosine level have been reached and maintained. The suggested guidelines are as follows:

Age in Months	Phenylalanine (mg/kg)	Protein (g/kg)	Energy (Kcal/kg)	Fluid (ml/kg)
Birth to 3	70 to 25	3.00 to 2.50	145 to 95	150 to 125
3 to 6	55 to 20	3.00 to 2.50	145 to 95	160 to 130
6 to 9	50 to 15	2.50 to 2.25	135 to 80	145 to 125
9 to 1 year	45 to 15	2.50 to 2.25	135 to 80	135 to 120

For further information and references for the individual with PKU refer to the sources at the end of this section.

Adequacy

The total daily nutritional intake in the recommended amounts of phe and utilize the appropriate medical foods should be adequate for growth. The vitamin and mineral content of the diet should be analyzed and if it does not meet the 1989 RDA, a supplement should be recommended.

References

University of Michigan Hospitals, Food and Nutrition Services, *Guidelines for Nutritional Care,* Ann Arbor, Michigan, 1995.

Acosta, P., *The Ross Metabolic Formula System Nutrition Support Protocols,* Ross Laboratories, Columbus, Ohio, pp. 1–27, 1989.

Williamson, M., Kock, R., Azen, C., Chang, C., Correlates of intelligence test results in treated phenylketonuric children, Pediatrics, 68(2), pp. 161–167, 1981.

Puckett, R.P. and Brown, S.M.: *Shands Hospital at the University of Florida Guide to Clinical Dietetics,* 5th ed., Dubuque: Kendall/Hunt Publishing Co., 1993.

▶ MEDICAL FOODS USED IN THE TREATMENT OF PHENYLKETONURIA ◀

Medical Food	Composition	Suggested For: Infants	Children	Adolescents	Adults
Mead Johnson					
Lofenalac®*	Corn syrup, solids, casein hydrolyzate, corn oil, modified tapioca starch, vitamin and mineral mix, supplemental L-amino acids	X	X		
Phenyl-Free®*	Sugar, L-amino acids, corn syrup solids, modified tapioca starch, corn oil, coconut oil, vitamin and mineral mix		X	X	X
PKU 1*	L-amino acids, vitamin and mineral mix	X			
PKU 2*	L-amino acids, vitamin and mineral mix		X		
PKU 3*	L-amino acids, vitamin and mineral mix			X	X
Ross Laboratories					
Analog XP*	Corn syrup solids, peanut oil, refined animal fat, coconut oil, L-amino acids, vitamin and mineral mix	X			
Maxamaid XP*	Sucrose, L-amino acids, vitamin and mineral mix		X		
Maxamaid XP*	L-amino acids, sucrose, vitamin and mineral mix			X	X

* Registered Trademarks: Brand names are used for clarification and do not consititute endorsement of product(s)

Resources and Educational Materials for the Individual with PKU

Newsletters

Association for Neuro-Metabolic Disorders, 5223 Brookfield Lane, Sylvania, OH 43560 (affiliated with Pediatric Neurology Metabolic Clinic, University of Michigan.

National PKU News, 7760 Ridge Dr. NE, Seattle, WA 98115.

Food Lists and Cookbooks

Low Protein Cookery for PKU, (2nd ed), V.E. Schuett, 1988. 374 pages of recipes with phenylalanine, protein, and calorie counts. $15.00. Send orders to: University of Wisconsin Press, 114 N. Murray Street, Madison, WI, 53713.

Cooking for a Low Protein Diet, D. Hammock. $4.00. Send orders to: Pediatric Metabolic Disease Center, New York University Medical Center, 550 1st Avenue, New York, New York, 10016.

Low Protein Food List, (4th ed), V.E. Schuett, 1986. 900 foods (including brand names) for which phenylalanine, protein, and calorie counts are given. $8.15. Send orders to: University of Wisconsin Press, 114 N. Murray Street, Madison, Wisconsin, 53713.

Food Lists for Low Protein and PKU Diets, Lis, Lindberg, Tuerck. Send orders to: March of Dimes Metabolic Birth Defects Center, Oregon Health Sciences University, 707 SW Gaines Road, Portland, Oregon, 97201.

Lo-Pro Diet Guide, (3rd ed), R. Roberts, B. Meyer, 1987. Send orders to: Metabolism Clinic, James Whitcomb Riley Hospital for Children, Department of Pediatrics, Indiana University School of Medicine, 702 Barnhill Drive, Indianapolis, Indiana, 46223.

Parent References

Living with PKU. Send orders to: Mead Johnson Nutritionals, Evansville, Indiana, 47721, 1-800-457-3550.

Parents Guide to the Child with PKU. 45 page booklet filled with information for parents of infants and preschoolers with PKU, information on development of feeding skills, and problems that may be encountered. $8.00. Send orders to: Center for Family Services, 103 Sandels Building, Tallahassee, FL, 32306.

The Child with PKU. A 45 page booklet filled with information for parents of infants and young children with PKU. Lists of support groups, newsletters, and other resources. $5.00. Send orders to: Lois Castiglioni, RD, PKU Section, Child Development Division C19, Department of Pediatrics, UTMB, Galveston, Texas, 77550.

Children References

All About PKU. D. Wyatt. A handbook for children developed by the Metabolism Clinic of Children's Hospital, Cincinnati, Ohio. Free. Send orders to: Division of Inborn Errors of Metabolism, The Children's Hospital Research Foundation, Elland and Bethesda Avenue, Cincinnati, Ohio, 45229.

ABC's of PKU. M. Noble. A coloring book explaining PKU to children. $3.00. Send orders to: Lois Castiglioni, RD, Child Development, Department of Pediatrics, UTMB, Galveston, Texas, 77550.

What is PKU? I.M. Crump. A coloring and reading book for children with PKU. Send orders to: San Diego Regional Center for the Developmentally Disabled, Children's Hospital and Health Center, 8001 Forest Street, San Diego, California, 92123.

You and PKU. M. Taylor, V.E. Schuett, 1978. Send orders to: Waisman Center on Mental Retardation and Human Development, 1500 Highland Avenue, Madison, WI, 53706.

A Journey Into the World of PKU. Imaginative story about a spaceship journey to the "land of good and healthy". Informative yet fun, with many illustrations. Send orders to: Kenneth W. Wessel, John Hopkins Hospital, Department of Pediatrics Genetics, CMSC 1004, 600 N. Wolfe Street, Baltimore, MD, 21205.

Formula Companies for Treatment of Inborn Errors

Mead Johnson, Evansville, IN 47721 1-800-457-3550

Ross Laboratories, Columbus, OH 43216 1-800-367-7677

Scientific Hospital Supplies, P.O. Box 117, Gaithersburg, MD 20884 1-800-365-7354

Maternal PKU References

Understanding Maternal PKU. 12 page booklet for women with PKU and their families. Basic background information. Single copy free. Send orders to: The Childrens Hospital, PKU Program, Gardner 650, 300 Longwood Avenue, Boston, MA, 02115.

Maternal PKU: One Woman's Experience. 20 minute videotape of a couple discussing their decision to begin the diet before conception, and reflecting on their experiences with diet throughout the pregnancy. $50.00. Send orders to: PKU and Metabolic Clinic, Children's Memorial Hospital, 2300 Children's Plaza, Chicago, IL 60614.

The Young Woman with PKU. 51 page booklet in a loose leaf folder for additions and updates. Explains PKU and its affect on pregnancy, stressing the importance of returning to diet prior to pregnancy. Includes many illustrations. Lists resources for further information, supplies, and treatment centers. $5.00. Send orders to: Lois Castiglioni, RD, PKU Section, Child Development Division, C-19, Department of Pediatrics, UTMB, Galveston, TX, 77550.

Women with PKU. 18 page booklet giving brief background information on PKU, the diet, and family planning. Designed to serve as a useful booklet for record keeping. Single copy free. Send orders to: California Maternal PKU Project, Genetic Disease Branch, California Department of Health Services, 2151 Berkley Way, Berkley, CA. 94704.

▶ DEVELOPMENTAL DISABILITIES ◀

Description

This diet is prescribed for the individual who has exhibited nutritional problems resulting from developmental disabilities (DD). In the terms of the Developmental Disabilities Assistance and Bill of Rights Act of 1990 (PL 101-496): "The term, developmental disability, means a severe chronic disability of a person 5 years of age or older which is attributable to a mental or physical impairment or combination of mental and physical impairments; is manifested before the person attains age twenty-two; is likely to continue indefinitely; results in substantial functional limitations in three or more of the following areas of major life activity: (i) self-care, (ii) receptive and expressive language, (iii) learning, (iv) mobility, (v) self-direction, (vi) capacity for independent living, and (vii) economic sufficiency; and reflects the person's need for a combination and sequence of special, interdisciplinary, or generic care, treatment, or other services which are of lifelong or extended duration and are individually planned and coordinated, except that such term, when applied to infants and young children means individuals from birth to age 5, inclusive, who have substantial developmental delay or specific congenital or acquired conditions with a high probability of resulting in developmental disabilities if services are not provided."

For the individual with cerebral palsy, Down Syndrome, cleft lip and palate, seizures complaints, mental retardation, autism, and myelomeningocele, nutrition intervention usually is necessary. Individuals with DD require the same nutrient guidelines as the normal individual, however they are at an increased risk for stunted growth, obesity, poor weight gain, constipation, dehydration, and various vitamin and mineral deficiencies. These problems become present due to inadequate feeding skills, genetic disorders, oral-motor dysfunction, and nutrient and drug interactions.

The eventual design of nutritional intervention for the DD individual is to assure the achievement of optimal growth and developmental potential. To meet these goals, the child requires an in-depth analysis of nutritional status achieved by anthropometrics, dietary recall, and an evaluation of feeding skills. A successful nutritional protocol requires a thorough training of all associated caregivers including the family, school, and social environments.

An altered growth pattern is usually associated with biological and genetic defects and can become more evident due to poor oral intake and excessive or insufficient inactivity. Growth assessments become more of a concern during maturity and changes in body composition.

For both normal and impaired children the length and weight measurements are the usual growth indicators. It may be difficult to obtain the length measurements due to spasticity or lack of cooperation so it is recommended to use the arm span to estimate linear height for children who cannot stand and tibia length for children with contractures in their arms. Measurements of height, weight and head circumference should be obtained to monitor the child's individual growth process. Refer to the appendix to the Physical Growth Percentile Charts by the National Center for Health Statistics to compare the child's growth over a certain time frame, on a height and weight basis to help determine individual trends. This assessment of height and weight should consider the level of disability and dependence. The 10th percentile may be a more obtainable goal for an immobilized child rather than the standard 50th percentile.

Other anthropometric measurements helpful to assess body mass include midarm circumference, triceps skinfold and midarm muscle circumference. These additional measurements should be obtained due to some of the growth retarded children may also indicate reduced muscle mass so that weight becomes a less meaningful statistic.

Frequently, in DD, the feeding skills and normal ingestion of food is seriously impaired. Feeding problems may result from neuromuscular dysfunction, physical deformities, obstructive lesions, or psychosocial factors. Neuromuscular dysfunction leads to problems such as absent or weak sucking reflexes, delayed chewing, poor lip closure, tongue trust, drooling, uncoordinated swallowing mechanism, and the lack of muscle control for hand to mouth skills leading to the inability to self feed. A feeding evaluation by an occupational therapist is usually recommended to assist in assessing feeding skills and behaviors that may influence nutritional status. Brief mealtimes, positioning during meals, early fatigue and offering food of low caloric density have also been identified as contributing factors to poor energy intake.

The infant with cleft palate presents the most difficult feeding problem. Although, these infants usually gain adequate weight by 4 to 6 weeks of age when the family is fully educated on appropriate feeding skills. Children with cerebral palsy and other neuromuscular disorders experience oral-motor problems and difficulty in self feeding. Other factors that may have some affect on nutritional adequacy include pica, anorexia, early satiety and allergies to certain foods. If the child's disabilities severely inhibit adequate intake, the initiation of tube feedings may become essential.

Dietary Intake Recommendations

Energy: Energy requirements need to be evaluated on an individual basis depending on the type of disability and the activity level. Children with certain disorders that may limit physical activity, such as Down syndrome, may have a weight gain if the caloric level is not individualized. Estimates of energy requirements can be established using a diet history together with an assessment of physical status and lab values. Refer to the following suggested guidelines for suggested caloric requirements for specific disabilities.

▶ Ambulatory without motor dysfunction, ages 5 to 12 years   14.7 Kcal/cm height
▶ Ambulatory with motor dysfunction, ages 5 to 12 years   13.9 Kcal/cm height
▶ Nonambulatory with motor dysfunction, ages 5 to 12 years   11.1 Kcal/cm height
▶ Cerebral palsy with severely restricted activity   10 kcal/cm height
▶ Cerebral palsy with mild to moderate activity   15 kcal/cm height
▶ Myelomeningocele or other neurological disorder/disease
    with inactivity   7 to 10 Kcal/cm height
▶ Down's syndrome
       Male, ages 1 to 14 year   16.1 kcal/cm height
       Female, ages 1 to 14 years   14.3 kcal/cm height

Protein: Protein requirements of DD children are equivalent to the needs of normal children. Use the RDA for height/age or the RDA for weight/age when estimating protein requirements.

Fluids: A common problem for individuals with DD is an inadequate fluid intake and dehydration. This is caused by a decreased thirst response, trouble swallowing, refusal to drink or the incapacity to respond to thirst or signify a need to drink. Offering foods that are liquid at room temperature like jello, sherbet or ice cream is recommended.

Fiber: Constipation is a common occurrence due to low fluid and low fiber intakes. Decreased chewing ability leads to reduced intake of fibrous foods such as raw fruits and vegetables. It is suggested to encourage whole grain cereals, unprocessed bran that has been well soaked, prunes, and prune juice may add the required fiber for the prevention of constipation.

Problems: The common problems that occur and the common causes for the problem in the nutritional management of DD individuals can be summarized the following way.

▶ Poor weight gain	Increased caloric requirements due to infections or hyperactivity
	Lack of appropriate self feeding skills
	Offering low caloric density foods
	Oral-motor dysfunction
	Brief mealtimes
▶ Obesity	Decreased energy needs due to immobility or spasticity
	Genetic disorders such as Down's syndrome
	Birth defects such as myelomeningocele
▶ Stunted growth	Genetic disorders such as Down's syndrome
	Birth defects such as cerebral palsy
▶ Constipation	Low fiber and fluid intake
	Immobility
	Anticonvulsants and muscle relaxant medications
▶ Dehydration	Refusal to drink
	Trouble swallowing
	Incapacity to respond to thirst or signify a need to drink
▶ Vitamin/Mineral Deficiencies	Anticonvulsant medications
	Low nutrient intake

Adequacy

No defined diet protocol is available specifically for DD, consequently, the actual nutrient intake depends upon the individual's appetite, food preferences and ability to eat. Assuming that the individual consumes a wide variety of food in adequate amounts or is fed adequately by tube feeding, the 1989 RDA for all nutrients should be met. In instances of reduced caloric requirement, certain drug interactions and inadequate intake, a vitamin-mineral supplement may be necessary.

References

Culley, W.J., Goyal, K., Jolly, D.H., Mertz, E.T., Calorie intake of children with Down's syndrome (mongolism), *Journal of Pediatrics,* 66(4), pp. 772–775, 1965.

Cully, W.J., Middleton, T.O., Calorie requirements of mentally retarded children with and without motor dysfunction, *Journal of Pediatrics,* 75(3), pp. 380–384, 1969.

Pemberton, C.M., Moxness, K.E., German, M.J., Nelson, J.K., Gastineau, C.F., *Mayo Clinic Diet Manual.* 6th ed. Philadelphia, PA. BC Decker, Inc; 1988:316–322.

Position of The American Dietetic Association: Nutrition in comprehensive program planning for persons with developmental disabilities, *Journal of the American Dietetic Association.* 1992;92:613–615.

Puckett, R.P. and Brown, S.M.: *Shands Hospital at the University of Florida Guide to Clinical Dietetics.* 5th ed., Dubuque: Kendall/Hunt Publishing Co., 1993.

University of Michigan Hospitals, Food and Nutrition Services, *Guidelines for Nutritional Care,* Ann Arbor, Michigan, 1995.

Cystic Fibrosis

Description

Cystic fibrosis (CF) is an autosomal recessive genetic syndrome characterized by viscid exocrine gland secretions which may obstruct the bronchi, pancreatic and bile ducts, and the intestines. Clinical features include chronic pulmonary disease with recurrent infections, exocrine pancreatic insufficiency, increased concentration of electrolytes in the sweat, azotorrhea, steatorrhea, and growth failure. CF has an incidence of 1 in 2,000 live births in Caucasians and 1 in 20,000 in African American births. Median age of survival is 21 years and 30 years in the US and Canada respectively.

Children born with CF usually have a low birth weight and a mean height and weight during their childhood period that is below the general population. Also, delayed bone age and puberty may be evident. The CF patient usually is malnourished and with growth failure due to insufficient food intake, malabsorption secondary to pancreatic insufficiency, and increased energy expenditure caused by chronic pulmonary disease, infections, fever and chest physical therapy. An appropriate nutrition therapy regimen can result in improved growth, increased body mass, improved feeling of self-esteem and decreased episodes of severe pneumonia.

The nutritional requirements for patients with CF are increased above the Recommended Dietary Allowances (RDA). Some of the conditions requiring the increase include malabsorption due to exocrine pancreatic insufficiency, increased work of breathing, and infections. The goal of nutritional support is a well-balanced diet with an energy intake of 120–150% of estimated normal needs using the RDA for children and the Harris Benedict Equation for adults. An inadequate energy intake can result in weight loss, lean tissue wasting, stunted growth and decreased total body immunity.

Suggested protein intake is 120–150% of the RDA for children and adults should be encouraged to attain a protein intake of at least 0.8g/kg actual body weight (ABW). Achieving adequate protein intake is usually not a problem even though protein losses occur due to malabsorption. Individuals with recurrent pulmonary infections and infants are the most at risk for protein deficiency.

Fat restrictions are no longer utilized, but suggested minimum is 35–40% of total caloric intake. A high-fat, high-calorie diet, as opposed to the traditional fat-restricted diet, results in an individual with improved nutrition, growth, and survival in individuals with CF.

Individuals with CF are encouraged to take twice the normal daily dose of water-soluble vitamins due to their higher energy requirements. Additional fat-soluble vitamins in an aqueous form are encouraged due to the compromised fat absorption which occurs even with the use of pancreatic enzyme supplements. The recommended dosage of these vitamins is:

Vitamin A	5,000–10,000 IU/day
Vitamin D	400–800 IU/day
Vitamin E	50 IU for infants
	100 IU for children < 10 years of age
	200 IU for individuals >10 years of age
Vitamin K	50–100 ug/day for infants
	5 mg/week for individuals on chronic antibiotics

Pancreatic enzyme supplementation is suggested for the individuals with CF that have exocrine pancreatic insufficiency. Common signs and symptoms of this condition include:
▶ Large, bulky, malodorous stools
▶ Frequent stools
▶ Abdominal discomfort or cramping
▶ Failure-to-thrive
A random fecal fat study helps in determining if there is exocrine insufficiency.

Enteric-coated enzyme therapy has replaced the use of conventional enzyme powders, bicarbonate, and other antacids. Enteric-coated encapsulated microspheres resist inactivation by the acidic gastric contents and allow the active form of the enzymes to be present in the duodenum or jejunum. The use of the microspheres results in absorption of up to 85–90% of the total fat ingested. Protein and other nutrients have an increased absorption rate as well. The goal in pancreatic replacement is to provide sufficient enzymes to alleviate signs and symptoms of malabsorption.

There is no specific dose of the enzyme based on weight or age. The dosage is adjusted by determining the fat content of the diet and the individual's bowel response. The criteria for determining the effective enzyme dose is as follows:

▶ one or two bowel movements daily
▶ no abdominal pain
▶ no observable fat in the stool
▶ sinking stool (absence of steatorrhea)
▶ minimal flatus
▶ weight gain

Guidelines for pancreatic enzyme therapy include the following:

▶ Swallow whole capsules no more than 15 minutes before meals and snacks. They may be taken with food but should not be taken after meals.
▶ If the tablets are difficult to swallow, open and shake the microspheres onto a small quantity of a soft food, ie gelatin, applesauce, that does not require any chewing. Swallow immediately after putting the food in your mouth.
▶ To protect the enteric coating, do not chew or crush microspheres.
▶ Contact of the spheres with food having a pH greater than 6.0 (milk, ice cream, custard and many dairy products) could possibly dissolve the enteric coating. Manufacturers of the microspheres recommend not to mix with these products.

Individuals with CF require increased sodium in the diet due to the high salinity of their sweat. Hot weather, fever and strenuous activity along with an inadequate sodium intake can cause dehydration, hyponatremia and shock. Especially in the summer months, breast fed infants will generally require supplementation with sodium chloride. The use of a salt shaker and salty foods are encouraged for children and adults with CF.

The selection of infant formula is an important consideration. Proprietary cow's milk-based infant formulas, such as Enfamil® and Similac®, can be given to infants without malabsortion. Casein hydrolysate formulas, which include Pregestimil® or Nutramigen®, are usually given to infants with pancreatic insufficiency. To meet the increased requirements, formulas are often concentrated to 24 Kcal/oz or higher. Breast feeding an infant with CF is a controversial topic, but a recent study shows that 77% of CF Center Directors recommend breast feeding alone or with the pancreatic enzyme supplements and/or hydrolyzed formula.

The following chart demonstrates the relative enzyme activity in commonly used pancreatic enzyme replacement preparations.

▶ PANCREATIC ENZYME THERAPY ◀

Name	Content (1,000 USP Units)			Manufacturer
	Lipase	Amylase	Protease	
Pancrease®*	4	20	25	McNeil Plarmaceutical
Pancrease® MT4*	4	12	12	
Pancrease® MT10*	10	30	30	
Pancrease® MT16*	16	48	48	
Entolase®*	4	20	25	A.H. Robbins
Entolase® HP*	8	40	50	
Zymase®*	12	24	24	Organon
Creon®*	8	30	13	Reid-Rowell
*Pancreatin				

*Registered Trademarks: Brand names are used for clarification and do not consititute endorsement of product(s)

Adequacy

The actual nutrient intake depends upon the individual's appetite, preferences, and ability to eat. The diet will meet the 1989 Recommended Dietary Allowances if a variety of foods are consumed. The RDA may not be adequate to meet the increased nutrient needs warranted by malabsorption, infection and chronic lung disease. Vitamin needs are met by daily vitamin supplementation.

References

Corey, M., McLaughlin, F.J., Williams, M., Levison, H., A comparison of survival, growth, and pulmonary function in patients with cystic fibrosis in Boston and Toronto, *J Clin Epidemiol.* 1988;41:583–591.

George, D.E., Mangos, J.A., Nutritional management and pancreatic enzyme therapy in cystic fibrosis patients: State of the are in 1987 and projections into the future, *Journal of Pediatric Gastroenterology and Nutrition 7,* (Suppl 1), pp. S49–S57, 1988.

Goodchild, M.C., Nutritional management of cystic fibrosis. *Digestion.* 1987; 37 (suppl 1): 61–67.

Hendricks, K.M., Walker, W.A., *Cystic Fibrosis. In Manual of Pediatric Nutrition.* 2nd ed. Philadelphia, PA: BC Decker Inc.; 1990: 203–211.

Puckett, R.P., and Brown, S.M.: *Shands Hospital at the University of Florida Guide to Clinical Dietetics.* 5th ed., Dubuque: Kendall/Hunt Publishing Co., 1993.

Ramsey, B.W., Farrell, P.M., Pencharz, P., and the Consensus Committee. Nutritional assessment and management in cystic fibrosis: a consensus report. *Am J Clin Nutr.* 1992;55:108–116.

University of Michigan Hospitals, Food and Nutrition Services, *Guidelines for Nutritional Care,* Ann Arbor, Michigan, 1995.

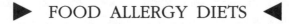

▶ FOOD ALLERGY DIETS ◀

Food allergy in the pediatric population is relatively common. The incidence in infants and children has been found to vary considerably in different studies from 0.3 to 38 percent. Allergic reactions range from mild transient symptoms to acute anaphalaxis. Some foods are highly allergenic; especially milk, eggs, cereal, nuts, fish and seeds. Food allergy seems to be more prevelant in the first month of life with the incidence declining in later childhood. Foods frequently are more allergenic in infants due to immaturity of digestive and immune processes of the gut. Foods have been reported to cause gastrointestinal allergy, acute uricaria, and atopic detmititis, and occasionally perennial allergic rhinitis and asthma. The frequency with which food allergens are responsible for persistent allergic symptoms is a controversial subject. Although many studies have been devoted to foods and their role in allergic reactions, only in the case of cod has the antigen been isolated and identified. Often there is no precise biochemical or symptomatic means of identifying the allergen. Allergy diets remain important as both diagnostic techniques and as therapy for infants, children and adults having food allergy. By analyzing a diet recall or history, a dietitian may be able to determine which foods cause allergic reactions. The trial and error method is often necessary because of imperfections in other diagnostic methods. When food allergy occurs, the parent or patient should be supplied with appropriate dietary instructions and probably should also be supplied with a list of related foods to avoid. For some patients, if all suspected foods are removed from the diet, it is effective to add foods back one at a time over 2–3 days intervals as improvement is demonstrated. This makes it possible to gradually achieve a dietary intake that does not contain offending foods, yet ensures an adequate intake of food. An unflavored elemental diet (such as Vivonex®) may be beneficial in diagnosis of multiple food allergies. It has the advantage of being a hypo-allergenic base to which foods can be added as challenges. The most frequently used allergy diets are presented in this manual, including:

Milk-Free: eliminates milk and milk products (cheese, butter, etc.).
Egg-Free: eliminates egg and egg products (egg noodles, commercial cookies, cakes, etc.).
Corn-Free: eliminates corn and corn products (corn starch, corn syrup, corn oil, etc.).
Wheat-Free: eliminates wheat and wheat products (bread, cake, gravies thickened with flour, etc.).
Soy-Free: eliminates soy and soy products (soy flour, soy oil, textured vegetable protein).

Other common food allergies and dietary treatments:

1. Cinnamon: eliminate almost all spiced foods: catsup, chili, apple products, etc.
2. Citrus: eliminate fruit juices of citrus family and carbonated beverages containing lemon or lime oil such as 7-Up® or Fresca®.
3. Chocolate
4. Fish
5. Pea
6. Strawberry
7. Tomato

▶ RELATED FOODS ◀

Family	Related Foods
Apple	Apple, pear, quince
Aster	Artichoke, chicory, dandelion, endive, lettuce, sunflower seeds, tarragon
Beef	Cow's milk
Beet	Beet, chard, lamb's quarters, spinach
Bird	All fowl and game birds including chicken, duck, fowl, goose, guinea pigeon, pheasant, quail, turkey, eggs
Blueberry	Blueberry, cranberry, huckleberry
Buckwheat	Buckwheat, rhubarb, garden sorrel
Cashew	Cashew, pistachio, mango
Chocolate	Both white and regular chocolate, cocoa, cola drinks
Citrus	Citron, lemon, lime, grapefruit, kumquat, orange, tangerine
Crustacean	Crab, lobster, shrimp
Fish	All fish either fresh or salt water including catfish, crappie, trout, tuna, sardine
Fungus	Antibiotics, molds, mushroom, yeast
Ginger	Cardamon, ginger, tumaric
Gooseberry	Currant, gooseberry

Family	Related Foods
Grape	Raisins
Grass	Bamboo sprouts, barley, cane, corn, millet, oats, rice, wild rice, sorghum, wheat
Laurel	Avocado, bay leaves, cinnamon, sassafras
Mallow	Cottonseed, okra
Melon (gourd)	Cantaloupe, cucumber, pumpkin, squash, watermelon, and other melons
Mollusk	Abalone, clam, mussel, oyster
Mustard	Broccoli, brussel sprouts, cabbage, cauliflower, chinese cabbage, collards, horseradish, kale, kohlrabi, kraut, mustard, radish, rutabaga, turnip, watercress
Myrtle	Allspice, clove, guavea, pimento
Onion	Asparagus, chives, garlic, leeks, onion, sarsaparilla
Palm	Date, coconut
Parsley	Angelica, anise, carrot, caraway, celery, celeriac, celery seed, coriander, cumin, dill, fennel, parsley, parsnip
Pea	Acacia, beans (navy, lima, pinto, string, soy, etc.), licorice, peas (green, field, black-eyed), peanuts, tragacath
Plum	Almond, apricot, cherry, wild cherry, nectarine, peach, plum
Potato	Eggplant, peppers (green, red, chili peppers, cayenne, and capscum but not black and white peppers), tomato, potato
Reptile	Frog, rattlesnack, turtle
Rose	Blackberry, boysenberry, dewberry, loganberry, strawberry, raspberry, youngberry
Walnut	Black walnut, butternut, English walnut, hickory nut, pecan

Milk-Free Diet

Cow's milk intolerance is primarily a disease of infancy, usually presenting in the first 3 months of life and resolving by age two. It is a relatively common allergy, wtih the incidence among the general pediatric population reported to be 0.3 to 7.0 percent; in children with diarrhea the occurrence is 14 to 30 percent.

Symptoms of allergy include diarrhea, vomiting, failure-to-thrive, eczema, wheezing, and malnutrition. Patients may also demonstrate protein-loosing enteropathy, fat malabsorption, sugar malabsorption, anemia (due to fecal blood loss), or enterocolitis. Diagnosis is confirmed by milk challenge after other etiologies have been ruled out. Patients should be placed on a non-antigenic formula or a milk-free diet until they demonstrate the ability to tolerate milk protein.

It should be noted that patients intolerant of cow's milk may also not tolerate other proteins including soy protein which is frequently utilized as a substitute for cow's milk. Soy protein has been found to be no less antigenic than cow's milk protein. Goat's milk is also not a suitable substitute since the protein in it "cross-reads" with cow's milk protein. In cases of soy and milk protein allergy, the use of protein hydrolysate formula (Nutramigen®), or an elemental formula (Pregestimil® or Vivonex®) is indicated.

Brand names have been used in these diets as they are necessary to provide the nutrition team the information needed to educate the patient and family. The authors are not endorsing the products or the companies who manufacture and/or distribute the products.

Nutritional Adequacy

This diet will meet the 1989 RDA for calories, protein, vitamins and minerals when types and amounts of foods approprite for age are included each day. If a milk substitute is not used, a calcium supplement is necessary.

Physician's Order

Milk-Free Diet (all milk and milk products omitted) or
No Milk Diet (milk only omitted); specify age

All milk and milk products are eliminated from the diet. ALL PRODUCT LABELS MUST BE READ to determine if a product contains milk or milk products. Possible sources of milk and milk products are:

Instant non-fat milk powder	Ice cream	Butter
Milk solids	Cheese	Whey
Casein hydrolysate	Casein	Cream
Lactoglobulin	Curd	Margarine
Lactoalbumin	Lactose	Caseinate

▶ MILK-FREE DIET ◀

Types of Food	Foods Allowed	Foods Not Allowed
Beverages	Water, tea, carbonated beverages, fruit drinks.	Milk beverages such as eggnog, cocoa, milkshakes, malts.
Milk 2–4 servings	Soy formulas: Isomil®, (Ross), Prosobee® (Mead Johnson), Nursoy® (Wyeth), Meat Base formula® (Gerber), Gasein Hydrolysate: Nutramigen® (Mead Johnson), Elemental: Pregestimil® (Mead Johnson)	Cow's milk, human breast milk, skim milk, nonfat dry milk, evaporated milk, condensed milk, yogurt, standard prepared infant formulas, Cocoa prepared with cow's milk, Ovaltine®, nondairy creamers containing caseinate.
Meat and meat substitutes 2–3 servings	Beef, lamb, chicken, ham, pork, kidney, liver, veal, turkey, fish, sausage and luncheon meats made without milk products, eggs, peanut butter.	Cheese, cottage cheese, sausage products such as weiners or bologna that contain milk products, breaded or creamed meat, fish or poultry, eggs cooked with milk or milk products, egg substitutes such as Egg Beaters®.
Bread and starches 4 or more servings	French, italian, or Vienna bread. Any bread made without milk (most breads contain non-fat dry milk), Ry-Krisp®, potato (white and sweet), macaroni, noodles, rice, spaghetti.	Any made with milk or milk products: doughnuts, pancakes, waffles, hot breads, biscuits, crackers, rolls rusk, zwieback, teething biscuits. Any prepared with milk or milk products such as mashed potatoes or macaroni or cheese.
Cereals 1 or more servings	Cooked cereals and ready to serve cereals prepared without milk or milk products.	All pre-cooked cereals prepared with added milk solids.
Vegetables 2 or more servings	All (include 1 serving dark green yellow vegetable daily for source of vitamin A).	Any prepared with milk or milk products such as creamed spinach.
Fruit 2 or more servings	All prepared and served without milk or cream (include 1 serving citrus fruit or juice for daily source of vitamin C).	None

Types of Food	Foods Allowed	Foods Not Allowed
Fats 3 or more servings (1 tsp each)	Kosher margarine, margarine wihtout added milk solids, vegetable oil, shortening, oil and vinegar, salad dressing, meat fat, lard, bacon, milk-free gravy.	Butter, cream, margarines containing milk solids. Salad dressings with mayonnaise containing milk or milk products. Milk gravy.
Desserts in moderation	Angel food cake, fruit ices, fruit whips, gelatin, meringues. Homemade products from allowed ingredients such as: cakes, pies, cookies and pudding.	Any prepared with ingredients not allowed. Commercial cakes, cookies, pies, pudding, ice cream, sherbet, prepared mixes
Miscellaneous	Salt, honey, sugar, corn syrup, hard candy, pure chocolate, pure cocoa, jelly, spices, herbs, pepper, catsup, mustard, nuts, olive, pickles, popcorn.	Milk chocolate, cream sauce, au gratin dishes, curd, whey. Foods fried in butter or batter, imitation chocolate chips.

▶ **MEAL PATTERN AND SAMPLE MENU** ◀
Milk-Free Diet (for child aged 1–3)

Breakfast	Snack	Lunch
¼ cup orange juice ½ cup oatmeal 2 tsp milk-free margarine ½ cup Isomil®	½ cup Isomil® 2 saltine crackers	1 tbsp creamy peanut butter on 1 slice French bread 4 carrot sticks ½ cup applesauce ½ cup Isomil®

Snack	Supper	Snack
½ cup apple juice 2 Ry-Krisp® crackers	2 oz hamburger ½ cup mashed potatoes ¼ cup green beans 1 slice French bread 2 tsp milk-free margarine ½ cup Isomil®	½ cup Isomil® ⅓ cup soy ice cream

Egg-Free Diet

Egg is a common food allergen. Allergies are usually to the white rather than the yolk. Egg white, which is principally albumin, is an extremely potent antigen and may provoke violent and sudden reactions upon ingestion in sensitive individuals. Egg allergy is more frequently seen in infancy and early childhood. It decreases with age and may even disappar in adult.

Nutritional Adequacy

This diet meets the 1989 RDA for calories, protein, vitamins and minerals when types and amounts of foods appropriate for age are included each day.

Physician's Order

Egg-Free Diet, specify age.

All egg and egg products are eliminated from the diet. All labels MUST BE READ for products containing egg or egg products such as:

Eggs	Egg yolk	Egg powder
Liveten	Dried egs	Albumin
Ovalbumin	Ovomucin	Ovomucoid
Ovoglobulin	Egg albumin	Globulin
Egg whites	Vitellin	Ovovitellin

Low cholesterol egg substitute products may contain eggs. The fat substitute *Simplesse* contains egg protein. Many vaccines, such as MMR are commonly based on egg. The use of these vaccines should be used on the advise of the physician.

▶ EGG-FREE DIET ◀

Types of Food	Foods Allowed	Foods Not Allowed
Beverages	Water as desired, fruit drinks, tea, carbonated beverages.	Coffee or wine cleared with egg white or egg shells, root beer to which egg is added as a foaming agent, Citrotein®.
Milk 2–servings	All milk, all infant formulas, Ensure®, Sustacal®	Eggnog, malted cocoa drinks, any milk beverages prepared with albumin, egg or dried egg.
Meat and meat substitutes 2–3 servings	Meat, poultry, cheese, fish, seafood (prepared without eggs), meats breaded with egg-free breading.	Any prepared using egg as a binding agent such as sausage, hamburger, meatloaf, croquettes or casseroles. Breaded foods with egg used in bread in cheese souffle, cheese fondue, cheese puffs.
Eggs	None	Eggs in any form: (poached, scrambled, baked, creamed, deviled, fried, hard or soft cooked, omelet, sourfles, egg salad, egg sauces, meringues. Dried or frozen eggs. Egg substitutes such as Egg Beaters®.
Breads and starches 4 or more servings	Plain enriched rye, white, and whole wheat bread, Ry-Krisp® hamburger and hot dog buns, biscuits made from egg-free baking powder, any homemade breads from egg-free receipes (many commercial breads have eggs, dried eggs, egg powder as an ingredient or are brushed with egg whites as a glaze). White or sweet potatoes, macaroni, rice and spaghetti.	Commercially prepared muffins, pan cakes, French toast, popovers, dough nuts or waffles. Prepared mixes for pancakes, muffins, waffles, etc., duchess potatoes, potato cakes, potato puffs, egg noodles.
Cereals 1 or more serving	All	None
Vegetables 2 or more servings	All fresh, frozen, dried or canned vegetables (include one serving dark green or deep yellow vegetable daily for source of vitamin A).	Vegetables in egg sauces (examples: Hollandaise, custards, souffles).

Types of Food	Foods Allowed	Foods Not Allowed
Fruits 2 or more servings	All (include one serving citrus fruit or juice as source of vitamin C).	Fruit served with custard sauces, fruit whip
Fats 3 or more servings	Butter, margarine, cream, gravy, vegetable oil, shortening, oil and vinegar salad dressing, eggless mayonnaise, French dressing, bacon.	Mayonnaise, commercial salad dressing, Thousand Island dressing, tartar sauce or any prepared with eggs.
Desserts	Homemade frosting, cakes, cookies, pastries, pies, puddings, ice cream, sherbet-all prepared without eggs. Gelatin, popsicles, fruit ices.	Commercially prepared frostings, cakes, cookies, pastries, pies, puddings, ice cream sherbet (check ingredient label some are egg-free), pie crust brushed with egg, custard, marshmallows, meringue.
Miscellaneous	Salt, sugar, honey, molasses, syrups, jam, jellys, hard candy, gumdrops, nuts, popcorn, coconut, vinegar, pepper, yeast, olives, pickles, catsup, chili sauce, herbs, spices, flavorings.	Baking powder that contains egg white or albumin; divinity, fudge, nougat, marshmallows. Read labels, many commercial candies are brushed with egg white to give them luster. All prepared mixes, frozen dinners, etc., unless egg is not an ingredient.

▶ **SAMPLE MEAL PATTERN AND SAMPLE MENU** ◀
Egg-Free Diet (for child aged 1–3)

Breakfast	Snack	Lunch
1 slice cheese 1 slice white bread ½ cup cornflakes ½ cup milk ½ cup orange juice	2 Ry-Krisp® ½ cup milk	1 tbsp creamy peanut butter 1 slice white bread carrot sticks ½ apple ¼ cup milk

Snack	Supper	Snack
½ banana ½ cup apple juice	1 chicken leg ½ cup mashed potatoes 4 tbsp green peas 1 piece white bread 2 tsp margarine ½ cup milk	½ cup milk ½ cup homemade pudding (no eggs)

Corn-Free Diet

Corn is a frequently described allergen from the cereal group. It is a common component of many foods due to the inclusion of cornstarch and corn syrup in cooking, baking, and commercial products.

Nutritional Adequacy

The diet will meet the 1989 RDAs when types and amounts of foods appropriate for each age group are included daily.

Physician's Order

Corn-Free Diet, specify age.

All corn products are eliminated from the diet. All labels MUST BE READ for products containing corn and corn products such as:

Corn syrup	Corn meal	Cornstarch
Corn sugars	Corn syrup	Popcorn
Maize	Modified food starch	Grits
Hominy	Vegetable oil, (mixed)	Corn flour
Dextrose, dextrin	Maltodextrins	Baking powder (unless corn free)
Fructose	Lactic acid	Alcohol
Vegetable gum	Sorbitol	Vinegar (read label)
Margarine		

Paper containers (boxes, cups, plates, milk cartons) may contain corn and the inner surface of plastic food wrappers may be coated with corn starch. Syrups for canned fruits, luncheon meats and some baking powders may contain corn. Some alcoholic beverages also contain corn or corn products as well as some over the counter cough syrups. **Read labels carefully.** The protein has been removed from "pure" corn oil, and may be safe to use. Before using check with the physician.

▶ CORN-FREE DIET ◀

Types of Food	Foods Allowed	Foods Not Allowed
Beverages	Water as desired, tea, coffee, diet soda.	American wines, whiskey, gin, carbonated beverages, 7-Up®, Coca-Cola®, ale beer, instant coffee, lemonade.
Milk 2–4 servings	Whole, low fat, skim milk, evaporated milk, nonfat dry milk, buttermilk, Cow's milk based infant formulas: SMA®, Similac®, Enfamil®, PM 60/40®, Pregestimil®; Soy: Isomil®, Neomullsoy®.	Chocolate milk, milkshakes, soy milks, eggnog
Meat and meat substitute 2–3 servings	Beef, lamb, liver, pork, veal, chicken, turkey, fish, cheese, eggs, dried beans and peas.	Peanut butter, cold cuts, ham, weiners, sausage, breaded foods, chili, chop suey, chow mein, fish sticks.
Breads and starches 4 servings	White or whole grain bread if no cornmeal used in baking process. Saltine crackers, white and sweet potatoes, macaroni, noodles and rice.	Any bread containing a corn product or dusted with corn meal. Graham crackers, baking powder biscuits, baking mixes, corn fritters, pancakes, English muffins, tacos, tamales, tortillas.
Cereals 1 or more servings	Cooked or ready to eat cereals made from wheat, oats, rye, barley or rice.	Cornflakes, corn cereals, grits, hominy, presweetened cereals, polenta.

Types of Food	Foods Allowed	Foods Not Allowed
Soups as desired	Broth, homemade soups prepared without corn.	Vegetable soup, commercial soups
Vegetables 2 or more servings	All except corn (include 1 serving dark green or deep yellow vegetable daily for source of vtamin A).	Corn hominy, mixed vegetables, succotash, harvard beets, canned peas, frozen vegetables, pork and beans, creamed vegetables.
Fruits and fruit juices	Fresh fruits or juices, unsweetened fruit juices (include 1 serving citrus daily as a source of vitamin C.	Canned or frozen fruits, orange juice with "sugar added", dates, confection.
Fats 3 or more servings	Butter, cream, soy oil, safflower oil, peanut oil.	Corn oil, vegetable oil, gravy Shortening, margarine, bacon, salad dressing.
Desserts	Homemade cakes, cookies, pies, artifically sweetened gelatin.	Ice cream, sherbet, gelatin, cakes, cookies, pies, pastries, puddings, frosting.
Miscellaneous	Beet or cane sugar, lactose, maltose, sucrose, fructose, honey, pure maple syrup, Baker® unsweetened and semi-sweet chocolate, spices, herbs, peppers, baking soda, pure extracts, unbleached flour, pure yeast, baker's yest, arrowroot.	Corn sugar, dextrose, corn syrup, Karo® syrup, powdered sugar, confectioner's sugar, pancake syrup, jelly, jam, candy, salt, white distilled vinegar, monosodium glutamate, cornstarch, baking powder, cake yeast, vanilla in bleached flour, chewing gum, catsup, popcorn, potato chips, corn curls, corn chips, pickles, gelatin capsules, adhesives (envelopes, stamps, stickers) toothpaste, vitami preparations, medications taken as tablets, capsules or liquids, laundry starch.

*Note: Some brands of foods listed under omitted column may be corn-free. Check with manufacturer for complete ingredient list.

▶ MEAL PATTERN AND SAMPLE MENU ◀
Corn-Free Diet (children aged 3–7)

Breakfast	Lunch	Afternoon Snack	Supper
½ cup orange juice ½ cup oatmeal 2 tbsp peanut butter* 1 slice toast* 1 tsp butter 6 oz milk	6 oz homemade tomato soup 1 oz cheese 2 slices bread* 2 tsp mayonnaise carrot sticks 1 medium peach 6 oz milk	5 saltine crackers 8 oz apple juice	2 oz hamburger 1 bun lettuce and tomato 15 homemade french fries 2 tsp mayonnaise 6 oz milk homemade sugar cookies

*Corn-free

Wheat-Free Diet

Wheat is a frequently reported allergen in the cereal group. It is common food ingredient and may be ingested in the raw or cooked state. Complete elimination is difficult, however, dietary management should attempt to provide a diet free of wheat and wheat products.

Nutritional Adequacy

This diet meets the 1989 RDA for all nutrients when age-appropriate types and amounts of foods are included daily.

Physician's Order

Wheat-Free Diet, specify age.

Eliminate all wheat and wheat products from the diet. All labels MUST BE READ for products or ingredients that contain wheat products such as:

Wheat flour	Whole wheat flour	Unbleached flour
Gluten flour	Bleached flour	Pastry flour
Cake flour	Wheat starch	Bran
Semolina	Graham flour	Wheat germ
Farina	Bread crumbs	Cracker meal
Mixed hot cereal	Dry cereal that contains wheat products	
Modified food starch	Malt or cereal extract	

The elimination of *all* wheat and wheat products from the diet is difficult but careful reading of label and using manufacturer's product information is beneficial. Many baked goods, pasta products may contain wheat products. Crackers, cookies, cake mixes, gravies, sauces, salad dressings (wheat is used as a thicken agency) should be avoided as should other foods that use wheat products as a filler such as bologna, luncheon meats, hot dogs, and breaded items. Beer as well as some other alcoholic beverages may contain wheat.

▶ WHEAT-FREE DIET ◀

Types of Food	Foods Allowed	Foods Not Allowed
Beverages	Water as desired, tea, carbonated	Postum®, beer, whiskey
Milk 2–4 servings	Whole, lowfat, skim, evaporated or dry milk powder, buttermilk all infant formulas.	None
Meats & meat substitutes 2–3 servings	Beef, ham, liver, veal, pork, lamb chicken, turkey, fish, cheese, peanut butter, "all meat" wieners or luncheon meats, dried peas and beans, eggs.	Floured or breaded meat or poultry, meats containing filler such as meat loaf, wieners, bologna, luncheon meats.
Breads and starches 4 or more servings	Breads made from arrowroot, corn, rice, rye, potato, barley, soy or oat flour, Ry-Krisp®, rice sticks, white or sweet potato, rice.	Bread or bread crumbs made from wheat flour, wheat crackers, pretzels, matzos, doughnuts, muffins, rolls, dumplings, biscuits, pancakes, frenchtoast, bread and cracker stuffing, rye or corn bread containing wheat flour.
Cereals 1 or more servings	Cereals made from corn, oats or rice	Cereals containing wheat

Types of Food	Foods Allowed	Foods Not Allowed
Vegetables 2 or more servings	Fresh, frozen or canned with allowed flours, (include 1 serving of dark green or deep yellow vegetable daily as source of vitamin A.)	Any breaded or prepared with wheat flour
Fruit and fruit juices 2 or more servings	All fresh, frozen or canned fruits. (include 1 serving citrus fruit or juice daily as source of vitamin C.)	None.
Fats 3 or more servings	Butter, margarine, cream, vegetable oil, shortening, lard, pure mayonnaise gravy made with corn starch.	Commercially prepared salad dressing thickened with wheat flour, commercial gravy, gravy made with wheat flour.
Desserts	Custard, fruit ice, gelatin, corn starch or rice puddings, homemade cookies, cake, pie from allowed ingredients, homemade ice cream and sherbet, popsicles.	All products made with wheat flour, cakes, cookies, pies, pastries, ice cream, sherbet frosting, prepared mixes packaged mixes.
Miscellaneous	Salt, honey, sugar, jelly, syrup, hard candy, chocolate, cocoa, catsup, mustard, pepper, spices, herbs, pickles, olives, popcorn, cornstarch, vinegar.	Sauces thickened with wheat flour, many commercial candies such as candies with cream centers and prepared chocolates containing wheat products. Some brands of yeast, soy sauce; Accent®

▶ MEAL PATTERN AND SAMPLE MENU ◀
Wheat-Free Diet (for a child aged 4–7)

Breakfast	Lunch	Afternoon Snack	Supper
½ banana 1 cup cornflakes 8 oz whole milk 4 oz orange juice	1 "all meat" wiener with corn breading 15 potato chips ½ cup cole slaw with pure mayonnaise 1 medium apple 8 oz whole milk	8 oz lemonade 2 Ry-Krisp® 1 tbsp peanut butter	2 oz roast beef ½ cup mashed potatoes ¼ cup broccoli 1 roll (non wheat) 2 tbsp gravy/1 tsp margarine Popsicle 8 oz whole milk

Soy-Free Diet

Soybean is a significant allergen due to its frequent use in an increasing number of dietary products. When manifested in infancy, gastrointestinal sensitivity to soy protein is described as short in duration, violent, and severe. Challenge with soy protein causes diarrhea, vomiting, hypotension, lethargy, dehydration, metabolic acidosis, fever and leukocytosis in sensitive individuals. Symptomatology disappears after discontinuation of soy milk.

Soy protein intolerance should be suspected in infants who have diarrhea resistant to dietary management with soy formulas. A soy-free diet is necessary to allow for symptomatic and intestinal muscosal recovery.

Nutritional Adequacy

When the types and amounts of food appropriate for age are included each day, this diet meets the 1989 RDAs for good nutrition for all groups.

Physician's Order

Soy-Free Diet, specify age.

Eliminate all soybean and soybean products from the diet. All labels MUST BE READ for products or ingredients that contain soy, such as:

Vegetable protein	Lecithin	Tofu
Vegetable oil	Soya flour	Defatted soy flour
Soy sauce	Soy miso	Tempeh
Soya protein concentrate	Vegetable shortening	
Textured vegetable protein (TVP)	Modified food starch	

Soy products are frequently used as fillers and may not be marked on the label. Soy fillers are used in many of the frozen dinners found in the grocery store, fast food restaurants *may use* soy products as a filler for hamburgers, hot dogs, commercial ice cream and baked products may also contain soy products. In doubt don't purchase/use. Check with the manufacturers for product information.

▶ SOY-FREE DIET ◀

Types of Food	Foods Allowed	Foods Not Allowed
Beverages	Water as desired, tea, carbonated beverages, fruit drinks, coffee.	Any containing soy.
Milk 2–4 servings	Whole milk, 2% milk, evaporated milk, nonfat dry milk. Infant formulas: SMA®, Similiac® Enfamil®, Similac PM 60/40® Nutramigen®, Pregestimil®, Portagen®.	Soy milk such as Isomil®, Prosobee® Neomullsoy®, Soyalac®, Nursoy®, commercial milkshakes.
Meat and meat substitutes 2–3 servings	Beef, ham, kidney, lamb, liver pork, chicken, turkey, veal, fish Sausage and luncheon meats made without soy filler. Eggs, peanut butter, cheese, cottage cheese,	Cold cuts or sausage containing soy additives, hamburger with soy protein. "vegburgers" made with textured vegetable protein, products fried in soy oil, fish canned in soy oil.
Breads and starches 4 or more servins	Breads, rolls, crackers prepared without soybean flours, white and sweet potatoes, marcaroni, noodles, rice, spaghetti.	Soy bread, "Cornell bread", breads containing soy oil, soy crackers, spaghetti made with soy flour, products cooked in soy oil or soy margarine.
Cereals 1 or more servings	Cooked or ready-to-eat cereals without soy as an ingredient.	Cereals containing soy flour, soy oil, vegetable protein.
Soups as desired	Soups prepared without any soy or soy products.	Soups containing soy or soy products
Vegetables 2 or more servings	Any canned, cooked, frozen or vegetables (include 1 serving dark green or deep yellow vegetable daily for vitamin A).	Soybeans, soybean sprouts, vegetables prepared with soy sauce.

Types of Food	Foods Allowed	Foods Not Allowed
Fruit and fruit juices 2 or more servings	All (include 1 serving citrus fruit or juice daily for source of vitamin C).	None
Fats 3 or more servings	Butter, cream, bacon, margarine, shortening or oils which do not contain soy.	Soy oil margarine or shortening, salad dressing containing soybean oil as an ingredient.
Desserts in moderation	Gelatin, custard, puddings, homemade ice cream, sherbet, cakes, cookies, pastries, pies.	Commercial ice cream, most commercial bakery products (soybean flour is often added to keep moist).
Miscellaneous	Salt, sugar, honey, jelly, syrup, chocolate, cocoa, catsup, mustard, olives, pickles, vinegar, pepper, herbs, spices.	Lecithin (derived from soybeans, often used in candy), soy sauce, steak sauce, toasted soybeans, caramel candy, Worcestershire sauce.

▶ **MEAL PATTERN AND SAMPLE MENU** ◀
Soy-Free Diet (for child aged 1–3)

Breakfast	Snack	Lunch
¼ cup orange juice ½ cup grits 1 scrambled egg 1 slice toast* 1 tsp butter ½ cup milk	½ cup milk	½ cup tomato soup* ½ grilled cheese sandwich* ½ medium apple ½ cup milk

Snack	Supper	Snack
2 saltines* ½ oz cheese	1 chicken leg ½ cup mashed potatoes ¼ cup green beans 1 roll* 2 tsp margarine ½ cup milk	½ cup Jello® ½ cup milk

*Made with products that do not contain soy

Gluten-Free Diet

Description

Gluten is removed from the diet of patients with non-topical sprue (celiac sprue or gluten-induced sprue). A component of gluten, gliaden, can damage the intestinal wall causing malabsorption of nutrients. All foods prepared with wheat, rye, oats, barley, millet, amaranth, quinoa, and buckwheat are eliminated along with many packaged and processed foods that may contain gluten in combination with stabilizers. Reading product labels is very important when following this diet.

Adequacy

This diet meets the 1989 Recommended Dietary Allowance for good nutrition as established by the Food and Nutrition Board of the National Research Council when the types of foods and amounts suggested are included daily.

▶ GLUTEN-FREE DIET ◀

Types of Food	Foods Allowed	Foods Not Allowed
Milk (2 or more cups daily)	All milk, yogurt	Ovaltine*, malted milk
Meat, Poultry, Fish and Meat Substitutes (6 ounces daily)	All plain baked, broiled, fried meat, poultry, fish or shellfish prepared without breadings, bastings, or sauces unless made from allowed flours and thickening agents	Canned, stuffed, creamed or breaded: meats, poultry, fish and shellfish made with restricted flours; frozen dinners which contain gluten stabilizer
	Cold cuts and hot dogs labeled as pure meat or no fillers	Cold cuts and hot dogs which contain gluten fillers/stabilizers
	Natural or aged ripened cheeses, cottage cheese, processed cheeses (made without gluten stabilizers), nuts, peanut butter	Processed cheese, products made with gluten stabilizers
Eggs	Fresh, fried, scrambled **Egg substitutes, souffles made with allowed flours	None
Fruits (2 or more servings-include citrus daily)	All fruits and fruit juices	None
Vegetables (3 or more servings-include a dark green leafy or deep yellow vegetable 3–4 weekly)	All plain vegetables, dried beans and peas, potatoes, sweet potatoes, yams	**Commercially prepared vegetables, salads and vegetable juices, canned baked beans
Bread, Cereal, Rice and Pasta (6 or more servings daily)	Breads or muffins made with allowed flours and thickening agents; rice wafers or sticks; pure corn meal tortillas, gluten free bread mix APROTEN* pasta products.	All bread, rolls, muffins doughnuts, crackers, snack foods and bread products containing wheat, rye, barley, oats, bran, buckwheat, graham, wheatgerm, malt or millet
		Regular macaroni, noodles, spaghetti, lasagna, and vermicelli
	Cornflakes*, puffed rice, Kellogg's Sugar Pops*, Post's Fruity* and Chocolate Pebbles*, pure cornmeal, grits, hominy and cream of rice cereal; rice, **packaged rice mixes	Cereals prepared with wheat, rye, oats, or barley
Desserts **Fats and Oil**	Homemade cakes, cookies, pastries, pies, puddings (cornstarch, rice, tapioca), ice cream, and custards prepared with allowed ingredients; gelatin desserts, meringues, fruit ices, and whips	Commercial cakes, cookies, pies, doughnuts, pastries, puddings, pie crust; ice cream cones, prepared mixes containing wheat, rye, oats or barley; icing mixes; **ice cream and sherbet containing gluten stabilizers

Types of Food	Foods Allowed	Foods Not Allowed
	Butter, margarine, vegetable oil, vegetable shortening, animal fat, pure mayonnaise, homemade salad dressing and gravies prepared with allowed ingredients; nuts, **sour cream, cream, and **non-dairy creamers, **cream cheese	**Commercially prepared salad dressings and gravies containing gluten stabilizers or thickened with gluten-containing flours
Soups	Homemade broth and soups made with allowed ingredients; some commercially **canned soup	Noodle soup, bouillon, and dehydrated soup mixes
Beverages	Sanka*, pure instant coffee, coffee, tea, root beer+, carbonated beverages+, rum and unfortified wine (consult with physician before using any alcoholic beverages)	Hot chocolate, some commercial chocolate drinks, ale, beer, gin, whiskey#, Postum*
Miscellaneous	Salt, pepper, spices, herbs, sugar, honey, corn syrup, molassss, jelly, jam, candy with no gluten stabilizers, wine and cider vinegar, olives and pickles	Gravy and **seasoning mixes, condiments that contain stabilizers and emulsifiers derived from or containing wheat, rye, oats or barley; distilled white vinegar#
Flour and Thickening Agents	Arrowroot Starch (A) Corn Flour (B,C,D) Corn Meal (B,C,D) Corn Starch (A) Potato Flour (B,C,E) Potato Starch Flour (B,C,E) Rice Bran (B) Rice Flours: Plain (B,C,D,E) Brown (B,C,D,E) Sweet (B,C,D,F) Rice Polish (B,C,G) Soy Flour (B,C,G) Tapioca (A,C,F)	Wheat Starch. All flours containing wheat, rye, oats and/or barley

(A) Good thickening agent
(B) Good combined with other flours
(C) Best combined with milk and eggs in baked product
(D) Grainy-textured products
(E) Drier product than with other flours
(F) Moister product than with other flours
(G) Add distinct flavor to product; use with moderation

* Registered Trademark:
Brand names are used for clarification and does not constitute endorsement of that product.
** Check Vegetable Gum used: avoid oat gum.
+ Some may be used if checked with manufacturer and found to be gluten free.
# Distilled white vinegar uses grain as a starting material. Whiskies, including "corn whiskey", use wheat, rye, oats or barley in the mash. It is advised that gluten-intolerant persons use cider and wine vinegar in food preparation. Avoid all whiskies.

Commercially prepared pickles, ketchup, mustard, mayonnaise, steak sauce and other condiments are usually made with distilled grain vinegar; however, the amount of gluten which would be present due to the vinegar would be insignificant. Thus, these items may be used in moderate amounts.

▶ SAMPLE MENU ◀

Breakfast	Lunch	Supper
Orange Juice	Roast Beef	Baked Chicken
Puffed Rice	Baked Potato	Rice
Scrambled Egg	Carrots	Green Beans
Gluten-Free Bread	Tossed Salad	Sliced Tomatoes
Margarine	Gluten-Free Bread	Cornbread
Jelly	Margarine	Margarine
Milk	Tapioca Pudding	Applesauce
Coffee–Sugar	Iced Tea–Sugar	Iced Tea–Sugar

References

American Dietetic Association: *Manual of Clinical Dietetics.* Chicago: 1988.

Mahan, K. and Arlin, M.: *Krause's Food, Nutrition and Diet Therapy,* 8th ed., Philadelphia: W.B. Saunders Company, 1992.

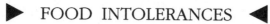

▶ FOOD INTOLERANCES ◀

Lactose-Free Diet

A lactose-free diet can be useful in the treatment of lactose malabsorption, caused by either a primary lactase deficiency which is the result of a congenital defect or prematurity, or a secondary lactase deficiency due to mucosal injury. There is also a third type of lactose malabsorption which is present in certain ethnic populations that manifests itself after weaning. The clinical symptoms of lactose malabsorption are associated with the fermentation of lactose in the intestinal lumen. These symptoms include abdominal cramping, increased intestinal motility and osmotic diarrhea.

Specifically, lactose malabsorption is defined as a rise in blood glucose of less than 26 mg/dl after a standard test dose of lactose. Other diagnostic tests for lactose malabsorption include barium-lactose roentgenographic study and analysis of breath hydrogen after lactose feeding. A more direct test involves assaying the lactase activity after a small intestinal biopsy.

Congenital lactase deficiency is rare and there is debate about whether it truly exists or is a result of some mucosal injury. Premature infants can be lactose malabsorbers because lactase activity between 26 and 34 weeks of gestation is approximately 30 percent of that found in a full term infant. A carbohydrate source other than lactose may be more appropriate for a 24–34 week gestational age infant.

Secondary lactase deficiency is associated with damage to the small intestine after such diseases as gastroenteritis, celiac disease and intractable diarrhea. Starvation and protein-calorie malnutrition can also result in a lactase deficiency. In these conditions, many other disaccharidases may be depressed but lactase activity appears to be the most sensitive to injury. In such cases, withdrawal of lactose eliminates the symptoms described above.

In some cases of lactose malabsorption a strict lactose-free diet may not be necessary for treatment but a moderate restriction may be indicated.

Nutritional Adequacy

Lactose-Free or Lactose-Restricted diets may not meet the 1989 RDA for calcium, vitamin D, and possibly riboflavin unless supplements or formulas (listed in Beverage List that follows) are included in the diet in appropriate amounts.

Physician's Order

Lactose-Free Diet or Lactose-Restricted Diet, specify age.

▶ LACTOSE-FREE DIET ◀

Types of Food	Foods Allowed	Foods Not Allowed
Formulas	Isomil®, Prosobee®, Pregestimil® Nutramigen®, Jevity®, Protagen®, Nursoy®, Osmolite®, Isocal®, Isocal HCN®, Vivonex®, Vivonex HN®, Sustacal®, Ensure®, Ensure Plus®, Glucerna®, Pulmocare®	All others
Beverages	Carbonated beverages, coffee tea, fruit juices, fruit drinks.	Milk and milk drinks of any kind, cream, Ovaltine®, hot chocolate.
Meat, fish, poultry	All fresh beef, lamb, pork, veal, poultry, seafood, kosher frankfurters	Any meat, seafood, or poultry prepared with batter or stuffing containing milk. Check package labels of sausage, weiners, luncheon meats, and bologna carefully.
Cheese	None	All
Egg	All throughly cooked	None
Vegetables	All prepared without milk or products.	Any vegetables that have lactose added during processing, i.e., butter or creamed vegetables.
Fruit	All throughly cooked	None
Potato or substitute	White or sweet potatoes, rice, corn, grits, dried peas and beans, macaroni, noodles.	Any creamed, breaded or buttered potatoes, french fries, potato chips, dehydrated potato product if lactose or milk has been added during processing.
Bread and cereal	Any made without milk or milk products, French bread, soda crackers.	All bread products containing milk or lactose, prepared mixes, muffins, biscuits, waffles, pancakes, pastries, cookies, cakes, crackers, etc., made with butter or margarine, some dry cereals, instant cream of wheat.

Lactose-Free Diet—(continued)

Type of Food	Foods Allowed	Foods Not Allowed
Desserts	Water and fruit ices, Jello®, angel food cake, homemade cakes, pies, cookies made from allowed ingredients.	All ice cream cream, sherbet, puddings cakes, cookies, pie crusts containing milk, commercial cakes, cookies and mixes, doughnuts.
Other sweets	Sugar, honey, syrups, jam, jelly, marmalade, preserves, hard sugar candy, corn syrup, molasses, any products	Candy containing lactose or milk, butterscotch toffee, caramels, chocolate, cocoa, peppermint.
Fats	Margarine not containing milk solids, vegetable oils, shortening, lard, bacon fat, mayonnaise, some nondairy creamers.	Butter, margarine containing milk solids. Commercial prepared salad dressings, sour cream, cream cheese.
Soups	Clear broth, bouillon, vegetable soup.	Milk and cream soups, soups containing margarine and butter.
Miscellaneous	Salt, vinegar, catsup, peanut butter, nuts, spices, mustard, flavoring extracts, herbs, olives, pickles, popcorn prepared with allowed margarine, chili powder, pepper.	Yogurt, sauces and gravies made with milk or milk products, chewing gum, some powdered soft drink mixes, artificial sweeteners containing lactose, flavored instant coffees.

▶ LACTOSE-FREE DIET FOR INFANTS ◀

Type of Food	Foods Allowed	Foods Not Allowed

Juices
  Heinz®
  Beechnut®
  Gerber®
	All	None

Formulas	Isomil®, Prosobee®, Pregestimil®, Nutramigen®, Portagen®, Nursoy®, Osmolite®, Isocal®, Isocal HCN®, Vivonex®, Vivonex HN®, LR®, HN®, Sustacal®, Sustacal HC®, Ensure®, Ensure Plus®	All others
Meats and meat substitutes Heinz Dinners®	Beef and egg noodles, egg noodles and beef; macaroni, tomatoes & beef; vegetables & bacon; vegetables & beef; vegetables & ham (strained); vegetables, dumplings & beef	Chicken noodle; macaroni, tomatoes & sauce & meat; turkey rice with vegetables; vegetables & ham (junior); vegetables & lamb; vegetables, egg noodles & chicken; vegetables, egg noodles & turkey
Heinz High Meat Dinner®	Beef with vegetables, beef with vegetables and cereal, chicken with vegetables	Turkey with vegetables

Lactose-Free Diet for Infants—(continued)

Type of Food	Foods Allowed	Foods Not Allowed
Heinz Meats®	All	None
Beechnut Dinners®	Beef & egg noodle, chicken noodle, turkey rice, chicken rice, vegetable bacon (strained only), vegetable beef, vegetable chicken, vegetable lamb, vegetable turkey	Cereal, egg yolk & bacon; macaroni, tomato & beef; spaghetti, tomato & beef; split pea & ham, vegetable bacon (junior), vegetable ham
Beechnut High Meat Dinners®	All	None
Beechnut Meats®	All	None
Beechnut Yogurts®	None	All
Gerber Vegetable & Meat Combinations®	Beef & egg noodles with vegetables, turkey & rice with vegetables, vegetables & bacon, vegetables & beef, vegetables & chicken, vegetables & lamb, vegetables & liver, vegetables & turkey, chicken & noodles (junior only)	Chicken & noodles (strained), macaroni & cheese, macaroni & tomato with beef, spaghetti, peas with ham
Gerber High Meat Dinners®	Beef with vegetables, chicken with vegetables, ham with vegetables, veal with vegetables	Turkey with vegetables
Gerber Meats & Egg Yolks®	All	None
Gerber Chunky foods	All	None
Gerber Finger Foods®	None	All
Vegetables		
Heinz®	Beets, carrots, green beans, mixed vegetables, squash sweet potatoes	Creamed corn, creamed green beans, creamed peas
Beechnut®	Carrots, green beans, garden vegetables, mixed vegetables, peas, peas & carrots, squash, sweet potatoes	Creamed corn
Gerber®	Beets, carrots, mixed vegetables, peas, squash, sweet potatoes, garden vegetables, green beans	Creamed corn, creamed green beans, creamed spinach
Fruit		
Heinz®	All	None
Beechnut Fruits®	All	None
Fruit Supremes®	All	None
Tropical Fruits®	All	None
Gerber®	All	None
Dry Cereals		
Heinz®	Barley, hi-protein, oatmeal, rice	Mixed
Beechnut®	All	None
Gerber® (ready-to-serve)	All	None
Jarred Cereal		
Heinz®	All	None

Type of Food	Foods Allowed	Foods Not Allowed
Beechnut®	Mixed cereal with applesause & bananas, oatmeal with applesauce & bananas	Rice cereal with applesauce & bananas
Gerber®	Mixed cereal with applesauce & bananas, oatmeal with applesauce & bananas	Rice cereal with applesauce & bananas, rice cereal with mixed fruit, cereal & egg yolk
Desserts Heinz®	Banana pudding, dutch apple dessert, fruit dessert, pineapple orange, peach cobbler	Custard pudding, tutti fruitti
Beechnut®	Fruit dessert, orange pineapple dessert, tropical fruit dessert, banana dessert apple betty, cottage cheese with pineapple juice, pineapple dessert, rice pudding	Vanilla custard pudding, banana custard pudding, chocolate custard pudding, apple custard pudding,
Gerber®	Banana apple dessert, cherry vanilla pudding, fruit dessert, peach cobbler with yogurt, vanilla custard pudding	Chocolate custard pudding, dutch apple dessert, Hawaiian Delight, orange pudding, raspberry dessert
Gerber Chunky Foods Fruit Desserts®	Bananas with tapioca, peach cobbler	Dutch apple dessert
Gerber Baked Goods®	Pretzels (animal), biscuits, zwieback toast	Arrowroot cookies, cookies

This diet based on information from Gerber®, Heinz®, Beechnut®. The manufacturers update this information periodically; the latest information should be requested.
Unless specified, items include strained and/or junior foods.

► SAMPLE MEAL PATTERN AND SAMPLE MENU ◄
Lactose-Free Diet

Breakfast	Lunch	Snack	Supper	Snack
½ cup orange juice 1 egg, scrambled 2 slices Vienna bread, toasted 2 tsp milk-free margarine 1 tbsp grape jelly 8 oz Ensure®	2 oz roast beef ½ cup rice ½ cup green beans 1 pear 2 slices Vienna bread 2 tsp milk-free margarine 1 tsp sugar 8 oz Ensure®	1 slice angel food cake with sliced peaches 8 oz Ensure®	2 oz round steak 1 small baked potato 2 tsp milk-free margarine ½ cup spinach 2 slices Vienna bread, toasted ½ cup fruit cocktail 1 tsp sugar 8 oz Ensure®	½ cup apricot nectar

Some Foods Companies from which Information Concerning Allergy Diets May be Obtained

Battle Creek Food Co. (vegetarian foods)
Battle Creek, Michigan

Campbell Soup Co.
Camden, New Jersey 08101

Chicago Dietetic Supply, Inc.
(Featherweight and Cellu products)
P.O. Box 529
Le Grange, Illinois 60525

Carnation Co. Research Labs.
8015 Van Nuyo Blvd.
Van Nuyo, Calif. 91412

E.J. Elwood, Inc.
Speciality Food Products
663 5th Avenue
New York, NY 10022

Standard Brands Sales Co. (specialty foods)
Standard Brands, Inc.
625 Madison Avenue
New York, NY 10022

General Foods Kitchens
250 North Street
White Plains, NY 10602

General Mills
4620 W. 77th Street
Minneapolis, Minn 55435

H.J. Heinz Co.
Box 57
Pittsburgh, PA 15230

Mead Johnson & Co.
Evansville, Ind. 47721

Kellogg's Co.
Battle Creek, Mich.

Loma Linda Foods
Riverside, Calif. or Mt. Vernon, Ohio

Nestle Company, Inc.
100 Bloomingdale, Road
White Plaines, NY 20605

Consumer Services Dept.
Quaker Oats Co.
Chicago, Ill. 60654

Pet, Inc.
Arcade Bldg.
St. Louis, MO 63166

Stokely-Van Camp, Inc.
Indianapolis, Ind. 46206

Ross Laboratories
Columbus, Ohio 43216

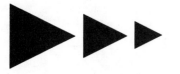

Modification for Test Diets

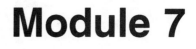

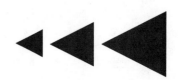

▶ TEST DIETS ◀

Renin Test

The Renin Test is used in the investigation of patients with renovascular, adrenal or primary hypertension. The physician should specify the sodium level and the number of days that the diet should be followed.

Reference

Manual of Clinical Dietetics: W.B. Saunders, Co.: Philadelphia, 1981.

Serotonin Test—(5-HIAA or 5-Hydroxyindoleacetic Acid)

The Serotonin Test is used to aid in establishing the diagnosis of carcinoid tumors. In patients with carcinomas, the tumor is the major body deposit of serotonin. Since elevated levels to 5-HIAA have been reported following ingestion of foods containing serotonin, this diet is given to avoid false positive results. The food items to avoid at least 24 hours prior to testing are:

Avocados	Plantains
Bananas	Plums
Eggplants	Tomatoes
Passion Fruits	Walnuts
Pineapples	

Reference

American Dietetic Association: *Manual of Clinical Dietetics.* Chicago: 1988.

Vanillylmandelic Acid (VMA) Test

The VMA test is used to diagnose the tumor, pheochromocytoma, in persons with unexplained hypertension. Failure to demonstrate significant changes in VMA excretion with various diets indicates that dietary restrictions are not necessary prior to determining VMA excretion. In place of the screening test for urine VMA, urine metanophrines are measured. The procedure is not affected by a varied diet.

Reference

American Dietetic Association: *Manual of Clinical Dietetics.* Chicago: 1988.

Fat-Free Test Meal

The fat-free test meal is used for gall bladder visualization x-rays. After fasting, the patient is given a light, fat-free meal prior to a gall bladder series.

Unless otherwise ordered the order is for ONE meal only. Meals may include:

Breakfast	Lunch/Supper
Fruit or Fruit Juice	Fruit or Fruit Juice
Toast	Fat-free Potatoes, Rice, or Pasta
Jelly	Bread-Jelly
Coffee or Tea	Gelatin
Salt-Sugar	Coffee or Tea
	Salt-Sugar

Reference

Manual of Clinical Dietetics: 2nd ed., Philadelphia: W.B. Saunders Co., 1981.

100 Gram Fat Test Meal

The diet is to provide 100 grams ± 10 grams of fat daily for a period of 3 days or 72 hours. The fecal fat test provides a means of measuring fecal fat for the diagnosis of cystic fibrosis or malabsorption problems. It is recommended that the fat remain constant in the diet.

The following foods should be included daily:

Food	Amount	gm Fat
Egg	1	5
*Meat	8 oz.	40
Whole Milk	3 cups	24
Fat	7 servings	35
		Total 104

Other foods may be used as desired.
* Medium Fat Meat

References

Mahan, K. and Arlin, M.: *Krause's Food, Nutrition and Diet Therapy.* 8th ed. Philadelphia: W.B. Saunders Company, 1992.

Pemberton, C., Moxness, K., German, M., Nelson, J., and Gastineau, C.: *Mayo Clinic Diet Manual: A Handbook of Dietary Practices.* 6th ed. Toronto: B.C. Decker, Inc., 1988.

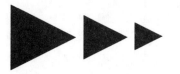

Appendices

▶ **APPENDIX A** ◀

Estimated Safe and Adequate Daily Dietary Intakes
of Selected Vitamins and Minerals[a]

Category	Age (years)	Vitamins	
		Biotin (µg)	Pantothenic Acid (mg)
Infants	0–0.5	10	2
	0.5–1	15	3
Children and adolescents	1–3	20	3
	4–6	25	3–4
	7–10	30	4–5
	11+	30–100	4–7
Adults		30–100	4–7

Category	Age (years)	Trace Elements[b]				
		Copper (mg)	Manganese (mg)	Flouride (mg)	Biotin (µg)	Pantothenic Acid (mg)
Infants	0–0.5	0.4–0.6	0.3–0.6	0.1–0.5	10–40	15–30
	0.5–1	0.6–0.7	0.6–1.0	0.2–1.0	20–60	20–40
Children and adolescents	1–3	0.7–1.0	1.0–1.5	0.5–1.5	20–80	25–50
	4–6	1.0–1.5	1.5–2.0	1.0–2.5	30–120	30–75
	7–10	1.0–2.0	2.0–3.0	1.5–2.5	50–200	50–150
	11+	1.5–2.5	2.0–5.0	1.5–2.5	50–200	75–250
Adults		1.5–3.0	2.0–5.0	1.5–4.0	50–200	75–250

[a]Because there is less information on which to base allowances, these figures are not given in the main table of RDA and are provided here in the form of ranges of recommended intakes.
[b]Since the toxic levels for many trace elements may be only several times usual intakes, the upper levels for the trace elements given in this table should not be habitually exceeded.

▶ **APPENDIX B** ◀

Median Heights and Weights and Recommended Energy Intake

Category	Age (years) or Condition	Weight (kg)	Weight (lb)	Height (cm)	Height (in)	REE[a] (kcal/day)	Multiples of REE	Average Energy Allowance (kcal)[b] Per kg	Per day[c]
Infants	0.0–0.5	6	13	60	24	320		108	650
	0.5–1.0	9	20	71	28	500		98	850
Children	1–3	13	29	90	35	740		102	1,300
	4–6	20	44	112	44	950		90	1,800
	7–10	28	62	132	52	1,130		70	2,000
Males	11–14	45	99	157	62	1,440	1.70	55	2,500
	15–18	66	145	176	69	1,760	1.67	45	3,000
	19–24	72	160	177	70	1,780	1.67	40	2,900
	25–50	79	174	176	70	1,800	1.60	37	2,900
	51+	77	170	173	68	1,530	1.50	30	2,300
Females	11–14	46	101	157	62	1,310	1.67	47	2,200
	15–18	55	120	163	64	1,370	1.60	40	2,200
	19–24	58	128	164	65	1,350	1.60	38	2,200
	25–50	63	138	163	64	1,380	1.55	36	2,200
	51+	65	143	160	63	1,280	1.50	30	1,900
Pregnant	1st Trimester								+0
	2nd Trimester								+300
	3rd Trimester								+300
Lactating	1st 6 months								+500
	2nd 6 months								+500

[a]Calculation based on FAO equations, then rounded.
[b]In the range of light to moderate activity the coefficient of variation is ;pm20%.
[c]Figure is rounded.

▶ **APPENDIX C** ◀

GIRLS: BIRTH TO 36 MONTHS
PHYSICAL GROWTH
NCHS PERCENTILES*

NAME_____ RECORD #_____

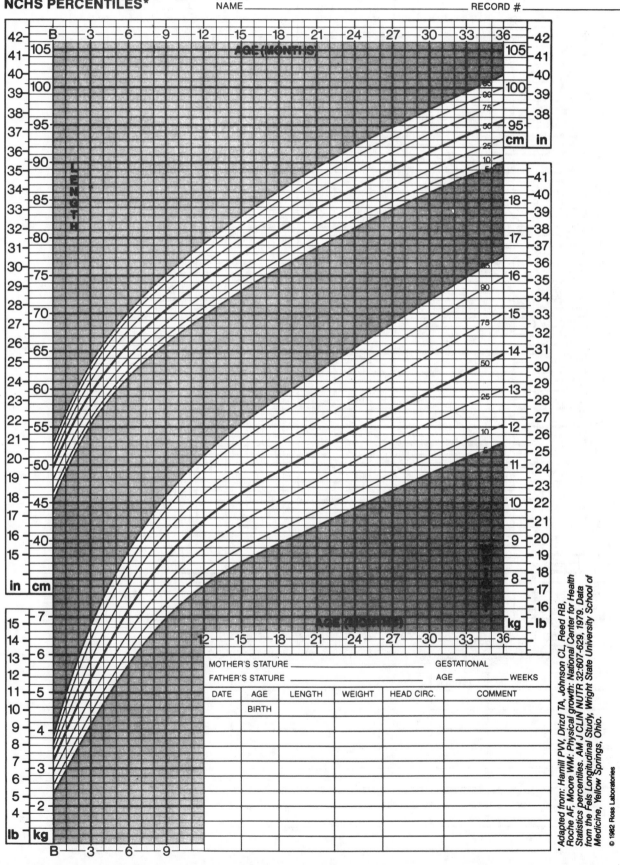

MOTHER'S STATURE _____ GESTATIONAL
FATHER'S STATURE _____ AGE _____ WEEKS

DATE	AGE	LENGTH	WEIGHT	HEAD CIRC.	COMMENT
	BIRTH				

* Adapted from: Hamill PVV, Drizd TA, Johnson CL, Reed RB, Roche AF, Moore WM: Physical growth: National Center for Health Statistics percentiles. AM J CLIN NUTR 32:607-629, 1979. Data from the Fels Longitudinal Study, Wright State University School of Medicine, Yellow Springs, Ohio.

© 1982 Ross Laboratories

GIRLS: BIRTH TO 36 MONTHS
PHYSICAL GROWTH
NCHS PERCENTILES*

NAME _____ RECORD # _____

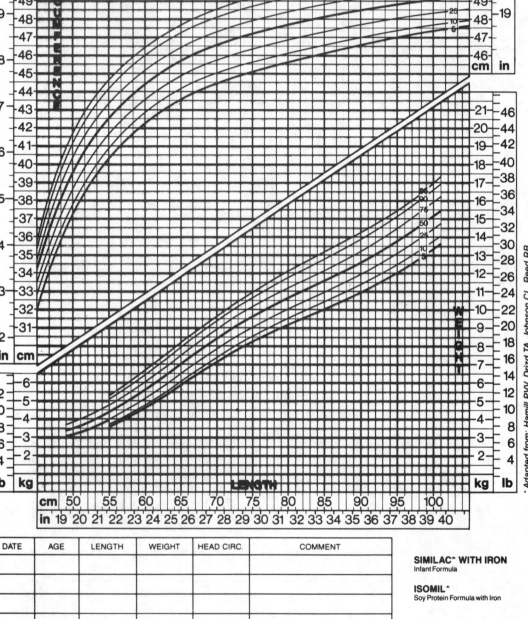

* Adapted from: Hamill PVV, Drizd TA, Johnson CL, Reed RB, Roche AF, Moore WM: Physical growth: National Center for Health Statistics percentiles. AM J CLIN NUTR 32:607–629, 1979. Data from the Fels Longitudinal Study, Wright State University School of Medicine, Yellow Springs, Ohio.

ⓒ 1982 Ross Laboratories

DATE	AGE	LENGTH	WEIGHT	HEAD CIRC.	COMMENT

SIMILAC® WITH IRON
Infant Formula

ISOMIL®
Soy Protein Formula with Iron

Reprinted with permission
of Ross Laboratories

▶ APPENDIX D ◀

GIRLS: 2 TO 18 YEARS
PHYSICAL GROWTH
NCHS PERCENTILES*

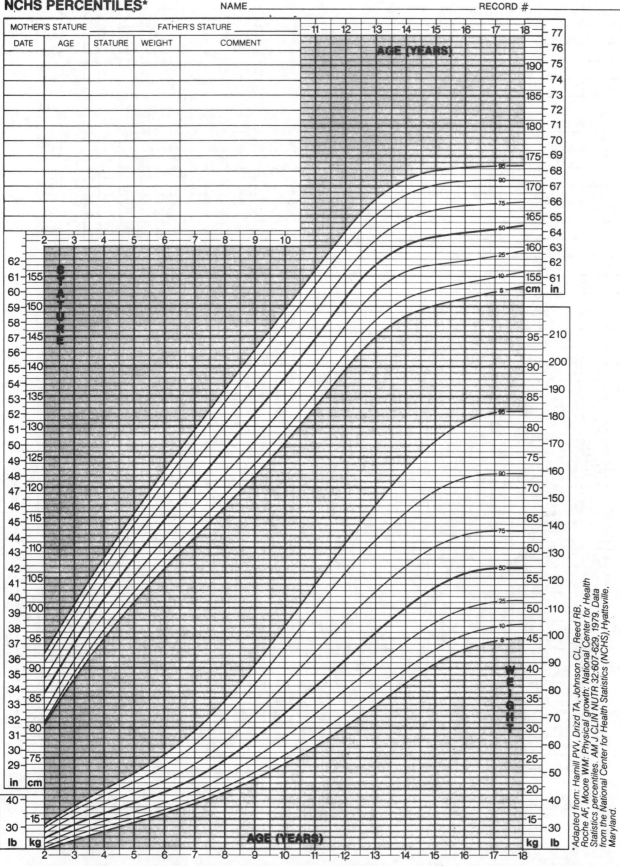

*Adapted from: Hamill PVV, Drizd TA, Johnson CL, Reed RB, Roche AF, Moore WM: Physical growth: National Center for Health Statistics percentiles. AM J CLIN NUTR 32:607-629, 1979. Data from the National Center for Health Statistics (NCHS), Hyattsville, Maryland.

© 1982 Ross Laboratories

GIRLS: PREPUBESCENT
PHYSICAL GROWTH
NCHS PERCENTILES*

NAME _____   RECORD # _____

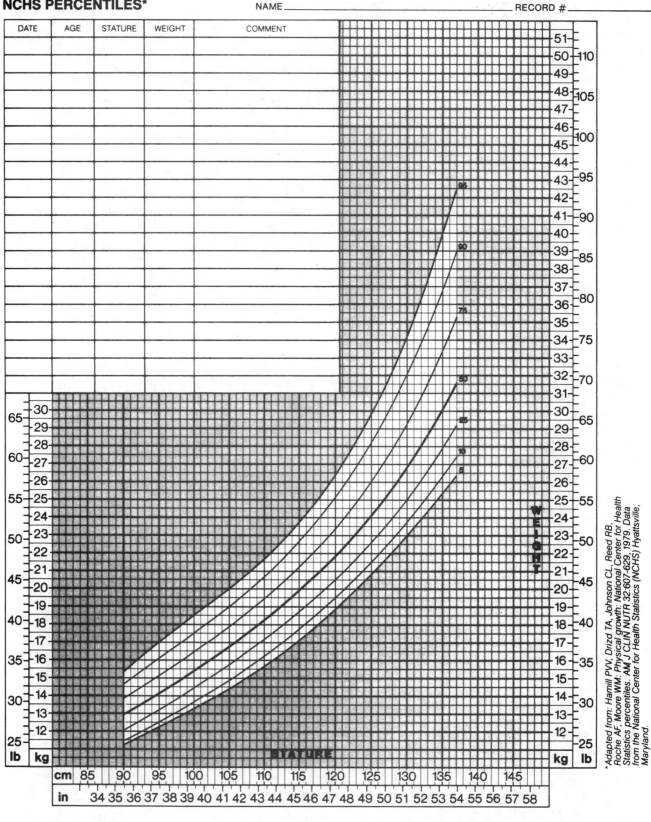

*Adapted from: Hamill PVV, Drizd TA, Johnson CL, Reed RB, Roche AF, Moore WM: Physical growth: National Center for Health Statistics percentiles. AM J CLIN NUTR 32:607-629, 1979. Data from the National Center for Health Statistics (NCHS) Hyattsville, Maryland.

© 1982 Ross Laboratories

SIMILAC® WITH IRON
Infant Formula

ISOMIL™
Soy Protein Formula with Iron

Reprinted with permission
of Ross Laboratories

► **APPENDIX E** ◀

BOYS: BIRTH TO 36 MONTHS
PHYSICAL GROWTH
NCHS PERCENTILES*

NAME _____ RECORD # _____

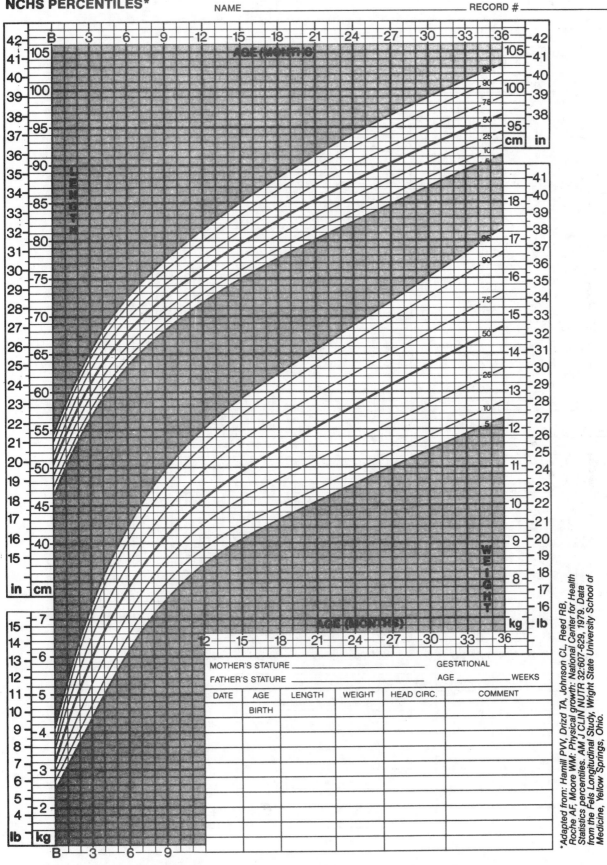

DATE	AGE	LENGTH	WEIGHT	HEAD CIRC.	COMMENT
	BIRTH				

MOTHER'S STATURE _____ GESTATIONAL

FATHER'S STATURE _____ AGE _____ WEEKS

*Adapted from: Hamill PVV, Drizd TA, Johnson CL, Reed RB, Roche AF, Moore WM: Physical growth: National Center for Health Statistics percentiles. AM J CLIN NUTR 32:607-629, 1979. Data from the Fels Longitudinal Study, Wright State University School of Medicine, Yellow Springs, Ohio.

© 1982 Ross Laboratories

BOYS: BIRTH TO 36 MONTHS
PHYSICAL GROWTH
NCHS PERCENTILES*

NAME _____ RECORD # _____

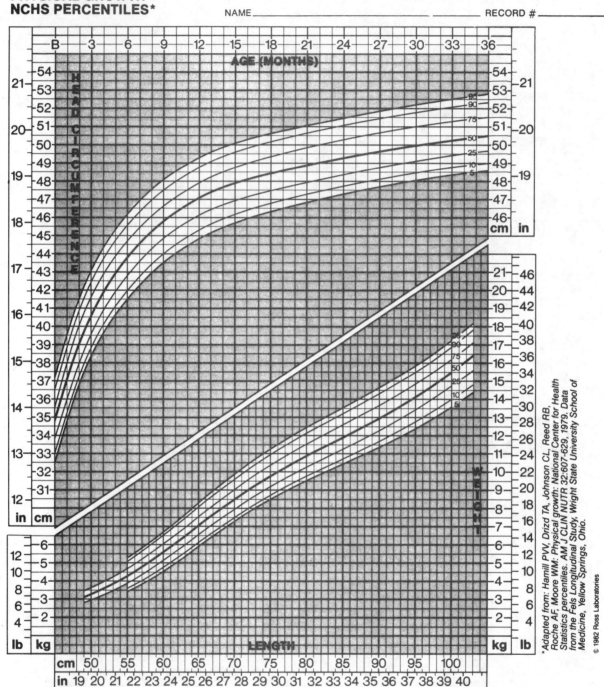

*Adapted from: Hamill PVV, Drizd TA, Johnson CL, Reed RB, Roche AF, Moore WM: Physical growth: National Center for Health Statistics percentiles. AM J CLIN NUTR 32:607-629, 1979. Data from the Fels Longitudinal Study, Wright State University School of Medicine, Yellow Springs, Ohio.

© 1982 Ross Laboratories

DATE	AGE	LENGTH	WEIGHT	HEAD CIRC.	COMMENT

SIMILAC® WITH IRON
Infant Formula

ISOMIL®
Soy Protein Formula with Iron

Reprinted with permission
of Ross Laboratories

▶ **APPENDIX F** ◀

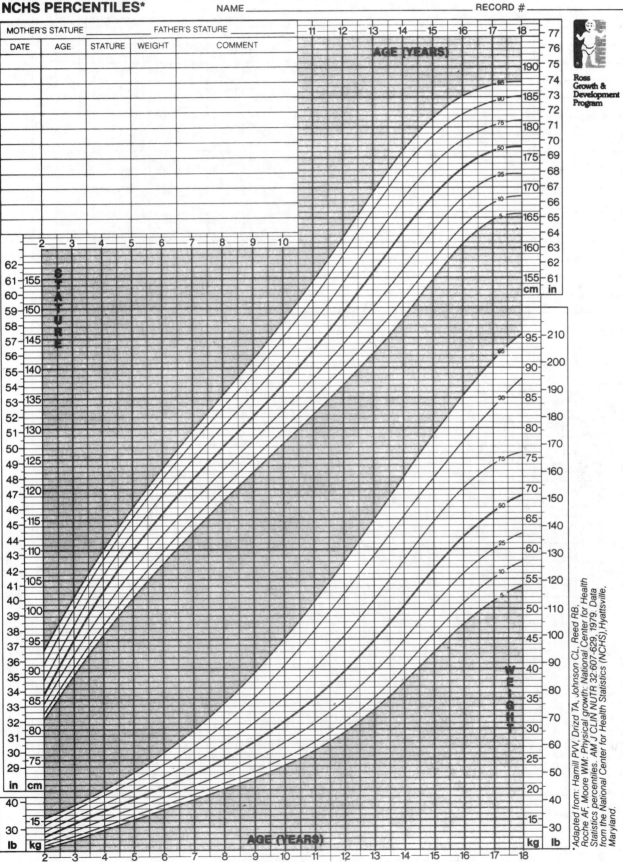

BOYS: 2 TO 18 YEARS
PHYSICAL GROWTH
NCHS PERCENTILES*

NAME _____ RECORD # _____

*Adapted from: Hamill PVV, Drizd TA, Johnson CL, Reed RB, Roche AF, Moore WM: Physical growth: National Center for Health Statistics percentiles. AM J CLIN NUTR 32:607-629, 1979. Data from the National Center for Health Statistics (NCHS), Hyattsville, Maryland.

© 1982 Ross Laboratories

Ross Growth & Development Program

BOYS: PREPUBESCENT
PHYSICAL GROWTH
NCHS PERCENTILES*

NAME _____ RECORD # _____

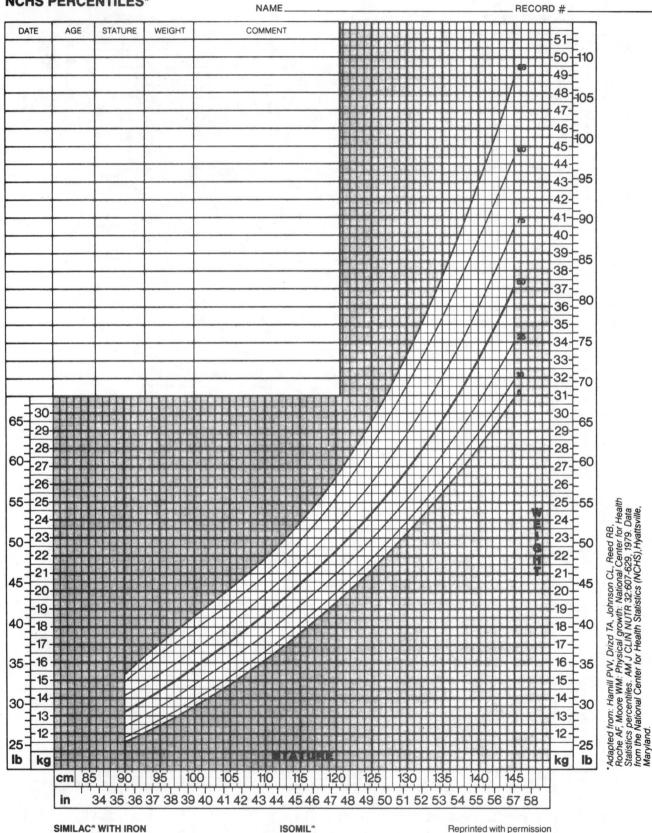

DATE	AGE	STATURE	WEIGHT	COMMENT

*Adapted from: Hamill PVV, Drizd TA, Johnson CL, Reed RB,
Roche AF, Moore WM: Physical growth: National Center for Health
Statistics percentiles. AM J CLIN NUTR 32:607-629, 1979. Data
from the National Center for Health Statistics (NCHS), Hyattsville,
Maryland.

© 1982 Ross Laboratories

SIMILAC* WITH IRON
Infant Formula

ISOMIL*
Soy Protein Formula with Iron

Reprinted with permission
of Ross Laboratories

▶ **APPENDIX G** ◀

The Warning Signs of poor nutritional health are often overlooked. Use this checklist to find out if you or someone you know is at nutritional risk.

Read the statements below. Circle the number in the yes column for those that apply to you or someone you know. For each yes answer, score the number in the box. Total your nutritional score.

DETERMINE YOUR NUTRITIONAL HEALTH

	YES
I have an illness or condition that made me change the kind and/or amount of food I eat.	2
I eat fewer than 2 meals per day.	3
I eat few fruits or vegetables, or milk products.	2
I have 3 or more drinks of beer, liquor or wine almost every day.	2
I have tooth or mouth problems that make it hard for me to eat.	2
I don't always have enough money to buy the food I need.	4
I eat alone most of the time.	1
I take 3 or more different prescribed or over-the-counter drugs a day.	1
Without wanting to , I have lost or gained 10 pounds in the last 6 months.	2
I am not always physically able to shop, cook and/or feed myself.	2
TOTAL	

Total Your Nutritional Score. If it's —

0-2   **Good!** Recheck you nutritional score in 6 months.

3-5   **You are at moderate nutritional risk.** See what can be done to improve your eating habits and lifestyle. Your office on aging, senior nutrition program, senior citizens center or health department can help. Recheck you nutritional score in 3 months.

6 or more   **You are at high nutritional risk.** Bring this checklist the next time you see your doctor, dietitian or other qualified health or social service professional. Talk with them about any problems you may have. Ask for help to improve your nutritional health.

These materials developed and distributed by the Nutrition Screening Initiative, a project of:

AMERICAN ACADEMY OF FAMILY PHYSICIANS

THE AMERICAN DIETETIC ASSOCIATION

NATIONAL COUNCIL ON THE AGING, INC.

Remember that warning signs suggest risk, but do not represent diagnosis of any condition. Turn the page to learn more about the Warning Signs of poor nutritional health.

Reprinted with permission of The Nutrition Screening Initiative. 2626 Pennsylvania Avenue, NW, Suite 301, Washington, DC 20037. A project of the American Academy of Family Physicians, the American Dietetic Association and the National Council on Aging, Inc. and funded in part by Ross Products Division, Abbot Laboratories.

**The Nutrition Checklist is based on the Warning Signs described below.
Use the word __DETERMINE__ to remind you of the Warning Signs.**

Disease

Any disease, illness or chronic conditions which causes you to change the way you eat, or makes it hard for you to eat, puts your nutritional health at risk. Four out of five adults have chronic diseases that are affected by diet. Confusion or memory loss that keeps getting worse is estimated to affect one out of five or more of older adults. This can make it hard to remember what, when or if you've eaten. Feeling sad or depressed, which happens to about one in eight older adults, can cause big changes in appetite, digestion, energy level, weight and well-being.

Eating poorly

Eating too little and eating too much both lead to poor health. Eating the same foods day after day or not eating fruit, vegetables, and milk products daily will also cause poor nutritional health. One in five adults skip meals daily. Only 13% of adults eat the minimum amount of fruit and vegetables needed. One in four older adults drink too much alcohol. Many health problems become worse if you drink more than one or two alcoholic beverages per day.

Tooth loss/mouth pain

A healthy mouth, teeth and gums are needed to eat. Missing, loose or rotten teeth or dentures which don't fit well or cause mouth sores make it hard to eat.

Economic hardship

As many as 40% of older Americans have incomes of less than $6,000 per year. Having less—or choosing to spend less–than $25-30 per week for food makes it very hard to get the foods you need to stay healthy.

Reduced social contact

One-third of all older people live alone. Being with people daily has a positive effect on morale, well-being and eating.

Multiple medicines

Many older Americans must take medicines for health problems. Almost half of older Americans take multiple medicines daily. Growing old may change the way we respond to drugs. The more medicines you take, the greater the chance for side effects such as increased or decreased appetite, change in taste, constipation, weakness, drowsiness, diarrhea, nausea, and others. Vitamins or minerals when taken in large doses act like drugs and can cause harm. Alert your doctor to everything you take.

Involuntary weight loss/gain

Losing or gaining a lot of weight when you not trying to do so is an important warning sign that must not be ignored. Being overweight or underweight also increases your chance of poor health.

Needs assistance in self care

Although most older people are able to eat, one of every five have trouble walking, shopping, buying and cooking food, especially as they get older.

Elder years above age 80

Most older people lead full and productive lives. But as age increases, risk of frailty and health problems increase. Checking your nutritional health regularly makes good sense.

► **APPENDIX H** ◄

Standards for Triceps Fatfold

These percentiles were derived from data obtained on all white subjects in the United States Ten-State Nutritional Survey of 1968–1970. In this survey, obesity in adults was defined as a fatfold greater than the 85th percentile.

Triceps Skinfold Percentiles (millimeters)

Age	Male					Female				
	5th	15th	50th	85th	95th	5th	15th	50th	85th	95th
0 to 5 mo	4	5	8	12	15	4	5	8	12	13
6 to 17 mo	5	7	9	13	15	6	7	9	12	15
1½ to 2½ yr	5	7	10	13	14	6	7	10	13	15
2½ to 3½ yr	6	7	9	12	14	6	7	10	12	14
3½ to 4½ yr	5	6	9	12	14	5	7	10	12	14
4½ to 5½ yr	5	6	8	12	16	6	7	10	13	16
5½ to 6½ yr	5	6	8	11	15	6	7	10	12	15
6½ to 7½yr	4	6	8	11	14	6	7	10	13	17
7½ to 8½yr	5	6	8	12	17	6	7	10	15	19
8½ to 9½yr	5	6	9	14	19	6	7	11	17	24
9½ to 10½yr	5	6	10	16	22	6	8	12	19	24
10½ to 11½ yr	6	7	10	17	25	7	8	12	20	29
11½ to 12½ yr	5	7	11	19	26	6	9	13	20	25
12½ to 13½ yr	5	6	10	18	25	7	9	14	23	30
13½ to 14½ yr	5	6	10	17	22	8	10	15	22	28
14½ to 15½ yr	4	6	9	19	26	8	11	16	24	30
15½ to 16½ yr	4	5	9	20	27	8	10	15	23	27
16½ to 17½ yr	4	5	8	14	20	9	12	16	26	31
17½ to 24½ yr	4	5	10	18	25	9	12	17	25	31
24½ to 34½ yr	4	6	11	21	28	9	12	19	29	36
34½ to 44½ yr	4	6	12	22	28	10	14	22	32	39

Adapted from Frisancho, A.: Triceps skin fold and upper arm muscle size norms for assessment of nutritional status, *American Journal of Clinical Nutrition,* 27, p. 1052, 1974.
Used by permission: Ann Grant and Susan DeHoog, from *Nutritional Assessment and Support,* 1991, published by Grant/DeHoog, 1991.

▶ APPENDIX I ◀

Standards for Arm Muscle Circumference

These percentiles were derived from data obtained on all white subjects in the United States Ten-State Nutritional Survey of 1968–1970.

Arm Muscle Circumference Percentiles (centimeters)

Age	Male					Female				
	5th	15th	50th	85th	95th	5th	15th	50th	85th	95th
0 to 5 mo	8.1	9.4	10.6	12.5	13.3	8.6	9.2	10.4	11.5	12.6
6 to 17 mo	10.0	10.8	12.3	13.7	14.6	9.7	10.2	11.7	12.8	13.5
1½ to 2½ yr	11.1	11.7	12.7	13.8	14.6	10.5	11.2	12.5	14.0	14.6
2½ to 3½ yr	11.4	12.1	13.2	14.5	15.2	10.8	11.6	12.8	13.8	14.3
3½ to 4½ yr	11.8	12.4	13.5	15.1	15.7	11.4	12.0	13.2	14.6	15.2
4½ to 5½ yr	12.1	13.0	14.1	15.6	16.6	11.9	12.4	13.8	15.1	16.0
5½ to 6½ yr	12.7	13.4	14.6	15.9	16.7	12.1	12.9	14.0	15.5	16.5
6½ to 7½ yr	13.0	13.7	15.1	16.4	17.3	12.3	13.2	14.6	16.2	17.5
7½ to 8½ yr	13.8	14.4	15.8	17.4	18.5	12.9	13.8	15.1	16.8	18.6
8½ to 9½ yr	13.8	14.3	16.1	18.2	20.0	13.6	14.3	15.7	17.6	19.3
9½ to 10½ yr	14.2	15.2	16.8	18.6	20.2	13.9	14.7	16.3	18.2	19.6
10½ to 11½ yr	15.0	15.8	17.4	19.4	21.1	14.0	15.2	17.1	19.5	20.9
11½ to 12½ yr	15.3	16.3	18.1	20.7	22.1	15.0	16.1	17.9	20.0	21.2
12½ to 13½ yr	15.9	16.9	19.5	22.4	24.2	15.5	16.5	18.5	20.6	22.5
13½ to 14½ yr	16.7	18.2	21.1	23.4	26.5	16.6	17.5	19.3	22.1	23.4
14½ to 15½ yr	17.3	18.5	22.0	25.2	27.1	16.3	17.3	19.5	22.0	23.2
15½ to 16½ yr	18.6	20.5	22.9	26.0	28.1	17.1	17.8	20.0	22.7	26.0
16½ to 17½ yr	20.6	21.7	24.5	27.1	29.0	17.1	17.7	19.6	22.3	24.1
17½ to 24½ yr	21.7	23.2	25.8	28.6	30.5	17.0	18.3	20.5	22.9	25.3
24½ to 34½ yr	22.0	24.1	27.0	29.5	31.5	17.7	18.9	21.3	24.5	27.2
34½ to 44½ yr	22.2	23.9	27.0	30.0	31.8	18.0	19.2	21.6	25.0	27.9

Adapted from Frisancho, A.: Triceps skin fold and upper arm muscle size norms for assessment of nutritional status, *American Journal of Clinical Nutrition,* 27, p. 1052, 1974.

Used by permission: Ann Grant and Susan DeHoog, from *Nutritional Assessment and Support,* 1991, published by Grant/DeHoog, 1991.

JUST THE FACTS

WHAT ARE PSYCHOACTIVE DRUGS?

AN EDUCATIONAL FACT SHEET FROM THE FLORIDA ALCOHOL & DRUG ABUSE ASSOCIATION

Psychoactive drugs affect the chemical and physical functioning of the brain. These drugs are often termed "mind-altering" because they change the perceptions and the behavior of the individual using them. There are six main classifications of psychoactive drugs: stimulants, depressants, narcotics, cannabis, hallucinogens and inhalants.

Stimulants

Stimulants are used primarily to relieve fatigue and increase alertness. The most widely used stimulants are nicotine, which is found in tobacco products, and caffeine, which is found in soft drinks, coffee and tea. Cocaine and amphetamines are more potent stimulants, People who use stimulants build up a tolerance, which means they have to take larger and larger quantities in order to maintain the desired effects. Greater levels of use in crease the likelihood of physical and psychological dependence.

Depressants

Depressants are often referred to as sedative-hypnotic drugs or downers because they depress the functioning of the central nervous system. Small amounts help relax muscles and produce calmness, while larger doses create difficulties with judgement, reflexes and speech. Depressants are often used for medical purposes to relieve anxiety, tension and insomnia. Nonmedical use of depressants has the potential for psychological and physical dependence which leads to abuse. Alcohol is the most widely used depressant followed by sedatives and tranquilizers.

Narcotics

Narcotics are drugs that dull the senses, induce sleep and become addictive with prolonged use. In medical use, the term narcotic refers to opium; narcotic analgesics are often referred to as opioids. The term analgesic refers to the pain-relieving effect of narcotics. Opium, morphine, heroin and codeine are the most commonly used narcotics. Opium is extracted from the seed pod of the opium poppy; morphine and codeine are derived from the substances found in opium. Heroin is a synthetic drug made by modifying the chemical sin opium.

Cannabis

Cannabis is a plant that grows mainly in tropical and subtropical climates and has been used as a drug for centuries. The main forms of cannabis are marijuana and hashish. Marijuana is produced by drying the tops and leaves of the cannabis plant. Hashish is a concentrated fro of marijuana made from the resin secretions of the cannabis plant. Tetrahydrocannabinol (THC) is the most significant psychoactive chemical ingredient found in cannabis. The level of THC determines the potency of the drug.

Hallucinogens

Hallucinogenic drugs are natural and synthetic drugs that distort the perception of reality and affect thought processes. The main forms of hallucinogenic drugs are phencyclidine (PCP), lysergic acid diethylamide (LSD), and organic drugs which include mescaline and psilocybin.

Inhalants

Inhalants are usually forms of aerosols or solvent that are inhaled and produce feelings of euphoria, excitation and light-headedness. The vapors from inhalants inter the bloodstream rapidly be way of the lungs and circulate throughout the body, often depressing body functions such as breathing and heart rate.

PSYCHOACTIVE DRUGS

DRUGS	MEDICAL USES	MEDICAL NAMES	SLANG NAMES	FORMS	USUAL ADMINISTRATION
STIMULANTS			**STIMULANTS**		
Nicotine	None	Nicotine	Butt, chew, smoke, cig	Pipe, tobacco, cigarettes, snuff	Sniff, chew, smoke
Caffeine	Hyperkinesis, Stimulant	Caffeine	None	Chocolates, tea, soft drinks, coffee	Swallow
Amphetamines	Hyperkinesis, Narcolepsy, Weight control, Mental disorders	Dexedrine, Benzedrine	Speed, bennies, dexies, pep pills	Capsules, liquid, tablets, powder	Inject, swallow
Cocaine	Local anesthetic	Cocaine	Coke, rock, crack, blow, toot, white blast, snow, flake	Powder, rock	Inject, smoke, inhale
DEPRESSANTS			**DEPRESSANTS**		
Alcohol	None	Ethyl alcohol	Booze	Liquid	Swallow
Sedatives	Anesthetic, Sedative hypnotic, Anticonvulsant	Secobarbital, Phenobarbital, Seconal	Barbs, reds, downers, sopors	Capsules, tablets, powder	Inject, swallow
Tranquilizers	Antianxiety, Sedative hypnotic	Valium, Miltown, Librium	Downers	Capsules, tablets	Swallow
NARCOTICS			**NARCOTICS**		
Opium	Analgesic, Antidiarrheal	Paregoric	None	Powder	Smoke, swallow
Morphine	Analgesic, Antitussive	Morphine, pectoral syrup	None	Powder, tablet, liquid	Inject, smoke, swallow
Heroin	Research	Diacetylmorphine	China white, smack, junk, H, horse	Powder	Inject, swallow, smoke
Codeine	Analgesic, Antitussive	Codeine, Empirin compound with codeine, Robitussin a-c	None	Capsules, tablet, liquid	Inject, swallow
CANNABIS			**CANNABIS**		
THC	Research, Cancer chemotherapy antinauseant	Tetrahydrocannabinol	THC	Tablets, liquid	Swallow
Hashish	None	Tetrahydrocannabinol	Hash	Solid resin	Smoke
Marijuana	Research	Tetrahydrocannabinol	Pot, grass, sinsemilla, dobie, ganja, dope, gold, herb, weed, reefer	Plant particles	Smoke, swallow
HALLUCINOGENS			**HALLUCINOGENS**		
PCP	None	Phencyclidine	Angel dust, zoot, peace pill, hog	Tablets, powder	Smoke, swallow
LSD	Research	Lysergic acid diethylamide	Acid, sugar	Capsules, tablets, liquid	Swallow
Organics	None	Mescaline, psilocybin	Mesc, mushrooms	Crude preparations, tablets, powder	Swallow
INHALANTS			**INHALANTS**		
Aerosols and Solvents	None	None	Glue, benzine, toluene, freon	Solvents, aerosols	Inhale

For more information contact the Florida Alcohol and Drug Abuse Association Resource Center, 1000 E. Lafayette St., Suite 100, Tallahassee, Florida 32301

IDENTIFICATION CHART

EFFECTS SOUGHT	POSSIBLE EFFECTS	OVERDOSE	LONG-TERM EFFECTS
STIMULANTS			**STIMULANTS**
Relaxation	Respiratory difficulties, fatigue, high blood pressure	None	Dependency, lung cancer, heart attack, respiratory ailments
Alertness	Increased alertness, pulse rate and blood pressure; excitation, insomnia, loss of appetite	Irritability	Dependency may aggravate organic actions
Alertness, activeness	Increased alertness, pulse rate and blood pressure; excitation, insomnia, loss of appetite	Agitation, increase in body temperature, hallucinations, convulsions, possible death	Severe withdrawal, possible convulsions, toxic psychosis
Excitation, euphoria	Increased alertness, pulse rate and blood pressure; excitation, insomnia, loss of appetite	Agitation, increase in body temperature, hallucinations, convulsions, possible death	Dependency, depression, paranoia, convulsions
DEPRESSANTS			**DEPRESSANTS**
Sense alteration, anxiety reduction	Loss of coordination, sluggishness, slurred speech, disorientation, depression	Total loss of coordination, nausea, unconsciousness, possible death	Dependency, toxic psychosis, neurologic damage
Anxiety reduction, euphoria, sleep	Loss of coordination, sluggishness, slurred speech, disorientation, depression	Cold and clammy skin, dilated pupils, shallow respiration, weak and rapid pulse, coma, possible death	Dependency, severe withdrawal, possible convulsions, toxic psychosis
Anxiety reduction, euphoria, sleep	Loss of coordination, sluggishness, slurred speech, disorientation, depression	Cold and clammy skin, dilated pupils, shallow respiration, weak and rapid pulse, coma, possible death	Dependency, severe withdrawal, possible convulsions, toxic psychosis
NARCOTICS			**NARCOTICS**
Euphoria, prevent withdrawal, sleep	Euphoria, drowsiness, respiratory depression, constricted pupils, sleep, nausea	Clammy skin, slow and shallow breathing, convulsions, coma, possible death	Dependency, constipation, loss of appetite, severe withdrawal
Euphoria, prevent withdrawal, sleep,	Euphoria, drowsiness, respiratory depression, constricted pupils, sleep, nausea	Clammy skin, slow and shallow breathing, convulsions, coma, possible death	Dependency, constipation, loss of appetite, severe withdrawal
Euphoria, prevent withdrawal, sleep,	Euphoria, drowsiness, respiratory depression, constricted pupils, sleep, nausea	Clammy skin, slow and shallow breathing, convulsions, coma, possible death	Dependency, constipation, loss of appetite, severe withdrawal
Euphoria, prevent withdrawal, sleep,	Euphoria, drowsiness, respiratory depression, constricted pupils, sleep, nausea	Clammy skin, slow and shallow breathing, convulsions, coma, possible death	Dependency, constipation, loss of appetite, severe withdrawal
CANNABIS			**CANNABIS**
Relaxation, euphoria, increased perception	Relaxed inhibitions, euphoria, increased appetite, distorted perceptions, disoriented behavior	Fatigue, paranoia, possible psychosis	Amotivational syndrome, respiratory difficulties, lung cancer, interference with physical and emotional development
Relaxation, euphoria, increased perception	Relaxed inhibitions, euphoria, increased appetite, distorted perceptions, disoriented behavior	Fatigue, paranoia, possible psychosis	Amotivational syndrome, respiratory difficulties, lung cancer, interference with physical and emotional development
Relaxation, euphoria, increased perception	Relaxed inhibitions, euphoria, increased appetite, distorted perceptions, disoriented behavior	Fatigue, paranoia, possible psychosis	Amotivational syndrome, respiratory difficulties, lung cancer, interference with physical and emotional development
HALLUCINOGENS			**HALLUCINOGENS**
Distortion of senses, insight, exhilaration	Illusions and hallucinations, distorted perception of time and distance	Longer and more intense "trips" or episodes, psychosis, convulsions, possible death	May intensify existing psychosis, flashbacks, panic reactions
Distortion of senses, insight, exhilaration	Illusions and hallucinations, distorted perception of time and distance	Longer and more intense "trips" or episodes, psychosis, convulsions, possible death	May intensify existing psychosis, flashbacks, panic reactions
Distortion of senses, insight, exhilaration	Illusions and hallucinations, distorted perception of time and distance	Longer and more intense "trips" or episodes, psychosis, convulsions, possible death	May intensify existing psychosis, flashbacks, panic reactions
INHALANTS			**INHALANTS**
Intoxication	Exhilaration, confusion, poor concentration	Heart failure, unconsciousness, asphyxiation, possible death	Impaired perception, coordination and judgement; neurologic damage

▶ APPENDIX K ◀

Alcohol, Kilocalorie, and Carbohydrate Content of Alcoholic Beverages

Beverage	Amount (oz)	Alcohol (g)	Calories	Carbohydrate (g)
Ale	8	8.9	98	8.0
Beer	12	13.1	148	13.2
Beer, light	12	11.5	100	4.8
Brandy	1	10.5	74	Trace
Champagne	4	11.9	98	3.6
Daiquiri	4	15.0	122	5.2
Gin, rum, vodka, whiskey, 86 proof	1.5	15.1	105	1.3
Highball	8	24.0	165	Trace
Martini	2.5	18.5	140	0.3
Sweet sherry, port, muscatel	2	9.4	94	7.0
Wine, California Red	4	10.0	85	0.5
Wine, California Sauterne	4	10.5	85	4.0
Wine coolers	12	15.0	192	22.0

References

Franz, M.J., *Exchanges for All Occasions—Meeting the Challenge of Diabetes,* Diabetes Center, Inc., Wayzata, Minnesota, p. 134, 1987.

Pennington, J.A., *Bowes and Church's Food Values of Portions Commonly Used,* (15th ed), J.B. Lippincott Company, Philadelphia, pp. 3–5, 1989.

Pennington, J.A., Church, H.N., *Bowes and Church's Food Values of Portions Commonly Used,* (14th ed), Harper and Row, New York, pp. 196–197, 1985.

▶ APPENDIX L ◀

Caffeine Content of Various Foods

Caffeine	Milligrams (mg)
CARBONATED BEVERAGES	
*Cherry, Coca-Cola–12 fl. oz. (370 g)	46
*Cherry Cola Slice–12 fl. oz. (360 g)	48
*Cherry RC–12 fl. oz. (360 g)	12
*Coca-Cola–12 oz fl. oz. (370 g)	46
*Coca-Cola Classic–12 fl. oz. (369 g)	46
*Dr. Pepper–12 fl. oz. (360 g)	41
*Jamaica Cola, Canada Dry–12 fl. oz. (360 g)	30
*Mello Yello–12 fl. oz. (372 g)	52
*Mr. Pibb–12 fl. oz. (369 g)	40
*Mountain Dew–12 fl. oz. (360 g)	54
*Pepsi Cola–12 fl. oz. (360 g)	38
*RC Cola–12 fl. oz. (360 g)	18
LOW CALORIE CARBONATED BEVERAGES	
*Diet Cherry, Coca-Cola–12 fl. oz. (354 g)	46
*Diet Cherry Cola, Slice–12 fl. oz. (360 g)	41
*Diet Coke, Cola-Cola–12 fl. oz. (354 g)	46
Diet Cola, Aspartame Sweetened–12 fl. oz. (355 g)	50
*Diet Dr. Pepper–12 fl. oz. (360 g)	41
*Diet Pepsi–12 fl. oz. (360 g)	36
*Diet Rite Cola–12 fl. oz. (360 g)	48
*Diet Soda, Sodium Saccharin Sweetened–12 fl. oz. (360 g)	39
*Pepsi Light–12 fl. oz. (360 g)	36
*Tab–12 fl. oz. (354 g)	46
COFFEE	
Brewed–6 fl. oz (177g)	103
*Ground Folgers–1 Tbsp. (6 g)	90
Instant Powder–1 rd. tsp. (1.8 g)	57
Decaffeinated–1 rd. tsp. (1.8 g)	2
*Folger's–1 tsp. (2.2 g)	75
with Chicory–1 rd. tsp. (1.8 g)	37
Prep from Instant Powder–6 fl. oz. water & 1 rd. tsp. Powder (179 g)	57
Amaretto, *General Foods–6 fl. oz. water & 11.5 g powder (189 g)	60
Amaretto, Sugar Free, *General Foods–6 fl. oz. water & 7.7 g powder (185 g)	60
Francais, *General Foods–6 fl. oz. water & 11.5 g powder (189 g)	53
Francais, Sugar Free, *General Foods–6 fl. oz. water & 7.7 g powder (185 g)	53
Irish Creme, *General Foods–6 fl. oz. water & 12.8 g powder (190 g)	58
Irish Creme, Sugar Free, *General Foods–6 fl. oz. water & 7.1 g powder (185 g)	48
Irish Mocha Mint, *General Foods–6 fl. oz. water & 11.5 g powder (189 g)	27
Irish Mocha Mint, Sugar Free, *General Foods–6 fl. oz. water & 6.4 g powder (184 g)	25
Orange Cappuccino, *General Foods–6 fl. oz. water & 6.7 g powder (191 g)	73
Orange Cappuccino, Sugar Free, *General Foods–6 fl. oz. water & 6.7 g powder (184 g)	71
Suisse Mocha, *General Foods–6 fl. oz. water & 11.5 g powder (189 g)	41
Suisse Mocha, Sugar Free, *General Foods–6 fl. oz. water & 6.4 g powder (184 g)	40
Vienna, *General Foods–6 fl. oz. water & 14 g powder (191 g)	56
Vienna, Sugar Free, *General Foods–6 fl. oz. water & 6.7 g powder (184 g)	55
With Chicory–6 fl. oz. water & 1 rd. tsp. powder (179 g)	38

Caffeine	**Milligrams (mg)**
HOT/ICED TEA	
Tea, Brewed, Black, 3 min.–6 fl. oz. water (178 g)	36
Tea, Iced, Prep from Instant Mix, *Crystal Light–8 fl. oz. (238 g)	11
Tea, Instant Powder–1 tsp. (0.7 g)	31
with Lemon Flavor–1 rd. tsp. (1.4 g)	25
with Sodium Saccharin & Lemon Flavor–2 tsp. (1.6 g)	36
with Sugar & Lemon Flavor–3 rd. tsp. (23 g)	29
CANDY	
Chocolate	
German Sweet, *Bakers–1 oz. square (28 g)	8
Semi-Sweet–1 oz. (28 g)	18
Semi-Sweet, *Bakers–1 oz. square (28 g)	13
Special Dark Sweet, *Hershey–1.45 oz. bar (41 g)	31
Sweet–1.45 oz. bar (41 g)	27
Chocolate Chips, Semi-Sweet–6 oz. pkg (170 g)	105
Milk Chocolate Chips–1 cup (170 g)	43

*Caffeine-Free *Coca-Cola contains 0 mg Caffeine
*Caffeine-Free Dr. Pepper Contains 0 mg Caffeine
*Caffeine-Free Diet Cola contains 0 mg Caffeine

*Caffeine-Free Diet Rite Cola contains 0 mg Caffeine
*Caffeine-Free Tab contains 0 mg Caffeine
*Decaffeinated Crystal Light Iced Tea Contains 0 mg Caffeine

*Registered Trademark: Brand names are used for clarification and do not constitute endorsement of that product.

Reference

Pennington, J.A. and Church, M.N.: *Bowes and Church's Food Values of Portions,* 16th ed., 1994.

► **APPENDIX M** ◄

Sodium Content of Selected Non-Prescription Drugs

Brand	Ingredients	Sodium Content/Single Dose (mg)
Alka-Seltzer®	Aspirin, sodium citrate	521 to 1,064
Amphogel®	Aluminum hydroxide	7
Aspirin	sodium salicylate	49
Basaljel®	aluminum carbonate	2.3
Bromo-Seltzer®	Acetaminophen, sodium citrate	717
Digel®	Aluminum hydroxide, magnesium hydroxide, simethicone	8.5
Fleet's Enema®	Sodium biophosphate, sodium phosphate	250 to 300 (absorbed)
Gaviscon®	Aluminum hydroxide, magnesium hydroxide	13
Maalox Plus®	Aluminum hydroxide, magnesium hydroxide, simethicone	1.3
Maalox TC®	Aluminum hydroxide, magnesium hydroxide	.08
Metamucil® (instant mix)	Psyllium, citric acid, sodium bicarbonate	250
Milk of Magnesia®	Magnesium hydroxide	.12
Mylanta II®	Aluminum hydroxide, magnesium hydroxide, simethicone	1.1
Riopan Plus®	Magnesium aluminum complex,	<0.1
Rolaids®	Aluminum carbonate	53
Sal Hepatica®	Sodium bicarbonate, sodium monohydrogen phosphate, sodium citrate	1,000
Soda Mint®	Sodium bicarbonate	89
Titralac®	Calcium carbonate	11
Tums®	Calcium carbonate	2.7

References

Food and Nutrition Services, Shands Hospital at the University of Florida, *Guide to Normal Nutrition and Diet Modification,* (3rd ed), Gainesville, Florida, P. 377, 1983.

Gilman, A.G., Rall, T.W., Nies, A.S., Taylor, P., *Goodman and Gilman's The Pharmacological Basis of Therapeutics,* (8th ed), Pergamon Press, New York, P. 985, 1990.

▶ APPENDIX N ◀

Sodium Values

Sodium Milligrams	Sodium Milliequivalents	Sodium Chloride Grams
393	17.0	1.0
500	21.8	1.3
800	34.7	2.0
1,000	43.5	2.5
1,500	75.3	3.8
2,000	87.0	5.0

To convert specific weight of sodium to sodium chloride: mg of sodium × 2.54 = mg of sodium chloride.
To convert specific weight of sodium chloride to sodium: mg of sodium chloride × 0.393 = mg of sodium.

▶ APPENDIX O ◀

Conversion of Milligrams to Milliequivalents

Ion	Approximate Atomic or Molecular Weight	Valence	Number of mg per mEq
Sodium Na+	23.0	1	23.0
Potassium K+	39.1	1	39.1
Ammonium NH4+	18.0	1	18.0
Magnesium Mg++	24.3	2	12.15
Calcium Ca++	40.0	2	20.0
Chloride Cl–	35.4	–1	35.5
Lactate $CH_3CH(OH)Coo-$	89.0	–1	89.0
Sulfate SO_4-	96.0	–2	48.0
Bicarbonate NCO_3-	61.0	–1	61.0
Monohydrogen phosphate HPO_4-	96.0	–2	48.0

To convert milligrams (mg) to millequivalents (mEq): (mg ÷ atomic weight) × valence = milliequivalents.

▶ APPENDIX P ◀

Types of Hyperlipoproteinemia

Fredrickson Type	Lipid Abnormality	Elevated Lipoproteins
I	Hyperchylomicronemia	Chylomicrons
IIa	Hypercholesterolemia	LDL
IIb	Combined hypercholesterolemia and endogenous hypertrigliceridemia	LDL, VLDL
III	Dysbetalipoproteinemia (broad beta pattern)	IDL (intermediate density lipoproteins)
IV	Hypertriglyceridemia	VLDL
V	Hypertriglyceridemia	VLDL, chylomicrons

Reference

National Heart and Lung Institute, *A Handbook for Physicians and Dieticians: Dietary Management of Hyperlipoproteinemia,* NIH Publication No. 80-110, Bethesda, MD, January, 1980.

▶ **APPENDIX Q** ◀

Foods High in Iron (More than 1.5 mg per Serving)

Food	Weight (g)	Approximate Measure	Per Serving	Per 100 grams
Apricots, dried	30	5 Halves	1.5	5.5
Beans, dry, cooked	30	½ cup	2.6	7.8
Beef, rib roast,	60	2 oz.	1.8	3.0
corned	60	2 oz.	2.6	4.3
dried	30	1 oz.	1.5	5.1
Bread, whole wheat	50	2 slices	1.6	—
Chocolate (bitter)	30	1 square	2.2	6.7
Clams	60	2 oz.	4.2	7.0
Dandelion greens	75	½ cup	2.3	3.1
Ham, smoked	60	2 oz.	1.7	2.9
Heart, beef	60	2 oz.	3.4	5.9
Kale	75	¾ cup	1.7	2.2
Kidney, beef	60	2 oz.	7.8	13.1
Lentils, dry, cooked	30	½ cup	2.2	6.8
Liver, beef	60	2 oz.	5.2	8.8
Liver sausage	30	1 slice	1.6	5.4
Molasses	20	1 Tbsp.	3.2	—
Oysters, raw	60	2 oz.	3.4	5.6
Peaches, dried	30	3 halves	1.9	6.9
Pork Loin	60	2 oz.	1.8	3.0
Prune Juice	128	½ cup	5.3	—
Raisins, dried	50	5 Tbsp.	1.7	3.3
Rice, enriched white, cooked	205	1 cup	1.8	—
Sardines	60	2 oz.	1.7	2.9
Shrimp, canned	60	2 oz.	1.9	3.1
Soybeans, dried	25	2 Tbsp.	2.0	8.0
Spinach	75	½ cup	1.5	2.0
Tongue, beef	60	2 oz.	1.7	1.7
Turkey	60	2 oz.	2.3	3.8
Turnip greens	75	½ cup	1.8	2.4
Veal roast	60	2 oz.	2.2	3.6
Yeast, compressed	30	1 oz.	1.5	4.9

Note: All measurements are for cooked food except where specified.

References

Nutritive Value of American Foods, Agriculture Handbook No. 456, 1975 Edition.

Watt, B.K., and Merrill, A.L., *Composition of Foods: Raw, Processed, Prepared,* USDA Handbook No. 8, Washington, DC, 1963.

▶ APPENDIX R ◀

Equivalent Weights and Measures

3 teaspoons	1 tablespoon
2 tablespoons	1 ounce
4 tablespoons	¼ cup
8 tablespoons	½ cup
16 tablespoons	1 cup
2 cups	1 pint
4 cups	1 quart
4 quarts	1 gallon
1 teaspoon	5 grams
1 tablespoon	15 grams
1 ounce, dry	28.35 grams
1 ounce, liquid	30 grams
½ cup	120 grams
1 cup	240 grams
1 pound	454 grams
1 gram	1 cc
1 teaspoon	5 cc
1 tablespoon	15 cc
1 ounce, fluid	30 cc
1 cup	240 cc
1 pint	480 cc
1 quart	960 cc
1 liter	1,000 cc

► **APPENDIX S** ◄

Metric System

US to Metric		Metric to US	
Length		*Length*	
1 inch	= 25.0 millimeters	1 millimeter	= 0.04 inch
1 foot	= 0.3 meter	1 meter	= 3.3 feet
Mass		*Mass*	
1 grain	= 64.8 milligrams	1 milligram	= 0.015 grain
1 ounce (dry)	= 28.0 grams	1 gram	= 0.035 ounce
1 pound	= 0.45 kilograms	1 kilogram	= 2.2 pounds
1 short ton	= 9.091 kilograms	1 metric ton	= 1.102 tons (short)
Volume		*Volume*	
1 cubic inch	= 16.0 cubic centimeters	1 cubic centimeter	= 0.06 cubic inch
1 teaspoon	= 5.0 milliliters	1 milliliter	= 0.2 teaspoon
1 tablespoon	= 15.0 milliliters	1 milliliter	= 0.07 tablespoon
1 fluid ounce	= 30.0 milliliters	1 milliliter	= 0.03 ounce
1 cup	= 0.24 liter	1 liter	= 4.2 cups
1 pint	= 0.47 liter	1 liter	= 2.1 pints
1 quart (liquid)	= 0.95 liter	1 liter	= 1.1 quarts
1 gallon (liquid)	= 0.004 cubic meter	1 cubic meter	= 264.0 gallons
1 peck	= 0.009 cubic meter	1 cubic meter	= 113.0 pecks
1 bushel	= 0.04 cubic meter	1 cubic meter	= 28.0 bushels
Energy		*Energy*	
1 calorie	= 4.18 joules (j)	1 joule (j)	= 0.24 calorie

▶ APPENDIX T ◀

Common Abbreviations

ad lib	as desired	Hct	hematocrit
ADA	American Dietetic Association	HDL	high density lipoprotein
	American Diabetic Association	Hgb	hemoglobin
AMA	American Medical Association	HOH	hard of hearing
	against medical advise	hs	hour of sleep
ASAP	as soon as possible	ht	height
as tol	as tolerated	Hx	history
BEE	basal energy expenditure	IBW	ideal body weight
b.i.d.	twice a day	ICU	intensive care unit
BP	blood pressure	IDDM	insulin dependent diabetes
C	cup		mellitus
c	with	i	one
Ca	calcium	ii	two
CA	cancer	iii	three
cal	calorie	IM	intramuscular
CBC	complete blood count	I&O	intake and output
cc	cubic centimeter	I.U.	international units
CMD	Certified Dietary Manager	IV	intravenous
CHO	carbohydrate	K	potassium
chol	cholesterol	Kcal	kilocalorie
Cl	chloride	Kg	kilogram
cm	centimeters	L	liter
COPD	chronic obstructive pulmonary	lb or #	pound
	disease	LDL	low density lipoproteins
CRF	chronic renal failure	lg	large
Cu	copper	mech	mechanical
CVA	cerbrovascular accident	mEq	milliequivalent
d/c	discontinue	mg	milligram
Diab	diabetic	MI	myocardial infarction
DTR	diet technician, registered	ml	milliliter
Dx	diagnosis	Na	sodium
ea	each	NaCl	sodium chloride
e.g.	for example	NIDDM	non-insulin dependent diabetes
EX	exchange		mellitus
FBS	fasting blood sugar	NKA	no known allergies
fdg	feeding	NPO	nothing by mouth
fl oz	fluid ounce	oz	ounce
GB	gall bladder	pc	after meals
GI	gastrointestinal	po	by mouth
gm	gram	prn	as necessary
GTT	glucose tolerance test	pro	protein

Common Abbreviations

q	every	TEE	total energy expenditure
qd	every day	tid	three times a day
qid	four times a day	TP	total protein
qod	every other day	Tx	treatment
RD	registered dietitian	UTI	urinary tract infection
RDA	Recommended Dietary	Vit	vitamin
	Allowances	VLDL	very low density lipoproteins
red	reducation	wk	week
ROM	range of motion	WNL	within normal limits
Rx	prescription	wt	weight
s	without	Zn	zinc
SOB	shortness of breath	>	greater than
t or tsp	teaspoon	<	less than
T or Tbs	tablespoon	=	equal

This is not an all inclusive list. Check the Medical Record/Patient Informational Services for the approved abbreviations used in your facility.

▶ APPENDIX U ◀

Normal Ranges for Laboratory Tests*

LAB Test	Normal Range
Albumin, Serum	3.5–5.0 gm/dl
Alakaline Phosphates	Adults 30–120 IU/L Puberty 120–540 IU/L
Asparlate Amino Transferase (GOT, AST, SGOT)	70–140 IU/L

Bilirubin
  Direct
  Total
	
	0.0–0.3 mg/dl
	0.1–1.0 mg/dl

Blood Urea Nitrogen BUN	Female 6–20 mg/dl Male 8–23 mg/dl
Calcium, Serum (Ca)	8.5–10.5 mg/dl
Chloride (Cl)	95–105 mEq/L
Cholestrol	desirable < 200 mg/dl High > 240 mg/dl
Creatinine, serum	0.7–1.6 mg/dl (varies with sex)
Folic Acid, red blood cell	140–369 mg/dl
Gamma glutamyl transpeptidase (GGT)	15–85 U/L
Glucose, blood	Adult: 65–110 mg/dl (fasting)
HDL Cholestrol	> 50 mg/dl–less risk of coronary heart disease < 35 mg/dl–high risk of coronary heart disease
Lactic dehydogenase serum (LDH)	< 130 mg/dl desirable 130–150 mg/dl borderline—high risk > 160 high risk
Magnesium, serum (Mg)	1.8–2.8 mg/dl
Osmolality, serum	280–350 mOsm/kg
Phosphorous serum (PO_4)	Adults 2.5–4.6 mg/dl Children 4.0–7.0 mg/dl
Potassium, serum (K)	3.5–5.0 mEg/L
Riboflavin serum	1.0–1.67 A/C
Sodium, Serum (Na)	135–145 mEq/L
Thiamine, serum	1.0–1.23 A/C acceptable 5.3–79 mcg/dl normal
Total lymphocyte count (TLC)	1200–2000 cells/mm < 1200 cells/mm significant delepetion
Total protein, serum	6.0–8.0 gm/dl
TRANS Ferrin	205–374 mg/dl
Triglycerides	<250 mg/dl desirable 500 mg/dl high

LAB Test	Normal Range	
Urinalysis		
pH	5–8	
Glucose	Negative	
Ketones	Negative	
Bilrubin	Negative	
Hemoglobin	Negative	
White blood count	0–2 HPF	
Red blood count	0–2 HPF	
Hemogram	*Adult Male*	*Adult Female*
White blood count (WBC)	$4.5–11.0 \times 10^3$/CU MM	same
Red blood count (RBC)	$4.5–5.9 \times 10^6$ CU MM	$4.0–5.2 \times 10^6$ CU MM
Hemoglobin (Hgb)	13.5–17.5 mg/dl	12.0–16.0 mg/dl
Hematocrit (Hct, PCV)	41–53%	36–46%
Mean Cell Volume	80–100 CU MIC	80–100 CU MIC
Mean Cell Hemoglobin	26–34 pg	26–34 pg

*A composite of a number of facilities.

▶ **APPENDIX V** ◀

General Information

Approx Body Composition

Water	55–65%
Protein	18–20%
Fat–	Men up to 20%
	Women up to 30%
Carbohydrates	0.5%
Minerals	4%
Vitamins	traces

1 can regular soft drink = 150 cals
150 × 30 = 4500 cals per month
1 kg fat = 7700 cals

1 ml alcohol = 5.6 kcal
Proof ÷ 2 = % of alcohol
86% proof whiskey = 43% alcohol
1 oz (30 ml) = 43 × 30 × 5.6 kcal = 78 kcal

1 kcal = 4.184 joules

Physiological Fuel Factors
CHO = 4 cal
FAT = 9 cal
Protein = 4 cal

► **APPENDIX W** ◄

Recommended Dietary Allowances (RDA), 1989[a]

Age (years)	Weight (kg)	Weight (lb)	Height (cm)	Height (inches)	Protein (g)	(RE) Vitamin A	(µg) Vitamin D	(mg) Vitamin E	(µg) Vitamin K	(mg) Vitamin C	(mg) Thiamin	(mg) Riboflavin	(mg equiv.) Niacin	(mg) Vitamin B$_6$	(µg) Folate	(µg) Vitamin B$_{12}$	(mg) Calcium	(mg) Phosphorus	(mg) Magnesium	(mg) Iron	(mg) Zinc	(µg) Iodine	(µg) Selenium
Infants																							
0.0–0.5	6	13	60	24	13	375	7.5	3	5	30	0.3	0.4	5	0.3	25	0.3	400	300	40	6	5	40	10
0.5–1.0	9	20	71	28	14	375	10	4	10	35	0.4	0.5	6	0.6	35	0.5	600	500	60	10	5	50	15
Children																							
1–3	13	29	90	35	16	400	10	6	15	40	0.7	0.8	9	1.0	50	0.7	800	800	80	10	10	70	20
4–6	20	44	112	44	24	500	10	7	20	45	0.9	1.1	12	1.1	75	1.0	800	800	120	10	10	90	20
7–10	28	62	132	52	28	700	10	7	30	45	1.0	1.2	13	1.4	100	1.4	800	800	170	10	10	120	30
Males																							
11–14	45	99	157	62	45	1000	10	10	45	50	1.3	1.5	17	1.7	150	2.0	1200	1200	270	12	15	150	40
15–18	66	145	176	69	59	1000	10	10	65	60	1.5	1.8	20	2.0	200	2.0	1200	1200	400	12	15	150	50
19–24	72	160	177	70	58	1000	10	10	70	60	1.5	1.7	19	2.0	200	2.0	1200	1200	350	10	15	150	70
25–50	79	174	176	70	63	1000	5	10	80	60	1.5	1.7	19	2.0	200	2.0	800	800	350	10	15	150	70
51+	77	170	173	68	63	1000	5	10	80	60	1.2	1.4	15	2.0	200	2.0	800	800	350	10	15	150	70
Females																							
11–14	46	101	157	62	46	800	10	8	45	50	1.1	1.3	15	1.4	150	2.0	1200	1200	280	15	12	150	45
15–18	55	120	163	64	44	800	10	8	55	60	1.1	1.3	15	1.5	180	2.0	1200	1200	300	15	12	150	50
19–24	58	128	164	65	46	800	10	8	60	60	1.1	1.3	15	1.6	180	2.0	1200	1200	280	15	12	150	55
25–50	63	138	163	64	50	800	5	8	65	60	1.1	1.3	15	1.6	180	2.0	800	800	280	15	12	150	55
51+	65	143	160	63	50	800	5	8	65	60	1.0	1.2	13	1.6	180	2.0	800	800	280	10	12	150	55
Pregnant					60	800	10	10	65	70	1.5	1.6	17	2.2	400	2.2	1200	1200	320	30	15	175	65
Lactating																							
1st 6 mo					65	1300	10	12	65	95	1.6	1.8	20	2.1	280	2.6	1200	1200	355	15	19	200	75
2nd 6 mo					62	1200	10	11	65	90	1.6	1.7	20	2.1	260	2.6	1200	1200	340	15	16	200	75

[a]The allowances are intended to provide for individual variations among most normal, healthy people in the United States under usual environmental stresses. Diets should be based on a variety of common foods in order to provide other nutrients for which human requirements have been less well defined. See the text for a more detailed discussion of the RDA and of nutrients not tabulated.
Source: *Recommended Dietary Allowances,* © 1989 by the National Academy of Sciences, National Academy Press, Washington, D.C.